HEMATOLOGY/ ONCOLOGY CLINICS OF NORTH AMERICA

Colorectal Cancer

GREGORY G. GINSBERG, MD, GUEST EDITOR

VOLUME 16 • NUMBER 4 • AUGUST 2002

W.B. SAUNDERS COMPANY
A Division of Elsevier Science
PHILADELPHIA   LONDON   TORONTO   MONTREAL   SYDNEY   TOKYO

W.B. SAUNDERS COMPANY
A Division of Elsevier Science

The Curtis Center • Independence Square West • Philadelphia, Pennsylvania 19106

http://www.wbsaunders.com

HEMATOLOGY/ONCOLOGY CLINICS
OF NORTH AMERICA   Volume 16, Number 4
August 2002   ISSN 0889-8588
Editor: Kerry Holland

The ideas and opinions expressed in *Hematology/Oncology Clinics of North America* do not necessarily reflect those of the Publisher. The Publisher does not assume any responsibility for any injury and/or damage to persons or property arising out of or related to any use of the material contained in this periodical. The reader is advised to check the appropriate medical literature and the product information currently provided by the manufacturer of each drug to be administered to verify the dosage, the method and duration of administration, or contraindications. It is the responsibility of the treating physician or other health care professional, relying on independent experience and knowledge of the patient, to determine drug dosages and the best treatment for the patient. Mention of any product in this issue should not be construed as endorsement by the contributors, editors, or the Publisher of the product or manufacturers' claims.

Hematology/Oncology Clinics of North America (ISSN 0889-8588) is published bi-monthly by W.B. Saunders Company. Corporate and editorial offices: The Curtis Center, Independence Square West, Philadelphia, PA 19106-3399. Accounting and circulation offices: 6277 Sea Harbor Drive, Orlando, FL 32887-4800. Periodicals postage paid at Orlando, FL 32862, and additional mailing offices. Subscription prices are $186.00 per year (US individuals), $242.00 per year (US institutions), $237.00 per year (foreign individuals), $295.00 per year (foreign institutions), $212.00 per year (Canadian individuals), and $295.00 per year (Canadian institutions). Foreign air speed delivery is included in all *Clinics* subscription prices. All prices are subject to change without notice. POSTMASTER: Send address changes to *Hematology/Oncology Clinics of North America*, W.B. Saunders Company, Periodicals Fulfillment, Orlando, FL 32887-4800. **Customer Service: 1-800-654-2452 (US). From outside the US, call 407-345-4000.** E-mail: hhspcs@harcourt.com

Hematology/Oncology Clinics of North America is covered in *Index Medicus, EMBASE/Excerpta Medica, and BIOSIS.*

Printed in the United States of America.

GUEST EDITOR

GREGORY G. GINSBERG, MD, Associate Professor of Medicine, Gastroenterology Division, University of Pennsylvania School of Medicine; Director, Endoscopic Services, Hospital of the University of Pennsylvania, Philadelphia, Pennsylvania

CONTRIBUTORS

DOUGLAS G. ADLER, MD, Department of Medicine, Division of Gastroenterology and Hepatology, Mayo Medical Center, Rochester, Minnesota

NUZHAT A. AHMAD, MD, Assistant Professor, Division of Gastroenterology, Department of Medicine, University of Pennsylvania Cancer Center, University of Pennsylvania School of Medicine, Philadelphia, Pennsylvania

TODD H. BARON, MD, FACP, Department of Medicine, Division of Gastroenterology and Hepatology, Mayo Medical Center, Rochester, Minnesota

ROBERT J. CANTER, MD, Assistant Instructor, Department of Surgery, University of Pennsylvania School of Medicine, Philadelphia, Pennsylvania

JAMES A. DiSARIO, MD, Associate Professor of Medicine, Huntsman Cancer Center, University of Utah Health Sciences Center, Salt Lake City, Utah

NORA DOBOS, MD, Department of Radiology, Hospital of the University of Pennsylvania, Philadelphia, Pennsylvania

RAYMOND N. DuBOIS, MD, PhD, Professor, Departments of Medicine/GI and Cell Biology; Mina Cobb Wallace Chair in Gastroenterology and Cancer Prevention; Associate Director of Cancer Prevention, Control, and Population Based Research; Director, Division of Gastroenterology, Vanderbilt University Medical Center, Nashville, Tennessee

JAMES W. FLESHMAN, MD, FACRS, FACS, Professor of Surgery; Chief, Section of Colorectal Surgery, Washington University and Barnes Jewish Hospital, St. Louis, Missouri

DOUGLAS L. FRAKER, MD, Jonathan E. Rhoads Associate Professor, Department of Surgery, University of Pennsylvania, Philadelphia, Pennsylvania

GREGORY G. GINSBERG, MD, Associate Professor of Medicine, Gastroenterology Division, University of Pennsylvania School of Medicine; Director, Endoscopic Services, Hospital of the University of Pennsylvania, Philadelphia, Pennsylvania

STEPHEN HAHN, MD, Department of Radiation Oncology, Division of Hematology Oncology, Department of Medicine, University of Pennsylvania School of Medicine, Philadelphia, Pennsylvania

DANIEL G. HALLER, MD, Professor, Hematology/Oncology Division, Department of Medicine, University of Pennsylvania Medical Center, Philadelphia, Pennsylvania

TIMOTHY C. HOOPS, MD, Clinical Assistant Professor, Division of Gastroenterology, Department of Medicine, University of Pennsylvania, Philadelphia, Pennsylvania

MICHAEL L. KOCHMAN, MD, FACP, Associate Professor, Division of Gastroenterology, Department of Medicine, University of Pennsylvania Cancer Center, University of Pennsylvania School of Medicine, Philadelphia, Pennsylvania

JOHN P. LYNCH, MD, PhD, Assistant Professor, Division of Gastroenterology, Department of Medicine, University of Pennsylvania, Philadelphia, Pennsylvania

JAMES M. METZ, MD, Department of Radiation Oncology, Division of Hematology Oncology, Department of Medicine, University of Pennsylvania School of Medicine, Philadelphia, Pennsylvania

DOUGLAS NELSON, MD, Staff Physician, Gastroenterology, Minneapolis VA Medical Center; Associate Professor of Medicine, University of Minnesota, Minneapolis, Minnesota

KATHRYN A. PETERSON, MD, Assistant Professor, Division of Gastroenterology, Department of Internal Medicine, University of Utah Health Sciences Center, Salt Lake City, Utah

SONIA L. RAMAMOORTHY, MD, Section of Colorectal Surgery, Washington University and Barnes Jewish Hospital, St. Louis, Missouri

STEPHEN E. RUBESIN, MD, Professor, Department of Radiology, Hospital of the University of Pennsylvania, Philadelphia, Pennsylvania

ROBERTO J. SANTIAGO, Department of Radiation Oncology, Division of Hematology Oncology, Department of Medicine, University of Pennsylvania School of Medicine, Philadelphia, Pennsylvania

MICHAEL SOULEN, MD, Associate Professor, Department of Radiology, University of Pennsylvania, Philadelphia, Pennsylvania

WEIJING SUN, MD, Assistant Professor, Hematology/Oncology Division, Department of Medicine, University of Pennsylvania Medical Center, Philadelphia, Pennsylvania

MARCO E. TURINI, Department of Nutrition, Nestlé Research Center, Lausanne, Switzerland

NOEL N. WILLIAMS, MD, Assistant Professor, Division of Gastro-Intestinal Surgery, Department of Surgery, University of Pennsylvania School of Medicine, Philadelphia, Pennsylvania

CONTENTS

Each year in the United States, colon cancer leads to the death of nearly 60,000 men and women. Because of its enormous impact, colon cancer has been the focus of intense investigation for many years. Research over the last decade has firmly established that the progression from normal colonic epithelium to colon cancer is in every case a step-wise process in which specific pathologic and molecular markers can be identified for study and clinical therapy. This neoplastic progression occurs along a limited set of pathways, in which specific tumor-suppressors are inactivated or oncogenes activated in a defined order. Although incomplete, our new understanding of the process of carcinogenesis in the colon has already significantly impacted patient care, and increasingly rapid research developments and technological advances will transform the way we prevent, diagnose, and treat this common and deadly form of cancer.

Because cancer usually develops over a 10- to 20-year period, true chemopreventive agents should be provided before or early on in the initiation steps of carcinogenesis to have beneficial effects. Other agents may be more suitable to limit colorectal cancer development if provided at a later stage of carcinogenesis.

neoadjuvant therapy. Those potential benefits include decreased local recurrence and increase in sphincter sparing surgery. Conversely, patients with superficial lesions may be spared surgery and cured with endoscopic mucosal resection.

in the United States. Based on the American Cancer Society's estimates, there will be 138,900 (68,800 in men and 70,100 in women) new cases diagnosed with colorectal cancer in 2001, and 57,200 deaths will be caused by this disease. Of the new cases, nearly 60% present with lymph node involvement or metastatic disease. Overall survival for colorectal cancer has improved over the past several decades. This is probably because of increased screening, resulting in stage migration with more patients being diagnosed with early, localized disease. Better preoperative staging, improved surgical techniques and pathologic evaluation of resected specimens have also contributed to the improvement of the overall outcome for these patients. Survival has also been improved by the use of adjuvant chemotherapy in colon cancer and combined modality therapy with chemotherapy and radiation in rectal cancer. Recent advances in chemotherapeutic approaches include novel cytotoxic chemotherapy agents. Biological and molecular targeting agents may impact survival even further.

The integration of radiotherapy to the adjuvant treatment of rectal cancer was prompted by the predominance of locoregional failures after curative surgery. This characteristic in the pattern of failure is one of the main reasons adjuvant radiotherapy plays a greater role in rectal cancer than in colon cancer. It has been demonstrated that local failure rates after surgery alone for rectal cancer are strongly dependent on the degree of bowel wall invasion, lymph node involvement, and margins of resection. These same locoregional factors are also predictive of distant metastasis and survival. In addition, local failure is associated with devastating symptoms that severely affect the quality of life of patients. For these reasons, locoregional control remains a major issue in the treatment of rectal cancer. This article summarizes the evidence that has established chemoradiotherapy as part of the standard of care for rectal cancer and the techniques used for its delivery.

Patients with colorectal cancer often present with advanced disease and are sometimes candidates only for palliative therapies. Many of these patients present with subtotal or complete colonic obstruction. Self-expanding metal stents are now available to palliate obstructing or near-obstructing lesions of the large intestine, and their use is becoming commonplace. In patients with malignant large bowel obstructions without widespread disease, the placement of a colonic self-expanding stent can allow preoperative decompression and bowel preparation to allow for a one-stage surgical procedure. In patients with large bowel obstruction from advanced or widespread malignancies, as is much more commonly seen, colonic stents can be placed as purely palliative devices. Lasers also can play a role in the palliation of colorectal cancer, but their use as a sole means of palliation is declining.

FORTHCOMING ISSUES

October 2002

Targeted Therapies
Manuel Hidalgo, MD, *Guest Editor*

December 2002

Health Policy and Law
Bryan Liang, MD, JD, *Guest Editor*

February 2003

Thrombosis and Thrombophilia: Diagnosis and Management
Rodger L. Bick, MD, PhD, FACP, *Guest Editor*

RECENT ISSUES

June 2002

Palliative Cancer
Paul Walker, MD, and
Eduardo Bruera, MD, *Guest Editors*

April 2002

Flow Cytometry and Its Applications in Hematology and Oncology
Roger S, Riley, MD, PhD, *Guest Editor*

February 2002

Pancreatic Cancer
Peter Kozuch, MD, and
Howard W. Bruckner, MD, *Guest Editors*

VISIT THESE RELATED WEB SITES

MD Consult—A comprehensive online clinical resource:
www.mdconsult.com

For more information about Clinics:
www.wbsaunders.com

Hematol Oncol Clin N Am
16 (2002) xi

HEMATOLOGY/
ONCOLOGY
CLINICS OF
NORTH AMERICA

Preface

Colorectal cancer

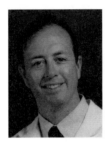

Gregory G. Ginsberg, MD
Guest Editor

Colorectal cancer is a leading cause of cancer and cancer death in North America. It affects men and women, young and old, ignoring socioeconomic and racial differences. This issue of *Hematology/Oncology Clinics of North America* provides a multidisciplinary and in-depth treatment of the dedicated subject matter. The authorship is drawn from experts in the fields of molecular biology, gastroenterology, colorectal and oncologic surgery, interventional radiology, and medical and radiation oncology. Readers will avail themselves of the current and future understanding of the development, prevention, detection, and treatment of early and advanced stages of colorectal cancers through which improved patient outcomes and professional satisfaction can be expected.

Gregory G. Ginsberg, MD
Associate Professor of Medicine
University of Pennsylvania School of Medicine
Gastroenterology Division
Director of Endoscopic Services
Hospital of the University of Pennsylvania
3400 Spruce Street, 3 Ravdin
Philadelphia, PA 19104, USA

Hematol Oncol Clin N Am
16 (2002) 775–810

HEMATOLOGY/
ONCOLOGY
CLINICS OF
NORTH AMERICA

The genetic pathogenesis of colorectal cancer

John P. Lynch, MD, PhD[a],*, Timothy C. Hoops, MD[a,b]

[a]Division of Gastroenterology, Department of Medicine, University of Pennsylvania,
415 Curie Boulevard, Philadelphia, PA 19104, USA
[b]Presbyterian Medical Center, 39th and Market Streets, Philadelphia, PA 19104, USA

Each year in the United States, colon cancer is diagnosed in nearly 140,000 men and women and leads to the death of nearly 60,000. As such, it is the second leading cause of cancer death. Because of its enormous impact, colon cancer has been the focus of intense research for many years. Twenty-five years ago, basic research in biology was revolutionized with the development and rapid dissemination of the techniques and methods now collectively referred to as molecular biology. In the 1980s, these techniques were first applied to the problem of colon cancer, yielding new insights and greatly improving our understanding of the process of colorectal tumorigenesis. During this period, the genetic basis of colorectal cancer was first fully appreciated.

Throughout the 1990s, the pace of discovery quickened. Our understanding of the genetic events underlying colon cancer development and progression has now evolved to the point where patient care is significantly impacted. Insights into the genetic basis of colorectal cancer (1) has provided a rational basis for primary prevention [1,2]; (2) has enhanced screening in familial colorectal cancer syndromes [2–4]; (3) may soon alter how we screen for sporadic colorectal neoplasias [5]; (4) has begun to affect the management of patients with colon cancer [6]; and (5) has identified potentially new therapeutic targets [7,8]. This article will attempt to summarize the most current concepts regarding the genetic basis of colon cancer, as well as review several of the more important regulatory pathways involved in this process.

Concepts of colorectal tumorigenesis

Adenoma-carcinoma sequence

It has long been recognized that human colon cancer rarely, if ever, arises directly from normal epithelium. Multiple areas of investigation have determined

---

* Corresponding author.
E-mail address: lynchj@mail.med.upenn.edu (J.P. Lynch).

0889-8588/02/$ – see front matter © 2002, Elsevier Science (USA). All rights reserved.
PII: S 0 8 8 9 - 8 5 8 8 (0 2) 0 0 0 2 9 - 1

that most human colorectal cancers arise from adenomas. Adenomas are dysplastic but nonmalignant masses in the colon [9–11]. They are characterized by their size, histologic type (tubular, tubulovillous, and villous), and degree of dysplasia. The hypothesis that colorectal tumorigenesis develops via the intermediate adenomatous polyp is supported by pathologic, epidemiologic, observational clinical, and animal studies. Early carcinomas are frequently seen in large adenomatous polyps, and often areas of adenomatous change can be found surrounding human colon cancers. Epidemiologic data indicates adenomas and carcinomas are found in similar distributions in the colon, and adenomas are typically observed 10–15 years prior to the onset of cancer in both sporadic and familial colon cancers. The pivotal National Polyp Study has determined that endoscopic removal of polyps reduces the subsequent incidence of colon cancer in treated patients [12]. Lastly, in animal models of colon cancer, adenoma development precedes carcinoma, and carcinomas develop uniformly in adenomatous tissues. The adenoma-carcinoma sequence describes this progression from normal mucosa to invasive carcinoma.

Adenomatous polyps form in the colon when normal mechanisms regulating epithelial renewal are disrupted [9]. Typically, surface cells of the colon are constantly lost to the lumen because of cell death (apoptosis) or mechanical exfoliation and must be replaced. Renewal depends on a continuous, regulated process of proliferation of stem and crypt base cells and differentiation of daughter cells. Proliferation normally occurs exclusively at the crypt base. Daughter cells ascend from the base, cease proliferating, and terminally differentiate. This highly ordered process is progressively disrupted in adenomas as they increase in size and degree of dysplasia. The proliferative zone shifts to include the whole crypt and surface epithelium. There is no increase in apoptosis to offset the elevated proliferation. The resulting increased numbers of epithelial cells lead to the irregular infolding and branching characteristic of adenomas. The degree to which the underlying mesenchyme proliferates to support the overgrowing epithelium helps determine polyp size and polyp histology (villous or tubulovillous).

Aberrant crypt foci (ACF), described first over 10 years ago [13], are believed to be the intermediate between normal colonic mucosa and the adenomatous polyp [14,15]. ACF are microscopic lesions, first identified in methylene-blue stained colons of azoxymethane-treated mice as crypts that appeared larger and thicker, with an increased luminal diameter and an opening that was often slitlike or serrated. ACF can be composed of as few as 1 crypt or as many as 200 or more, and the surface can be flat, bulge slightly, or appear concave. Most ACF are hyperplastic (65–95%); however, a significant proportion are dysplastic and similar to adenomas [16,17]. The dysplastic ACF are on average larger, contain more crypts, and are characterized by pleomorphic, stratified nuclei, decreased mucin staining, increased proliferation, and extension of proliferation to the upper crypt [17,18]. In humans, ACF, like adenomas, are found in greater numbers in the left colon, in older patients, and in patients with colon cancer or familial colon cancer syndromes [15]. ACF are monoclonal lesions [19], and severe dysplasia, including carcinoma in situ, has been reported [20]. Genetic analysis of ACF has identified several mutations seen also in adenomatous polyps [15,16,21–26]. Lastly, ACF are the earliest precursor lesions observed in animal models of carcinogenesis. They are specifically induced by known carcinogens in a dose-dependent fashion and precede the development of frank polyps and cancer [13,14,27,28]. Because ACF are considered to be the earliest precursor lesions in the progression to colon cancer, they are being used as early biomarkers for neoplasia in both animal and human studies. But there remains some concern with their use until a better understanding of the natural history of ACF is obtained. In particular, the question as to whether hyperplastic ACF can progress to adenoma and cancer needs to be fully explored.

The multistep process of cancer development

Carcinogenesis had long been thought to be a step-wise process [29]; the advent of molecular biology provided the tools to clearly establish this. These methods determined that cancer is caused by an accumulation of multiple somatic mutations in a cell's DNA. With each step along the process, more mutations are acquired until malignant transformation has occurred. Common mutational events observed in human cancers include point mutations, altered DNA methylation, and gene rearrangements, amplifications, and deletions. The results of these mutations fall into one of three broad classes: (1) gain-of-function events, generally activation of growth-promoting pathways including oncogenes; (2) loss-of-function events, primarily inactivation of tumor suppressors and apoptotic pathways; and (3) epigenetic alterations (DNA methylation patterns), which can lead to both aberrant gene expression and silencing [30]. More than a decade ago, it was first observed that carcinogenesis progresses along a limited set of pathways; certain gene mutations are commonly acquired in a fairly specific order. This has been demonstrated in a variety of human cancers, but one of the best and earliest models for this was colon tumorigenesis. This hypothesis was first proposed by Fearon and Vogelstein [31] in 1990, and studies carried out in the past decade have served only to improve and refine this model.

Fundamental to the multistep hypothesis is the clonal nature of neoplasms, with each neoplastic cell derived from a single progenitor [10,32]. This progenitor experiences one or more mutational events that endow it with survival advantages. When one of the daughter cells acquires another mutation providing it with an additional advantage, a wave of clonal expansion follows. This process is repeated, and, as further beneficial mutations accrue, a mass is formed. Ultimately, a daughter cell will accumulate the right set of mutational events and undergo malignant transformation characterized by unregulated cell growth, evasion of apoptosis, induction of angiogenesis, severe genomic instability, local invasiveness and, eventually, distant metastases [33].

This progression to carcinogenesis is by no means absolute. Although colonic epithelial cells are constantly acquiring somatic mutations, the development of neoplasia is still exceedingly infrequent. Mutational events are more likely to be silent, or be detrimental to the survival of the cell, rather than promote neoplasia.

Mechanisms exist within the cell to identify and repair mutations or, if the mutations are too extensive to repair, initiate apoptotic cell death. It is likely that these processes, as well as local environmental and systemic functions, provide continuous selective pressures on the neoplastic cells. This would explain why colon cancer strikes predominantly late in life, why most polyps never progress to adenocarcinoma, and why it typically can be 10–15 years or more before an adenoma transforms into a carcinoma [34,35]. It also explains why there are a limited number of genetic pathways leading to carcinogenesis—the vast majority of mutational events direct the cell along an evolutionary 'dead-end' [36].

The identification of these genetic pathways was greatly assisted by the study of familial cancer syndromes and the long, difficult work carried out to identify the inherited genetic mutations. Typically, genes identified in familial cancer syndromes were often found to be involved in the genesis of sporadic cancers [37]. This observation has led to the concept of "gatekeepers" and "carertakers" [38]. Gatekeepers are genes that directly regulate growth by inhibiting proliferation or promoting cell death. Each tissue type has a small number of gatekeepers responsible for limiting growth; loss or inactivation of the gatekeeper(s) dramatically increases tumor initiation. Caretaker genes are responsible for maintaining genetic stability. Inactivation of a caretaker promotes carcinogenesis indirectly by increasing the rate of accumulation of mutations. When a caretaker gene function is lost, all genes experience increased mutation rates, but ultimately a gatekeeper is mutated in both alleles, and tumor initiation is greatly enhanced.

Although the inherited colon cancer syndromes familial adenomatous polyposis (FAP) and hereditary nonpolyposis colorectal cancer syndrome (HNPCC) together account for only about 5% of all colon cancers, identification of the predisposing inherited mutations illuminated the predominant gatekeeper and caretaker genes whose mutation is critical in the development of nearly all colorectal cancers [37]. The central role played by these genes in colon cancer development is illustrated by Fig. 1. Two genetic pathways appear to be largely responsible for human colorectal tumorigenesis [37,39]. Pathway I is predominant, accounting for 80–85% of all human colon neoplasms. It is characterized by aneuploidy and chromosomal instability (CIN), and early inactivation of the gatekeeper APC (adenomatosis polyposis coli). Neoplasia in FAP progresses along this pathway, initiated by a germline mutation of the APC gene in one allele. Pathway II is responsible for 15–20% of colon cancers and is characterized by loss of a caretaker function, the inability to recognize and repair the many nucleotide mismatches that commonly occur during DNA replication. This function is termed mismatch-repair (MMR). Germline inactivation of a MMR gene is responsible for HNPCC [40].

Though these pathways describe the most common genetic events observed, not all events are found in every neoplasm. Flat adenomas and cancers tend to be more dysplastic than similarly sized polypoid adenomas and progress more quickly to cancer, but they are much less likely to have acquired an activated K-ras mutant [41–44]. Similarly, patients with inflammatory bowel disease are at risk for colon cancer via an alternate pathway, colitis associated cancer (CAC)

Pathway I

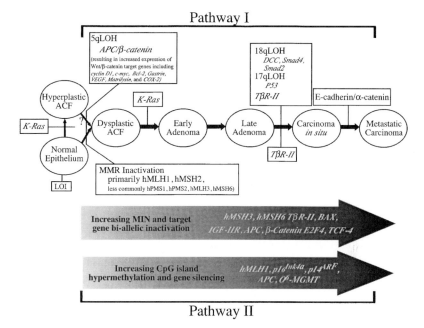

Fig. 1. Primary genetic pathways in the development of human colon cancer [37,39]. Primary morphologic and genetic events occurring during the progression to cancer in the human colon. Dysplastic ACF is the earliest recognized precursor; it is not known if hyperplastic ACF can progress to dysplastic ACF. Pathway I, which includes FAP as well as the majority of sporadic colon cancers, accounts for 80–85% of all human colon neoplasms. It is characterized by aneuploidy, CIN, and early inactivation of the gatekeeper APC. The timing of other significant genetic events is indicated, along with the genes affected. Pathway II is largely responsible for the remainder of colon cancers. Cancers arising along this pathway tend to occur proximally, be poorly differentiated, diploid, associated with an improved survival for patients, and have MIN. The primary genetic event is early inactivation of MMR, either by germline mutation of a MMR gene followed by loss of the second allele (as in HNPCC), or aberrant hMLH1 promoter hypermethylation in both alleles, resulting in hMLH1 gene silencing, occurring in sporadic MIN cancers. MIN and aberrant promoter hypermethylation are responsible for the inactivation of a number of other tumor-suppressors (*arrows*). The timing of their inactivation during carcinogenesis is unknown for all except the TGF-β receptor II (TβR-II). ACF, aberrant crypt foci; APC, adenomatosis polyposis coli; CIN, chromosomal instability; FAP, familial adenomatous polyposis; HNPCC, hereditary nonpolyposis colorectal cancer syndrome; MIN, microsatellite instability; MMR, mismatch repair.

[45,46]. These alternate pathways are clinically important and will likely further our understanding of tumorigenesis. We will focus for the remainder, however, on the genetic events critical to Pathways I and II.

Genetic instability and epigenetics

A cardinal feature of cancer cells is their genetic instability [32,47,48]. This instability has been observed in the earliest stages of tumorigenesis, the ACF [21,49]. It is not uncommon for the rate of instability to increase during the progression to carcinoma [47,48]. We now recognize there exist several distinct forms of genetic instability [36,47]. At present, our understanding of these forms is limited; as we learn more, it is likely their importance to models of tumorigenesis will increase.

The vast majority of human tumors are aneuploid, with an abnormal chromosome and DNA content. Aneuploidy is marked by gains or losses of whole chromosomes, a phenotype described as chromosomal instability (CIN) [47]. An important feature of CIN is loss of heterozygosity (LOH), the loss of one allele of a gene. Thus, only one copy of a gene need be somatically mutated with the loss of the wild-type allele by LOH. Other features of CIN tumors include gene amplification and chromosomal translocations. The causes of CIN are currently unknown, but DNA damage checkpoints and spindle checkpoints appear to have a critical role in this process [48]. Human genes involved in the DNA damage checkpoint known to play important roles in tumorgenesis include the breast-cancer related BRCA1 and BRCA2 genes, and P53 [48]. The mitotic spindle, which equally segregates chromosomes between daughter cells during cell division, is monitored by spindle checkpoints [50]. Our understanding of mammalian spindle checkpoints is limited, but abnormalities in them can be demonstrated in CIN colon cancers. In two colon cancer cell lines, inactivating mutations in the human homologue of the yeast spindle checkpoint Bub1 gene were identified [51]. Recently, several studies have shown that the APC protein, in addition to its central role as a gatekeeper in FAP and sporadic carcinogenesis, is also critically involved in chromosome segregation [52,53]. APC links microtubules to the chromosomal kinetochores during mitosis by binding kinetochore-anchored Bub1 and Bub3. APC mutants, like those commonly found in colon cancers, lack these binding sites and produce chromosomal segregation defects in vitro. Mechanisms governing chromosomal translocations and gene amplifications remain to be determined, although several studies suggest these features may be caused by the same defect in chromosomal segregation [48,54].

Perhaps the best understood of the genetic instabilities involved in colon cancer progression is MMR [55–58]. The MMR system recognizes the base-base mismatches and short insertion/deletion mispairings that occur with DNA replication and homologous recombination. These errors, if not corrected prior to DNA replication, would be passed on to daughter cells. The MMR system recognizes these areas of mismatch and signals for repair [59]. Short repetitive DNA segments found throughout the genome, referred to as microsatellites, are particularly vulnerable to this type of error and are frequently mutated in cells deficient for MMR [48,58]. Hence, the phenotype is often referred to as microsatellite instability (MSI or MIN). Genes that contain these repetitive sequences in their coding regions are particularly susceptible to inactivating mutations during DNA replication in MIN neoplasms [60–62]. MIN cancers, unlike CIN neoplasms, tend to be diploid [48]. MIN is present infrequently, occurring in about 15% of colon, endometrial, and gastric cancers [48].

Lastly, epigenetic regulation of gene expression is proving to play an important role in carcinogenesis [63–65]. Epigenetic mechanisms include DNA methylation, gene imprinting, and histone acetylation. DNA methylation is an important mediator for gene silencing and repressing viral and transposon transcription. CpG dinucleotides, present in the promoters of many genes, are targeted for methylation [63]. Methylated CpG is bound by a family of proteins known as methyl-CpG binding domain proteins (MBDs), which in turn form a multi-protein complex that alters chromatin conformation and silences gene expression [64,65]. Normally, methylation of these CpG islands within promoters is tightly regulated; fully methylated CpG islands are rare and are found only in the promoters of genes on the inactivated X-chromosome in females and genes regulated by imprinting [64]. Imprinting refers to the process whereby the alleles of certain genes are differentially methylated [66]. This pattern is set in the zygote and gamete prior to fertilization, and maintained during development to suppress expression of the maternal or paternal copy of an allele. It now appears that disordered promoter methylation and loss of imprinting (LOI) are both involved in the pathogenesis of some colorectal cancers.

The aberrant hypermethylation of CpG islands is likely acquired gradually [63]. Therefore, gene silencing can be detected early in the pathway to cancer and is often progressive. In colon cancer, p16^{Ink4a} (regulates cyclin D activity), MLH1 (a MMR gene), p14^{ARF} (upregulates P53 activity), APC, and O^6-MGMT (repairs guanine to adenosine mutations, the kind that activate K-ras) have been identified as common targets for silencing by promoter methylation [67–72]. LOI of the insulin-like growth factor II gene (IGF2) has been highly associated with MMR colon cancer, accounting for 33–91% of MMR colon cancers across several studies [73–75]. Perhaps the most surprising finding was that this LOI could be detected in normal colonic mucosa of affected patients, as well as the blood of affected and, to a lesser degree, unaffected individuals [73]. This would suggest the disordered methylation might be a predisposing condition rather than a somatically acquired event. In fact, a DNA "methylator" phenotype, the "CpG island methylator phenotype" (CIMP) [76,77], has been hypothesized as a possible cause of sporadic and some familial colon cancers. The clinical and molecular characterization of this phenotype is an area of active investigation.

Gene pathways commonly mutated in colorectal carcinogenesis

The wingless type/APC/β-catenin pathway

Perhaps the most critical gene target in the progression to colorectal cancer is the APC tumor suppressor. APC mutations occur early in sporadic colon cancer development and with great frequency, and germline transmission of a single mutant APC allele is the cause of FAP [78]. APC mutations are so common largely because of the important role played by APC in regulating the wingless signaling pathway. The Wingless-type (Wnt) signaling pathway is an evolutionarily conserved cascade of protein interactions whose purpose is to transduce a signal from a cell surface receptor to the nucleus and alter gene expression [79–82]. This pathway is necessary for patterning and axis formation during early embryonic development. It has also surprisingly been found to play a central role in supporting the process of intestinal epithelial renewal. The most current model for Wnt/APC/β-catenin signaling is presented in Fig. 2 [79–82]. In the unstimulated state, free β-catenin is rapidly recruited from the cytoplasm and the nucleus

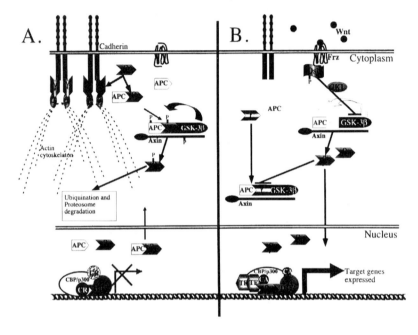

Fig. 2. Regulation of Wnt/APC/β-catenin pathway signaling [79–82]. Mechanisms regulating this signaling pathway are presented. (A) In the absence of Wnt signaling, free β-catenin (β) is rapidly sequestered (ie, cadherin adhesion complexes) or recruited from the cytoplasm and the nucleus into a multi-protein complex with APC, axin, and GSK-3β. APC possesses nuclear import and export functions and shuttles β-catenin from the nucleus to the cytoplasm where it joins the multiprotein complex. GSK-3β actively phosphorylates target proteins APC, axin, and β-catenin. Phosphorylation of APC and axin significantly increases their binding with β-catenin; axin phosphorylation also promotes axin protein stability. Phosphorylated β-catenin is marked for destruction via the ubiquitin/proteosome pathway. This reduces β-catenin levels overall and effectively blocks the Wnt signaling cascade. The expression of the Wnt/APC/β-catenin targeted genes is tightly restricted; in the absence of β-catenin, TCF/LEF factors recruit CR to silence these genes. α: α-catenin; γ: γ-catenin. (B) When present, secreted Wnt protein binds its receptor, Frz, thereby activating it. The activated receptor phosphorylates Dsh that, in conjunction with CK I, inactivates GSK-3β. Once GSK-3β is inactivated, axin is actively dephosphorylated, and the multi-protein complex itself breaks down. Axin levels fall, and both axin and APC bind β-catenin less effectively when dephosphorylated. With the breakdown of the complex, β-catenin is no longer phosphorylated by GSK-3β. This results in unphosphorylated β-catenin accumulating in the cytoplasm, which then translocates to the nucleus. In the nucleus, β-catenin complexes with T-cell and LEF transcription factors to form a bipartite transcription factor able to reverse the active repression and instead attract CA to enhance gene transcription and expression. Plakoglobin, also known as γ-catenin (γ), can compete with β-catenin for APC binding. This may lead to increased free β-catenin levels and activate Wnt/APC/β-catenin nuclear signaling. Ca, coactivators; CK, casein kinase; CR, corepressor proteins; Dsh, disheveled; Frz, frizzled; GSK, glycogen synthase kinase; LEF, lymphoid-enhancing transcription factors.

into a multi-protein complex with APC, axin, and glycogen synthase kinase (GSK)-3β. APC possesses nuclear import and export functions; it is in fact required for the shuttling of β-catenin from the nucleus to the cytoplasm [83,84] where it joins the multi-protein complex. Axin serves as the scaffolding protein, recruiting the other factors of the complex. GSK-3β actively phosphorylates target proteins APC, axin, and β-catenin, among others [80,82,85,86]. Phosphorylation of APC and axin significantly increases their binding with β-catenin; axin phosphorylation also promotes axin protein stability and thereby promotes formation of the multi-protein complex. Phosphorylated β-catenin is marked for destruction via the ubiquitin/proteosome pathway. This reduces β-catenin levels overall and effectively blocks the Wnt signaling cascade.

Normally, the secreted Wnt protein binds and activates its receptor, encoded by the frizzled (Frz) gene [79–82]. The activated receptor phosphorylates the disheveled (Dsh) protein which, in conjunction with another kinase, casein kinase I (CK I) [87], inactivates GSK-3β. Once GSK-3β is inactivated, axin is actively dephosphorylated, and the multi-protein complex itself breaks down [88]. Axin levels fall, and both axin and APC bind β-catenin less effectively when dephosphorylated. With the breakdown of the complex, β-catenin is no longer phosphorylated by GSK-3β. This results in unphosphorylated β-catenin accumulating in the cytoplasm, which then translocates to the nucleus [79–82]. In the nucleus, β-catenin complexes with T-cell (TCF) and lymphoid-enhancing (LEF) transcription factors to enhance the transcription of genes now known for their role in cell growth and tumorigenesis.

The expression of the TCF/LEF targeted genes is tightly restricted; in the absence of β-catenin, TCF/LEF factors recruit repressor proteins to silence these genes [81,89–93]. But in the presence of β-catenin, the TCF/LEF-β-catenin proteins form a bipartite transcription factor able to reverse the active repression and instead attract proteins that enhance gene transcription and expression. Many of the genes activated by TCF/LEF-β-catenin are known to be important for tumor development and progression, which may explain why this pathway is so often targeted early in colon tumorigenesis. TCF/LEF-β-catenin targeted genes have been observed to be inappropriately expressed in colon polyps as well as cancers, and include cMyc, cyclin D1, the multi-drug resistance 1 gene (MDR1), gastrin, matrilysin, peroxisome proliferator-activated receptor δ (PPARδ), and, COX-2 [94–99]. In summary, somatic mutations that lead to increased β-catenin levels can promote tumor progression by enhancing TCF/LEF target gene expression.

In the past several years, other mechanisms to regulate the Wnt/APC/β-catenin signaling pathway have been observed. Some involve "crosstalk" between signaling pathways (TGF-β, RAS, MAPK) [89,100]; others directly block the interaction between TCF/LEF and β-catenin by acetylation of TCF/LEF [89]; and still others sequester free β-catenin from TCF/LEF (eg, E-cadherin, vitamin D) [89,101–104]. Some modifiers appear to work by reducing the activity of important Wnt/APC/β-catenin targets such as COX-2 (eg, cytosolic phospholipase A_2) [105], whereas the mechanism for others remains uncertain (eg, secretory phospholipase A_2) [106]. One modifier, protein phosphatase 2A

(PP2A), is likely another tumor suppressor that is targeted during carcinogenesis in certain cancer types [107]. In general, it is unclear what roles these modifiers play in regulating the normal process of epithelial renewal in the intestine, or if they are at all involved in the progression to colon cancer.

The role of APC in colorectal cancer

APC and familial adenomatous polyposis syndromes

FAP is a dominantly inherited syndrome characterized by the development of hundreds to thousands of colorectal polyps by the second and third decade of life [81]. Inevitably, some of these polyps progress to cancer. Genetic studies of FAP kindreds linked inheritance of this syndrome to chromosome 5q21. Subsequent efforts identified APC as the tumor-suppressor responsible for FAP [78]. Nearly 80% of FAP families have identifiable germline mutations in one allele of APC in effected individuals. Similar high rates of germline mutations were seen in the FAP varient Gardner syndrome. MIN mice with a mutated APC allele, and transgenic mice with a truncated APC protein ($APC^{\Delta 716}$), develop numerous adenomatous polyps in their small intestine and colon [108,109]. In both humans and mice, the earliest premalignant lesions, dysplastic ACF and small adenomatous polyps, are characterized by loss of the second APC allele either by somatic mutation or LOH. The method by which the second allele is lost appears to depend on the germline genotype. Primary mutations within a region of APC known as the mutation cluster region (MCR) are predisposed to LOH of the second allele, whereas all other primary mutations preferentially acquire a somatic mutation of the other APC allele within the MCR [110].

Nearly all of the germline mutations in APC are nonsense or frameshift mutations that result in a truncated protein. The APC protein is a large protein containing 2843 amino-acids and more than a dozen functional domains. One third of these mutations are located in a small region between amino-acid codons 1061 and 1309, the mutation cluster region [81]. The remainder largely occur between codons 200 and 1600. The MCR is located just above the domains required for β-catenin downregulation and axin binding, and therefore proteins truncated here cannot promote β-catenin destruction. Loss of the second functional APC allele would therefore lead to unregulated β-catenin levels, causing induction of TCF/LEF-induced gene expression, and unregulated growth [111,112]. This effect on β-catenin levels is entirely caused by the mutant APC; restoration of wild-type APC protein expression in colon cancer cell lines reduces free β-catenin levels and abrogates TCF/LEF target gene transcription [111]. In addition to loss of axin and β-catenin downregulating domains, all truncated APC forms lose the microtubule/EB-1 binding and the hBub1/hBub3 binding domains as well. This appears to promote the chromosomal instability that is a characteristic feature of FAP colon cancer as well as most sporadic colon cancers [52,53].

The FAP phenotype expressed in an individual depends in part on the site of the germline APC mutation. Severe polyposis is seen in those with the mutation between codons 1250 and 1464, whereas attenuated FAP, characterized by fewer than 100 polyps, is often caused by mutations at the extreme ends of the APC coding sequence [81]. Congenital hypertrophy of the retinal pigment epithelium (CHRPE), a condition present at any age in 60% of FAP families, is associated with germline mutations between codons 457 and 1444. Desmoid tumors are limited to those individuals with mutations between 1403 and 1578. In addition, extracolonic manifestations of FAP and hepatoblastomas associated with FAP have likewise been associated with germline mutations in specific clusters. The mechanisms by which these different APC mutants give rise to the associated phenotypes are not known.

APC and sporadic colorectal cancers

The study of APC mutations in FAP has provided tremendous insight into the role of this protein in sporadic colon carcinogenesis, by far a more common condition. Nearly 80% of sporadic cancers have identifiable mutations of the APC gene. MIN tumors may have a slightly lower frequency of APC mutations, and they tend to have one and two base deletion/insertions rather than nucleotide transition and transversions as the mutational event [113,114]. These somatically acquired mutations are distributed in patterns similar to the germline mutations in FAP, including a preference for mutations within the MCR [81]. As with FAP, these mutations largely lead to premature truncation of the APC protein and loss of the β-catenin regulatory domains. Thus, much of what has been learned about APC function, mutations, and its role in FAP colon cancer is directly applicable to sporadic human colon cancers.

APC mutations are seen as frequently in the smallest adenomatous polyps as in colon cancer [26,81]. This strongly implicates mutational inactivation of APC as one of the earliest events in sporadic tumorigenesis in the colon. Not all colon cancers have identifiable mutations in APC, though. A rare few silence APC expression by an epigenetic mechanism, promoter methylation [81]. About 15% of colon cancers express full-length APC [115]. Half of these express β-catenin mutants that cannot be phosphorylated by GSK-3β leading to unregulated β-catenin levels.

The role of other Wnt pathway members in colorectal cancer

Wnt receptors/ligands

At least 16 different members of the Wnt family of secreted glycoproteins have been identified. Although some family members can promote transformation in experimental systems in vitro and in vivo, to date no compelling evidence has been found directly implicating Wnt proteins in human carcinogenesis [82,91]. Similarly, 11 different frizzled receptor genes have been identified; however, not all frizzled receptors activated β-catenin signaling when bound by the Wnt protein [82,91]. In addition to the receptors, there exists a family of secreted proteins with homology to the frizzled receptor, called secreted frizzled-related proteins (sFRP). The sFRPs may act to antagonize Wnt signaling by sequestering Wnt proteins or, alternatively, some sFRPs may in fact activate Wnt signaling. In any event, neither the frizzled receptors nor the sFRPs have yet been observed to play a role in colorectal tumorigenesis.

Disheveled

The disheveled protein inactivates GSK-3β when stimulated by the frizzled receptor. Mutations that activate disheveled could in theory continuously suppress GSK-3β activity, thereby maintaining elevated β-catenin levels and induction of TCF/LEF target genes [82,91]. No activating mutations in disheveled have been observed in human cancers, however.

β-catenin

Mutations that stabilize the β-catenin protein are a common mechanism for activation of the Wnt signaling pathway in human cancers. Most frequently, these mutations are targeted to exon 3, where the GSK-3β regulatory domain is located [112,116,117]. Some cancers have single base missense substitutions, changing a regulatory serine or threonine to another base [112,117]. Other cancers have complete internal deletions of exon 3, removing this regulatory domain entirely [116]. These stabilizing mutations in β-catenin are able to immortalize intestinal epithelial cells in culture, and transgenic mice expressing only the stabilized form develop a polyposis phenotype virtually identical to the one seen with APC germline mutations [118].

Despite the fact that stabilizing β-catenin mutations can largely substitute for APC inactivation in a number of experimental models, the distributions of these mutations in human cancers is quite different. Stabilizing mutations are infrequent in colorectal cancers, only occurring in up to one half of the cancers without APC mutations [119]. β-catenin mutations may be seen more frequently in small adenomas than in carcinomas, suggesting this mutation may be less likely to progress to carcinoma than APC inactivation [120]. Stabilizing β-catenin mutations are seen with greater frequency in other human cancers including hepatocellular carcinoma (20%), sporadic desmoid tumors (50%), and intestinal-type gastric cancer (27%) [91]. Similar mutations have been observed at a lower frequency in medulloblastomas, endometrial and ovarian cancers, and anaplastic thyroid cancers [91]. APC mutations are rarely observed, or not seen at all, in many of these cancer types.

In addition to its role in Wnt signaling, β-catenin is an important component of the cell-cell adherens junctions. These junctions form between cells and are calcium-dependent. Cadherins are primarily responsible for the cell-cell junction, and the cadherins in turn are linked to the cell's actin cytoskeleton by catenin proteins, including β-catenin. It has been demonstrated that free β-catenin can be sequestered by the cell-cell adhesion proteins, resulting in reduced TCF/LEF target gene expression, suppression of cell transformation, and promotion of cancer cell differentiation [101,102,104]. It is not expected, however, that this would be an early mechanism in tumorigenesis. E-cadherin or α-catenin mutations, both of which inactivate cell-cell adhesion and are found with some frequency in colon cancer, occur late in cancer development and could only contribute to late progression. Other mechanisms of sequestration have been described in different organisms; whether these are also present in humans, and their role in cancer progression, is unknown.

γ-catenin

Also known as plakoglobin, γ-catenin is another component of the cell-cell adhesion complex, with a role in both adherens and desmosomal junctions. γ-catenin shares significant homology with β-catenin. Similar to β-catenin, γ-catenin binds to and its levels are regulated by APC [79,121]. When APC function is lost, both β- and γ-catenin levels rise. γ-catenin is likewise translocated to the nucleus, where it activates TCF/LEF target gene expression [79,121]. γ-catenin overexpression can induce an oncogenic transformation of cells in vitro, and this transformation is dependent on TCF/LEF activity [122]. In contrast with β-catenin, γ-catenin cannot activate the same set of TCF/LEF target genes, and its actions may be primarily mediated by increasing β-catenin levels rather than direct interaction with the TCF/LEF transactivators [123]. γ-catenin does not appear to be frequently mutated in colon cancer [82,91,119]. Thus, at present γ-catenin appears to play a supporting but not critical role in colon tumorigenesis.

Protein phosphatase 2A

Protein phosphatase 2A (PP2A) is a serine-threonine phosphatase that binds axin and has a complex regulatory role in Wnt signaling. Although it might be expected to dephosphorylate axin and thereby promote Wnt signaling, the precise role of PP2A in Wnt signaling has not been fully established [91]. PP2A is a holoenzyme consisting of a catalytic subunit PP2A-C, a variable regulatory subunit PP2A-B, and a structural subunit PP2A-A. In addition, each subunit has multiple isoforms, undoubtedly adding to the complexity and difficulty in understanding its role in Wnt signaling. PP2A can dephosphorylate axin in vitro, and the catalytic subunit can in some experimental models promote Wnt-pathway signaling [123]. But in other experimental models, PP2A expression with its regulatory subunit is required for β-catenin degradation. Over expression of one subunit PP2A-B56 in human colon cancer cells reduces β-catenin levels [124,125]. Lastly, the structural subunit PP2A-Aβ isoform is somatically mutated in one allele of 15% of colon and lung cancers, with frequent LOH of the other allele [106]. It seems likely that PP2A subunits perform opposing roles in regulating Wnt/APC/β-catenin signaling, and that some of the subunits serve a tumor-suppressor function that is targeted during colon tumorigenesis.

GSK-3β

Like APC and axin, GSK-3β is an essential member of the multi-protein complex that targets β-catenin for destruction in the absence of Wnt signaling. It would therefore be expected to behave as a tumor suppressor, and possibly be targeted for disruption during tumor development. Despite its role, no inactivating mutations in GSK-3β have been detected in one survey of colorectal cancer [82,

91,119]. A GSK-3β inhibitor, Frat-1, enhances the development of lymphoma in a mouse model; however, this factor is not known to play a role in colorectal cancer.

Axin

The axin protein is another important component of the multi-protein complex regulating Wnt signalling. It readily binds the other three, APC, β-catenin, and GSK-3β, and may therefore serve as the scaffolding to bring the other proteins in close proximity and promote GSK-3β phosphorylation and β-catenin destruction. Axin would therefore be expected to behave as a tumor suppressor. Although no inactivating mutations in Axin have been identified in human colon cancers, biallelic inactivation of axin has been observed in human hepatocellular carcinomas (HCC) [126]. All of the identified mutations were predicted to truncate the axin protein, eliminating the β-catenin binding sites. Most importantly, these mutations were observed in HCCs without APC or β-catenin mutations, further emphasizing the tumor-suppressing role of axin in HCC.

TCF/LEF

The TCF/LEF transcription factors play a critical role in Wnt signal transduction. Although no activating mutations in the TCF/LEF factors have been observed in human cancers, increased β-catenin levels, either by Wnt signaling or cancer-associated mutations in APC, axin, or β-catenin, lead to TCF/LEF activation and increased expression of TCF/LEF target genes. These target genes, as has been discussed, have long been associated with cell proliferation and tumor progression. The importance of the TCF/LEF factors in regulating intestinal epithelial proliferation is best demonstrated by a mouse model in which the TCF-4 gene has been "knocked out." These mice die shortly after birth because of complete failure of the stem-cell compartment of the small intestine to renew [127]. β-catenin-activated TCF/LEF is also important for the cancer phenotype. This is best evidenced by the use of dominant-negative TCF mutants that lack the β-catenin binding domain and therefore cannot induce TCF/LEF target genes. In fact, these mutants actively suppress TCF/LEF target gene expression even in the presence of wild-type TCF/LEF. In human colon cancer cell lines, these mutants can induce a more differentiated phenotype including restoration of a columnar, polarized cell morphology and new expression of genes associated with intestinal differentiation including intestinal fatty-acid binding protein and alkaline phosphatase [128,129].

Although TCF/LEF is not a target for mutation during carcinogenesis, an interesting story is emerging about the expression of these factors in colon cancer. LEF1 is not expressed in normal colonocytes [130]. In the thymus, where LEF1 is typically seen, two forms of LEF1 are expressed, a full-length form, and a truncated LEF1 lacking the β-catenin binding domain, a naturally occurring dominant-negative form. In human colon cancers, we see a selective expression of the full-length LEF1 only; the natural dominant-negative form remains silenced [130]. The advantage of this selective activation to tumor growth is obvious. How the cancer cells achieve this level of selection is unknown at present.

DNA MMR pathway

The duplication of DNA is a process carried out with great fidelity in all organisms from bacteria to humans. The reproductive success of an organism depends on its ability to maintain genetic integrity. Evolution has provided the means significantly to reduce the occurrence of errors during DNA replication. Each strand of DNA serves as a template during duplication. DNA polymerase and the replication machinery accurately synthesize a complementary DNA strand based on the template. Because of this fidelity, as well as intrinsic proofreading functions, nucleotide incorporation errors are estimated to be rare, on the order of 1 error per 10,000,000 bases [131]. Despite this very low rate of mistakes, enough errors could eventually accumulate to disrupt cellular function. Therefore, mechanisms have evolved to correct the errors that occur during DNA replication. A DNA sequence-repair mechanism would be predicted to have the several features. First, it must be able to recognize common errors of DNA replication, such as single base-base mispairings and small insertion/deletion loops (IDL). Second, it must be able to differentiate the template strand from the newly synthesized complimentary strand. Finally, it must be able to remove the sequence in error and replace it with the correct nucleotides [55].

Investigations into replication repair mechanisms have been ongoing for some time and have yielded great insight into the process. Foremost among these has been the study of the Mutator pathway present in the bacteria *Escherichia coli*. Genetic and biochemical studies with this organism have defined a repair mechanism possessing all of the above features, and this has served as a model for studies in eukaryotic cells from yeast to humans [55–57,59]. In *E coli*, the MutS protein recognizes and binds mispaired nucleotides. This binding promotes interaction with the MutL protein, which then stimulates ATP-dependent translocation of the complex until it reaches a MutH protein bound to a hemimethylated DNA sequence GATC (template DNA is fully methylated by the DAM methylase; recently synthesized DNA is unmethylated). MutH cleaves the unmethylated DNA strand and recruits exonucleases to remove the incorrect sequence. The strand is then resynthesized by DNA polymerase III. Inactivation of the genes involved in this repair pathway results in a mutator phenotype that is quite similar to that observed in MIN human cancers.

Studies in eukaryotic cells, primarily human and yeast, have identified proteins homologous in structure and function to the prokaryotic MutS and MutL proteins. These factors are called MutS homologues (MSH) or MutL homologues (MLH) [55,56,59]. In humans, there are at present nine known homologues; five MSH (hMSH2–hMSH6) and four MLH (hMLH1, hMLH3, hPMS1, and hPMS2) [59,132]. All are involved in maintaining the fidelity of the DNA sequence, although they do not all function to correct the errors occurring during nuclear DNA replication. Some function to maintain genetic integrity of organellular DNA, and others play prominent roles correcting errors from recombination events in the postmeiotic nuclei [133,134]. Classic MutS function in eukaryotes is performed by heterodimeric proteins with overlapping, but not identical, roles. The dimer hMSH2–hMSH6 recognizes with greatest affinity single base-base mispairings and single base IDLs. Single-base as well as larger IDL mispairings are both identified by the hMSH2–hMSH3 heterodimer [56,134].

The MSH proteins possess two functions critical to their role in DNA MMR. In addition to their recognition of DNA mispairings, they also contain highly conserved adenosine-5′-triphosphate (ATP) binding domains and intrinsic ATPase activity [55,56,59]. In the inactive state, MSH dimers are bound to adenosine-5′-disphosphate (ADP) and possess increased affinity for DNA mispairings. Once bound to mispaired DNA, the MSH heterodimers exchange ADP for ATP. Two models have been proposed for the subsequent repair steps. One model suggests ATP hydrolysis powers translocation/looping of the DNA by the MSH heterodimers, much like the process described for *E. coli* DNA repair [135]. The other model is based on observations with G-protein signaling and guanosine-5′-disphosphate/guanosine-5′-triphosphate (GDP/GTP) exchange. It has been suggested that the ADP/ATP exchange promotes a conformational change in the MSH heterodimer, releasing it from the DNA mispair and converting it into a "sliding clamp" [59,136]. This sliding clamp diffuses along the DNA, acting possibly to signal for sequence repair. ATP hydrolysis releases the heterodimer from the DNA and recycles the protein to a state ready to bind DNA mispairings once again. With either model, mispair recognition and ATP hydrolysis are both necessary functions for initiating MMR.

MutL activity in eukaryotes is also provided by heterodimers [55,56]. The heterodimers hMLH1–hPMS2 and hMLH1–hMLH3 have been demonstrated to complement mismatch deficient cell extracts in experimental systems. Currently, it is believed the MLH heterodimers function to recruit other proteins involved in DNA repair to the MSH-mismatch recognition complex. These other proteins are involved in strand identification, mismatch excision, and replacement. The identity of these other factors is unknown, although several candidates are currently under investigation. MED1, a protein identified by its ability to bind hMLH1, is a methyl-CpG binding protein with endonuclease activity that has been hypothesized to be a eukaryotic MutH [137]. Expression of a mutant MED1 protein led to induction of microsatellite instability in a dominant fashion, suggesting it may play an important role in MMR, possibly in strand identification. Proliferating cell nuclear antigen (PCNA) is another leading candidate for determining template strand identification [55,56]. PCNA interacts with eukaryotic MutS and MutL homologues, is required for MMR, and its mutation in yeast induces genetic instabilities similar to that seen in human MIN cancers. Most importantly, PCNA interacts directly with the DNA replication complex and could therefore serve to couple the MMR complex with the DNA replication fork. PCNA could simply assist in template-strand identification or even help recruit DNA polymerase to the repair site. Genetic studies in yeast have indicated mismatch excision, and repair depends on the exonuclease activity of several proteins, EXO1 and DNA polymerases δ and ε [55,56]. Combined inactivation of these proteins in yeast induces a MIN-like instability. But until mutations in these proteins are described in familial or sporadic human colon cancers, their specific role in promoting colon carcinogenesis will remain unknown.

In addition to a role in repairing mismatches that occur normally during DNA replication, these same factors appear essential to other surveillance and repair functions present in the nucleus. The MMR pathway is involved in the identification of mispairings and DNA damage from a variety of processes, not just those arising from DNA replication. DNA damage from chemical injury (alkylating agents), ionizing radiation, oxidation damage, and meiotic recombinations are all sensed by the repair pathway [55,56,138–140]. Once sensed, cell-cycle checkpoint arrest and/or apoptosis is activated in the cells by the MMR system through both P53-dependent and independent pathways [139,140]. This expanded role for the MMR in DNA surveillance has significant clinical implications. Cancers deficient in MMR are less responsive to chemotherapeutic agents [141–143]. Additionally, treatment of tumors with chemotherapeutic agents could select for the outgrowth of clones insensitive to DNA damage. Thus, our growing understanding of the MMR pathway is likely to continue to impact colon cancer therapy in the future.

DNA MMR and colon cancer phenotypes

Hereditary nonpolyposis colon cancer

HNPCC (or Lynch syndrome) is a common form of familial cancer, responsible for up to 5% of all colon cancers [40,144]. Clinically, HNPCC is a dominantly inherited disorder characterized by the development of colon cancer at an early age (mean 45 years), and nearly 90% are found to have microsatellite instability [144]. Colon cancers in HNPCC kindreds have a preference for proximal sites, are associated with an improved survival, multiple colorectal cancers, and a histology that is poorly differentiated, more frequently mucinous, and with a marked lymphocytic infiltrate. Colonic adenomas in these families can vary from one to a few, have a greater frequency of villous and dysplastic components, and likely progress more rapidly to cancer than adenomas in non-HNPCC kindreds [144]. The original criteria (Amsterdam I, 1990) [145] defined HNPCC families as having colon cancer in three close relatives in two successive generations, one individual being a first-degree relative of the other two; and one of the cancers should occur before the age 50. Advances in the genetic basis of HNPCC led to the realization that extraintestinal cancers may be predominant in some kindreds, and therefore the criteria were modified. In the new criteria, HNPCC is defined by familial clustering (three close relatives in two successive generations) of colorectal and/or endometrial cancers [144]. Other malignancies that can qualify as an HNPCC defining cancer [144] include gastric, ovarian, ureter/renal pelvis, brain (primarily glioblastome multiforme—also known as Turcot's syndrome) [146], small bowel, hepatobiliary, and skin (sebaceous gland malignancies—Muir-Torre syndrome) [147].

Microsatellite instability was first recognized to be an important feature of HNPCC colon cancers in 1993. Early reports utilized a variety of markers and definitions for MIN cancers; however, a recent National Cancer Workshop has recommended a consensus panel of five mononucleotide and dinucleotide markers be used [148]. Instability in two or more markers was defined as a high degree of instability, known as Microsatellite-High (MSI-H). Instability in one marker was termed MSI-Low (MSI-L), and absence of instability was termed microsatellite-stable (MSS). Inactivating germline mutations in hMLH1 or hMSH2 are observed in nearly 60% of the HNPCC families, particularly those with MSI-H cancers [149]. These mutations are distributed throughout the hMLH1 and hMSH2 genes, and they do not appear to cluster within specific domains [150]. Germline mutations have been described for hPMS1, hPMS2, hMSH6, and hMLH3 [149,151–156], but these are not common amongst classic HNPCC kindreds. Germline mutations in the hMSH6, hPMS2, and possibly hPMS1 genes are more likely to be manifest in nonclassic HNPCC families; those with later onset of colonic malignancies or those with extra-intestinal cancers. For instance, endometrial cancer is more common in female carriers of hMSH6 germline mutations than colon cancer [157]. Therefore, a significant proportion of HNPCC families have no identifiable germline mutation to explain their cancer predisposition.

Individuals with predisposing germline mutations in one of the MMR genes must inactivate the second allele in order to progress to cancer along this pathway. Generally, this occurs by LOH or somatic mutation of the normal allele. Epigenetic inactivation of the normal allele may also play a role; hMLH1 promoter silencing by CpG island hypermethylation has been described [158]. Lastly, dominant mutations in MMR genes have been described both experimentally as well as in human families [159,160]. These dominant mutations do not require inactivation of the normal allele and are in fact associated with widespread microsatellite instability in normal, non-neoplastic cells. Once the MMR gene is effectively inactivated in both alleles, MMR function is compromised and sequence errors begin to accumulate in the genomes of daughter cells. This occurs early in the progression to colon cancer, as microsatellite instability has been commonly demonstrated in the aberrant crypt foci isolated from HNPCC patients [21,22]. Targeted disruptions ("knockouts") of various MMR pathway members in mice has been helpful in confirming cancer phenotypes associated with loss of specific MMR genes [161].

Studies of MIN cancers have begun to describe the spectrum of genes inactivated in this manner. In the colon, there is progressive biallelic inactivation of a variety of genes involved in critical processes such as growth regulation, differentiation, apoptosis, and DNA surveillance and repair. APC or β-catenin are frequently mutated by frameshift mutations in nearly 70% of HNPCC colon cancers [113,114]. These mutations inactivate APC but activate β-catenin by removal of the regulatory domain. Other tumor suppressors commonly mutated include the TGF-βRII and insulin-like growth factor-II receptors (IGFIIR). The TGF-βRII receptor is inactivated in close to 90% of MIN colon cancers, and this mutation is believed to occur with the transformation of an MIN adenoma to carcinoma [60,162]. The IGFIIR receptor is less frequently affected; about 20% of

HNPCC colon cancers mutate this gene [163]. The p53 tumor suppressor itself is infrequently mutated in HNPCC colon cancers [164,165]; however, an important p53 pro-apoptotic effector, the BAX gene, is inactivated in 55% of these cancers [61,166]. Thus p53-mediated apoptosis is effectively blunted. The mutS and mutL homologues hMSH3, hMSH6, and hMLH3 are frequently inactivated by frame-shift mutations within microsatellite sequences [62,167], as are other gene products important for DNA replication and repair like MED1 [168], ATM [169], and the DNA helicase BLM [170]. These events may further diminish DNA repair functions and promote mutagenesis. This may in part explain why MIN has been noted to increase during the adenoma-carcinoma sequence. Lastly, the transcription factors E2F-4 [171] and TCF-4 [172], as well as the candidate tumor-suppressor RIZ gene product [173], and caspase-5 [174], also frequently acquire frameshift mutations in HNPCC colon cancers. In summary, inhibition of DNA MMR promotes the accumulation of frameshift mutations that inactivate tumor-suppressors, promote growth, and accelerate malignant transformation of colonic epithelial cells.

Sporadic colon cancers

Sporadic colon cancers with microsatellite instability constitute about 10–15% of all colon cancers [58]. Sporadic MIN colorectal cancers share some features with HNPCC cancers; however, new studies are suggesting the genetic events underlying their genesis may be quite different. In contrast with MSS cancers, sporadic MIN colon cancers tend to occur proximally, have a greater mucinous component, be poorly differentiated, diploid, and associated with an improved survival for patients [175–177]. When compared with HNPCC cancers, sporadic MIN tumors are more frequently MSI-L. Microsatellite instability in sporadic cancers behaves as it does in HNPCC; many of the same tumor-suppressor genes containing microsatellite sequences are inactivated by frameshift mutations, although the frequencies of inactivation can differ from HNPCC [60,168,178]. Though somatic mutations in hMLH1, hMSH2, and hPMS2 have all been implicated as a cause of sporadic MIN cancers [179,180], the frequency with which these mutations have been identified has been quite low. Somatic mutations in hMLH1 and hMSH2 occur with frequencies of only 10–20% each. Biallelic inactivating hPMS2 mutations have been described in a single case of sporadic colon cancer. Somatic hMSH6 and hPMS1 mutations have not been observed in sporadic colon carcinogenesis.

Further studies with sporadic MIN colon cancers revealed that, though coding sequences for hMLH1 were wild-type, hMLH1 protein levels were markedly diminished. A careful analysis revealed that the lack of protein was caused by specific silencing of the gene [71,72,158]. The hMLH1 promoter contains CpG islands found to be heavily methylated in many of the sporadic MIN colon cancers. Promoter methylation commonly is biallelic; thus, both alleles are potentially inactivated by this process. Also, reversal of the methylation by demethylating agents has led to hMLH1 re-expression in MIN colon cancer cell lines [72]. Together, these observations clearly provide a role for hMLH1 promoter hypermethylation in inducting the MIN phenotype in a subset of sporadic colorectal cancers. One study, comparing somatic mutations and LOH with hMLH1 protein levels and promoter hypermethylation, found strikingly that 83% of the sporadic colon cancers had significant hMLH1 promoter hyper-methylation [181]. In this same series, LOH and somatic mutations of hMLH1 occurred in 24% and 13% of sporadic cancers, respectively. When somatic mutation and LOH occurred together in a single cancer, however, promoter hypermethylation was noticeably absent. More commonly, a somatic mutation or LOH occurred with hMLH1 promoter hypermethylation, suggesting the epigenetic silencing may be the predominant event or, in the least, serve as the second hMLH1 inactivating "hit".

One larger question remains; what is driving this CpG island hypermethyla-tion? That is presently unknown, but the promoters of several genes with CpG islands are commonly affected in the same sporadic cancer [76,77]. This has led to the hypothesis of a "methylator" pathway as a separate genetic pathway in colon carcinogenesis with distinctive features and gene expression patterns. Sporadic MIN colon cancers thus may largely arise from a genetic process quite distinct from that in HNPCC colon cancers, although phenotypically the cancers are similar.

The TGF-β signaling pathway

TGF-β is one of several members of a superfamily of signaling molecules that play a critical role in the control of cell growth, differentiation, and development. Other family members include bone morphogenic protein (BMPs), Mullerian-inhibiting substance, inhibins, and activins [182]. TGF-β is expressed in a variety of tissues including cells of both mesenchymal and epithelial origin. The effects of this ligand are quite pleomorphic, with specific effects determined by the cell type to which the factor binds. TGF-β was originally identified as one of two growth factors present in the conditioned media of transformed fibroblasts [182]. In cells of mesenchymal origin, TGF-β signaling promotes a proliferative response; however, in epithelial cells, including colonocytes, TGF-β is primarily a growth inhibitor [182,183]. Numerous observations, both experimental and clinical, now indicate loss of sensitivity to the growth-inhibitory effects of TGF-β is frequently associated with malignant progression of a number of cancers including those of the breast, pancreas, and colon [182–185]. The TGF-β signalling pathway is thus frequently targeted for silencing during carcinogenesis. Studies of this pathway in colon and other cancers have recently identified previously unknown tumor-suppressor genes; their role in signaling and tumori-genesis will be discussed.

TGF-β initiates signaling in a cell by binding and activating a conserved set of receptors (Fig. 3) [182–187]. There are three classes of receptor molecules, type I (TβR – I), type II (TβR – II), and β-glycan type III (TβR – III). Types I and II are structurally similar and are the principle effectors of TGF-β signaling. Both classes of receptor have an extracellular ligand-binding domain, a single transmembrane

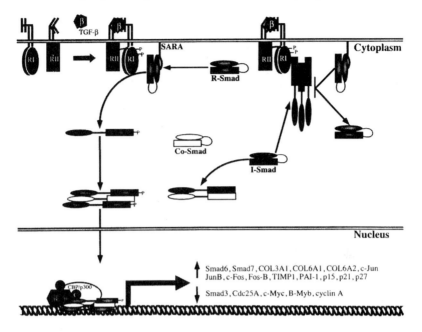

Fig. 3. The TGF-β signaling pathway [182–187]. TGF-β homodimer (β) initiates signaling by binding and activating a conserved set of receptors TβR − I (RI) and TβR − II (RII). TβR − II receptor phosphorylates TβR − I, activating its intrinsic kinase activity. The TβR − I kinase in turn phosphorylates and activates downstream targets, the principle ones being the Smad proteins. In the unstimulated state, R-Smads are localized to the cytoplasm where they are in an autoinhibitory conformation. R-Smads are maintained at the cell-membrane, near the TGF − β receptors by the cell-membrane anchored SARA protein. TGF-β mediated receptor activation leads to phosphorylation of the SARA-associated R-Smads. This releases the R-Smads from their autoinhibitory conformation and from the SARA protein. The activated receptor Smads associate with Co-Smads, and this complex then translocates to the nucleus where it specifically targets a number of growth-related genes to alter expression levels. TGF-β signaling via Smads can produce opposite effects on different genes in the same cell. Some genes are induced by TGF-β/Smad signaling, and other genes are actively repressed. The Smad factors achieve this varied effect because of their prolific interactions with a great variety of transcription factors (TF) and cofactors (C). Inhibitory Smads compete with the receptor Smads for binding to TGF-β receptors and Co-Smads, inhibiting receptor Smad signaling. C, cofactor; Co-Smad, common Smad; R-Smads, receptor Smads; SARA, Smad anchor for receptor activation; TF, transcription factors.

domain, and cytoplasmic serine/threonine kinase domains. In the unstimulated state, they likely exist as homodimers [183]. TGF-β, which itself is naturally a homodimer, binds both TβR − I and TβR − II and stabilizes the formation of a heterotetrameric complex. The TβR − II receptor then phosphorylates TβR − I, activating its intrinsic kinase activity. The TβR − I serine/threonine kinase in turn phosphorylates and activates downstream targets, the principle ones being the Smad proteins [182–187].

Smad proteins share two conserved domains, the amino-termininal MH1 domain (important for DNA binding and autoinhibition) and the carboxy-terminal MH2 domain (containing receptor binding, stimulatory phosphorylation, transcriptional activation, and oligomerization sites) [183,186]. There are three broad classes of Smad proteins, the receptor Smads 1, 2, 3, 5 and 8, the common mediator Smad4, and the inhibitory Smads 6 and 7 [183,184,186]. Smads 2 and 3 are the receptor Smads specific for TGF-β signaling. Inhibitory Smads compete with the receptor Smads for binding to TGF-β receptors, inhibiting receptor Smad phosphorylation and activation.

In the unstimulated state, receptor Smads are in an autoinhibitory conformation. Receptor Smads maintained close to the cell-membrane, near the TGF-β receptors, by binding to the cell-membrane anchored Smad anchor for receptor activation (SARA) protein or microtubule proteins [183,186] (see Fig. 3). TGF-β mediated receptor activation leads to phosphorylation of the SARA-associated Smads 2 and 3 in their MH2 domain. This releases the Smads from their autoinhibitory conformation and from the SARA protein. The activated receptor Smads associate with Smad4, and this complex then translocates to the nucleus where it specifically targets a number of growth-related genes to alter expression levels.

TGF-β signaling via Smads can produce opposite effects on different genes in the same cell. Some genes are induced by TGF-β/Smad signaling, like the inhibitory Smads 6 and 7, oncoproteins c-Jun, Jun-B, c-Fos, and Fos-B [184], proteins involved in extracellular matrix formation including, collagen, fibronectin, PAI-I and TIMP-1 [182,188], and the cell cycle inhibitors p15, p21, and p27 [182,184,189]. Other genes are actively repressed by it, including Smad3, the oncoproteins c-Myc and B-Myb, and the cell cycle proteins Cdc25A, and cyclin A [184,189]. These altered patterns of gene expression promote growth inhibition and cell differentiation, the hallmarks of TGF-β signaling. The activated Smad factors achieve this varied effect because of their prolific interactions with a great variety of transcription factors and cofactors. The Smad protein complex binds a specific DNA sequence called the Smad binding element (SBE), located in the promoters of TGF-β responsive genes [184,187]. Smads bind the SBE and synergize with other bound transcription factors, such as AP-1, ATF-2, β-catenin/TCF/LEF, Mixer, and FAST among others to recruit transcriptional coactivators that promote gene expression [184,186,187]. Smads interact with other transcription factors such as the glucocorticoid receptor or the TGIF factor to recruit corepressors and actively suppress gene transcription. Thus, the local promoter and cellular environment are important determinants of the response to TGF-β signaling.

TGF-β signaling is also modified by a number of other signaling pathways, some of which are very important in carcinogenesis. The MAPK pathway can both promote or block TGF-β signaling, depending on the stimulus [184]. In fact, there is evidence for a non-Smad TGF-β receptor signaling pathway that may involve MAPK intermediates [184]. Several growth factors and inflammation mediators directly inhibit TGF-β/Smad signaling. Tumor necrosis factor-α (TNF-α), interlukin 1a, and interferon-γ all induce the inhibitor Smad7 to suppress activation of the pathway [183,186,190]. Another inhibitory mechanism involves blocking nuclear translocation of activated Smads. Phosphorylation of receptor Smads in their linker region leads to their retention in the cytoplasm by an unknown mechanism [183]. K-ras activation, either by growth factor stimulation or the acquisition of an activating mutation, can induce Smad linker phosphorylation and cytoplasmic retention, most likely by activation of the ERK kinases [191]. This obviously has important implications in carcinogenesis.

The role of TGF-β in colorectal cancer

Observations both clinical and experimental now clearly implicate loss of TGF-β growth control as a critical event in colorectal tumorigenesis [182–185]. Studies with a number of colon cancer cell lines found nearly 75% had lost responsiveness to TGF-β growth control [192]. The complexity of the TGF-β signaling has provided cancer cells a number of ways to inactivate the pathway. But in practice, it seems only a few are favored by the process of carcinogenesis.

One of the primary means of pathway inactivation involves mutation of the TβR–II receptor. Microsatellite unstable colon cancers have been found to have extremely high rates of TβR–II inactivation in both alleles, approaching 90% in some studies [60,193]. This high rate is caused by the presence of two microsatellite regions within the coding sequence of the TβR–II receptor. These regions are frequently mutated in MIN colon cancers; 1–2 base-pair deletions and insertions within this sequence result in a truncated, nonfunctional receptor protein. Inactivating mutations of the TβR–II are a late event in colorectal tumorigenesis (see Fig. 1). They have been detected in MIN adenomas but are nearly universally present in MIN colon cancers of all stages and thus are associated with progression to carcinoma [162,194]. Mutations of the this receptor are sufficient for the TGF-β resistance phenotype, as MIN colon cancer cell lines can have their TGF–β responsiveness restored by expression of a nonmutated TβR–II receptor [195].

The TβR–II is also inactivated by mutations within its serine/threonine kinase domain. These mutations have been reported in both MIN and CIN colon cancers [192]. It has been estimated that approximately 15% of microsatellite-stable CIN colon cancers may harbor inactivating mutations within the receptor's kinase domain. Because most MIN colon cancers have TβR–II mutations, as many as 30% of all human colon cancers may acquire TGF-β resistance by inactivating mutations of the TβR–II [192]. Suprisingly, TβR–I mutations have not been widely reported as a mechanism for TGF-β resistance in human colon cancers. TβR–I mutations are well described in other cancers, most notably ovarian [185]. The reason for this apparent preference in the different cancers is not known.

Mutations that inactivate the Smad proteins are the other common mechanism for acquiring TGF–β resistance. Smad4 was initially identified as DPC4, a possible tumor-suppressor gene located on chromosome 18q21 [196]. 18q21 is a region with high rates of LOH and chromosome deletion in both pancreatic and colorectal cancer, typically occurring late in the progression from adenoma to carcinoma. Though nearly 50% of pancreatic cancers were found to have lost or functionally inactivated Smad4, only about 25% of colon cancers studied had similarly inactivated this protein [197]. The inactivating mutations included deletions as well as somatic mutations. This resulted in protein truncations or missense substitutions of highly conserved amino acids in the MH1 or MH2 domains. Suprisingly, the Smad2 gene is also located in the chromosome 18q21 region [198], along with the gene for deleted in colon cancer (DCC). Smad2 is inactivated in only 5–10% of all colon cancers studied [198,199]. Mutations were similar in nature to those found in Smad4. Thus, the frequent deletion of 18q in colorectal cancer is not fully explained by the losses of either Smad2 or Smad4. Transgenic mice with deletions of Smads 2, 3, 4, or 5 have been generated. Homozygous deletion of Smads 2, 4, or 5 result in embryonic lethality and have not been informative with respect to colon cancer [200,201]. Compound heterozygote mice with mutations in APC and Smad4 suggest, however, that there may be a synergism between these genes [201]. The mice acquired polyps with a more malignant and invasive phenotype than APC mutant mice alone.

Other Smad factors have been studied for loss or inactivation in colon cancer, but to date none have been described [202]. This is in contrast with the observation in transgenic mice that homozygous deletion of Smad3 is associated with colon cancer by 3–6 months of age [203]. It seems likely then that Smad3 mutations will eventually be identified in human colon cancers, but the frequency of these mutations may be quite small. Lastly, oncogenic activation of Ras has been associated with induction of TGF-β resistance in colon cancer cell lines by blocking nuclear translocation of Smads 2 and 3 [191]. As K-ras activation is a common early event in the adenoma-carcinoma sequence, TGF-β resistance is likely present early as well. The role this resistance plays in the process of carcinogenesis, as opposed to the late TβR-II and Smad 2/4 mutational events, is not known.

Despite these compelling observations, many questions remain regarding the role of TGF-β signaling in colorectal tumorigenesis. Though TGF-β signaling is a frequent target for mutagenesis, many primary cancers express high levels of the TGF-β ligand, and this has been correlated with clinically advanced disease [204,205]. It has been speculated that the tumor-expressed TGF-β ligand promotes tumor progression by enhancing angiogenesis or suppressing immune surveillance [183,204], but this has not been proven. It has also been reported that TGF-β signaling is necessary for the induction and maintenance of a metastatic phenotype in human colon carcinoma cells [206]. For these reasons, the clinical implications of TGF-β resistance must remain an area of active study.

p53, K-ras signaling, and other genes involved in colorectal carcinogenesis

As one of the oldest-known and best-studied tumor-suppressors, p53 plays a critical role in limiting the progression to carcinogenesis in the colon [207]. p53 is a sequence-specific transcription factor that is induced and activated by the same signals and stresses promoting neoplastic transformation including DNA damage, oncogene activation, hypoxia, telomere shortening, and loss of normal growth-regulatory signals [208–211]. Once activated, p53 induces a variety of growth-limiting responses including cell cycle arrest, apoptosis, senescence, differentiation, and antiangiogenesis. The specificity of the response depends on the nature of the stimulus, the type of cell or tissue affected, and other factors not understood at present. p53 produces a response largely by altering the expression of a growing number of target genes [212], including p21^{WAF1}, bax, Fas, KILLER/DR5, and 14-3-3σ, as well as others, although transcription-independent effects of p53 have been reported. Mice deleted or null for p53 develop normally, although they are cancer-prone as adults [213,214]. Similarly, Li-Fraumeni syndrome is a human condition caused by a germline mutation of p53 [215]. Patients with this syndrome frequently develop carcinomas, sarcomas, and leukemias, but colon cancer is rare. Because of its central role in responding to DNA damage and neoplastic signals, p53 has been called by some the "Guardian of the Genome" [216].

Inactivation of the p53 response pathway is a late event in the majority of human colon cancers, with colitis-associated cancers (CAC) being the most prominent exception [45,217]. In 50–70% of colon cancers, this occurs by inactivating mutation of one allele followed by loss of the remaining wild-type gene [10,207,210]. The remainder of colon cancers with wild-type p53 expression are believed to have blunted p53-responses [211]. These include induction of p53 inhibitors like MDM2 [208], silencing by methylation of activators such as p14^{ARF} [63], mutation of effector genes such as BAX in MIN cancers [166], or alterations of other components of the complex pathways normally present to regulate p53 activity [211]. p53 mutations have been reported in ACF [23,24,218] and adenomatous polyps [219,220], but their reported frequency is considerably reduced in comparison with adenocarcinomas. Identification of p53 status in carcinomas will have a growing role in patient care. At present, p53 mutations confer a poorer prognosis with reduced survival and increased rates of tumor recurrence [221,222]. Several new therapies seek to treat cancer by targeting p53-mutant cells, however. Viruses lethal only to cells with mutant p53 have been described and are being tested for therapeutic utility [223,224]. Immunotherapy using mutant p53 as a specific tumor antigen is under investigation [225]. Other therapies to correct p53 mutations directly or restore normal p53 responses are being studied [226,227]. These investigators hope p53 may prove to be a highly selective and effective target for future cancer therapies.

The Ras genes (h-Ras, n-Ras, and k-Ras) encode a family of small guanosine triphosphate hydrolases (GTPases) with potent transforming abilities that functionally behave as a "molecular switch" [228,229]. These proteins cycle between an inactive GDP-bound state and an active GTP-bound one. This cycle is regulated directly by a diverse number of guanine nucleotide exchange factors (GEFs) and GTPase activating proteins (GAPs), which are themselves regulated by a great number and variety of cell-surface receptors. Once in the active state, Ras responds by stimulating a varied array of different effector pathways including Raf/MAPK, PI3K/Akt, and Mekk/JNK, among others. This ability to stimulate a large number of diverse pathways may explain Ras's potent trans-forming ability, and why it is one of the most frequently mutated oncogenes in human cancer [228].

Ras mutations in cancer typically are point mutations at codons 12, 13, and 61 that leave the protein resistant to GAP-mediated GTP hydrolysis [229]. This results in a Ras protein constitutively in the active state. Of the three Ras genes, k-Ras is most commonly mutated in human colon cancer [228]. K-Ras mutations have been observed in the earliest neoplastic lesions of the colon, the ACF [23,26,218,230]. Sporadic, FAP-associated, and CpG island methylating color-ectal neoplasms have the highest rates of activating mutations (50–80%) [26,77,207,231], although k-Ras mutations may occur at a later stage in FAP carcinogenesis [26]. But activating k-Ras mutations were infrequently reported in flat colorectal and HNPCC cancers [41–44,164,165]. Because of its promiscuous effector pathways, activated Ras can inhibit tumor-suppressor pathways such as p53 [232] and TGF-β [191] to promote growth. For these and other reasons, mutant Ras is actively being investigated as a potential therapeutic target [7] and marker for noninvasive screening [7].

A number of other genes with importance for colon cancer progression, prognosis, staging, and therapeutics are the focus of intense investigation by a number of researchers. A few of these are listed in Table 1.

Table 1
Genes important for the progression, staging, and therapy of colon cancer

Gene name	Role in colorectal carcinogenesis
Src	Nonreceptor tyrosine kinase; elevated activity in most adenomas and colon carcinomas associated with tumor progression. Activating mutations described in a subset of advanced colon cancers [233].
COX-2	Inducible cyclo-oxygenase; actions include inhibiting intestinal epithelial differentia-tion, reducing apoptosis, and promoting angiogenesis. A possible therapeutic target for cancer prevention as well as chemotherapy [8].
CD44	Cell surface glycoprotein involved in matrix adhesion and lymphocyte activation and homing. Promotes growth and metastasis of tumors in vitro and in vivo [234].
DCC	Deleted in colon cancer; cell adhesion molecule closely related to NCAM. The DCC gene is located in a chromosomal region frequently lost in colon cancer (18q21) and its loss predicts greater mortality. Its role in colon cancer progression remains unclear, however [10].
PPARδ	Peroxisome proliferator-activated receptor δ; a nuclear hormone receptor that may be a receptor for COX-2 prostaglandins. A downstream target gene of the Wnt/APC/β-catenin pathway [235]. A possible therapeutic target.
PPARγ	Peroxisome proliferator-activated receptor γ; functions similar to PPARδ. Conflicting observations regarding its role in carcinogenesis have been reported [236]. A possible therapeutic target.
GC-C	Guanyl cyclase C receptor, specifically expressed in intestinal epithelium and colorectal adenocarcinoma. May be used clinically to identify microscopic metastases for staging [237].

APC, adenomatous polyperis coli; DCC, deleted in colon cancer; NCAM, Wnt, wingless type.

Summary

Research over the past decade has established that the progression from normal colonic epithelium to colon cancer is in every case a step-wise process in which specific pathologic and molecular markers can be identified for study and clinical therapy. Genetic and epigenetic instability appears fundamentally important to this process. We have now determined that this neoplastic progression occurs along a limited set of pathways, in which specific tumor suppressors are inactivated or oncogenes activated in a defined order. Although incomplete, our new understanding of the process of carcinogenesis in the colon has already significantly impacted patient care and will continue to do so for the foreseeable future. Increasingly rapid research developments and technologic advances will transform the way we prevent, diagnose, and treat this common and deadly form of cancer.

References

[1] Janne PA, Mayer RJ. Chemoprevention of colorectal cancer. N Engl J Med 2000;342:1960–8.

[2] Torrance CJ, Jackson PE, Montgomery E, et al. Combinatorial chemoprevention of intestinal neoplasia. Nat Med 2000;6:1024–8.

[3] American Gastroenterological Association medical position statement. Hereditary colorectal cancer and genetic testing. Gastroenterology 2001;121:195–7.

[4] Giardiello FM, Brensinger JD, Petersen GM. AGA technical review on hereditary colorectal cancer and genetic testing. Gastroenterology 2001;121:198–213.

[5] Ahlquist DA, Skoletsky JE, Boynton KA, et al. Colorectal cancer screening by detection of altered human DNA in stool: feasibility of a multitarget assay panel. Gastroenterology 2000;119: 1219–27.

[6] Watanabe T, Wu TT, Catalano PJ, et al. Molecular predictors of survival after adjuvant chemotherapy for colon cancer. N Engl J Med 2001;344:1196–206.

[7] Adjei AA. Blocking oncogenic Ras signaling for cancer therapy. J Natl Cancer Inst 2001;93: 1062–74.

[8] Dempke W, Rie C, Grothey A, et al. Cyclooxygenase-2: a novel target for cancer chemotherapy? J Cancer Res Clin Oncol 2001;127:411–7.

[9] Carethers JM. The cellular and molecular pathogenesis of colorectal cancer. Gastroenterol Clin North Am 1996;25:737–54.

[10] Hoops TC, Traber PG. Molecular pathogenesis of colorectal cancer. Hematol Oncol Clin North Am 1997;11:609–33.

[11] Kim EC, Lance P. Colorectal polyps and their relationship to cancer. Gastroenterol Clin North Am 1997;26:1–17.

[12] Winawer SJ, Zauber AG, Ho MN, et al. Prevention of colorectal cancer by colonoscopic polypectomy. The National Polyp Study Workgroup. N Engl J Med 1993;329:1977–81.

[13] Tudek B, Bird RP, Bruce WR. Foci of aberrant crypts in the colons of mice and rats exposed to carcinogens associated with foods. Cancer Res 1989;49:1236–40.

[14] Roncucci L, Pedroni M, Vaccina F, et al. Aberrant crypt foci in colorectal carcinogenesis. Cell and crypt dynamics. Cell Prolif 2000;33:1–18.

[15] Takayama T, Katsuki S, Takahashi Y, et al. Aberrant crypt foci of the colon as precursors of adenoma and cancer. N Engl J Med 1998;339:1277–84.

[16] Nucci MR, Robinson CR, Longo P, et al. Phenotypic and genotypic characteristics of aberrant crypt foci in human colorectal mucosa. Hum Pathol 1997;28:1396–407.

[17] Siu IM, Pretlow TG, Amini SB, et al. Identification of dysplasia in human colonic aberrant crypt foci. Am J Pathol 1997;150:1805–13.

[18] Shpitz B, Bomstein Y, Mekori Y, et al. Aberrant crypt foci in human colons: distribution and histomorphologic characteristics. Hum Pathol 1998;29:469–75.

[19] Siu IM, Robinson DR, Schwartz S, et al. The identification of monoclonality in human aberrant crypt foci. Cancer Res 1999;59:63–6.

[20] Konstantakos AK, Siu IM, Pretlow TG, et al. Human aberrant crypt foci with carcinoma in situ from a patient with sporadic colon cancer. Gastroenterology 1996;111:772–7.

[21] Heinen CD, Shivapurkar N, Tang Z, et al. Microsatellite instability in aberrant crypt foci from human colons. Cancer Res 1996;56:5339–41.

[22] Pedroni M, Sala E, Scarselli A, et al. Microsatellite instability and mismatch-repair protein expression in hereditary and sporadic colorectal carcinogenesis. Cancer Res 2001;61:896–9.

[23] Shivapurkar N, Huang L, Ruggeri B, et al. K-ras and p53 mutations in aberrant crypt foci and colonic tumors from colon cancer patients. Cancer Lett 1997;115:39–46.

[24] Shpitz B, Bomstein Y, Shalev M, et al. Oncoprotein coexpression in human aberrant crypt foci and minute polypoid lesions of the large bowel. Anticancer Res 1999;19:3361–6.

[25] Smith AJ, Stern HS, Penner M, et al. Somatic APC and K-ras codon 12 mutations in aberrant crypt foci from human colons. Cancer Res 1994;54:5527–30.

[26] Takayama T, Ohi M, Hayashi T, et al. Analysis of K-ras, APC, and beta-catenin in aberrant crypt foci in sporadic adenoma, cancer, and familial adenomatous polyposis. Gastroenterology 2001;121:599–611.

[27] Erik Paulsen J, Steffensen IL, Loberg EM. et al. Qualitative and quantitative relationship between dysplastic aberrant crypt foci and tumorigenesis in the Min/+ mouse colon. Cancer Res 2001;61:5010–5.

[28] Moen CJ, van der Valk MA, Bird RP, et al. Different genetic susceptibility to aberrant crypts and colon adenomas in mice. Cancer Res 1996;56:2382–6.

[29] Vogelstein B, Kinzler KW. The multistep nature of cancer. Trends Genet 1993;9:138–41.

[30] Ponder BA. Cancer genetics. Nature 2001;411:336–41.

[31] Fearon ER, Vogelstein B. A genetic model for colorectal tumorigenesis. Cell 1990;61:759–67.

[32] Cahill DP, Kinzler KW, Vogelstein B, et al. Genetic instability and darwinian selection in tumours. Trends Cell Biol 1999;9:M57–60.

[33] Hanahan D, Weinberg RA. The hallmarks of cancer. Cell 2000;100:57–70.

[34] Muto T, Bussey HJ, Morson BC. The evolution of cancer of the colon and rectum. Cancer 1975; 36:2251–70.

[35] O'Brien MJ, Winawer SJ, Zauber AG, et al. The National Polyp Study. Patient and polyp characteristics associated with high-grade dysplasia in colorectal adenomas. Gastroenterology 1990;98:371–9.

[36] Breivik J, Gaudernack G. Genomic instability, DNA methylation, and natural selection in colorectal carcinogenesis. Semin Cancer Biol 1999;9:245–54.

[37] Kinzler KW, Vogelstein B. Lessons from hereditary colorectal cancer. Cell 1996;87:159–70.

[38] Kinzler KW, Vogelstein B. Cancer-susceptibility genes. Gatekeepers and caretakers. Nature 1997;386:761–3.

[39] Chung DC. The genetic basis of colorectal cancer: insights into critical pathways of tumorigenesis. Gastroenterology 2000;119:854–65.

[40] Lynch HT, Smyrk T. An update on Lynch syndrome. Curr Opin Oncol 1998;10:349–56.

[41] Hasegawa H, Ueda M, Watanabe M, et al. K-ras gene mutations in early colorectal cancer. Flat elevated vs polyp-forming cancer. Oncogene 1995;10:1413–6.

[42] Olschwang S, Slezak P, Roze M, et al. Somatically acquired genetic alterations in flat colorectal neoplasias. Int J Cancer 1998;77:366–9.

[43] Saitoh Y, Waxman I, West AB, et al. Prevalence and distinctive biologic features of flat colorectal adenomas in a North American population. Gastroenterology 2001;120:1657–65.

[44] Yashiro M, Carethers JM, Laghi L, et al. Genetic pathways in the evolution of morphologically distinct colorectal neoplasms. Cancer Res 2001;61:2676–83.

[45] Itzkowitz SH. Inflammatory bowel disease and cancer. Gastroenterol Clin North Am 1997;26: 129–39.

[46] Walsh S, Murphy M, Silverman M, et al. p27 expression in inflammatory bowel disease-associated neoplasia. Further evidence of a unique molecular pathogenesis. Am J Pathol 1999;155: 1511–8.

[47] Lengauer C, Kinzler KW, Vogelstein B. Genetic instability in colorectal cancers. Nature 1997; 386:623–7.

[48] Lengauer C, Kinzler KW, Vogelstein B. Genetic instabilities in human cancers. Nature 1998;396: 643–9.

[49] Augenlicht LH, Richards C, Corner G, et al. Evidence for genomic instability in human colonic aberrant crypt foci. Oncogene 1996;12:1767–72.

[50] Murray AW. The genetics of cell cycle checkpoints. Curr Opin Genet Dev 1995;5:5–11.

[51] Cahill DP, Lengauer C, Yu J, et al. Mutations of mitotic checkpoint genes in human cancers. Nature 1998;392:300–3.

[52] Fodde R, Kuipers J, Rosenberg C, et al. Mutations in the APC tumour suppressor gene cause chromosomal instability. Nat Cell Biol 2001;3:433–8.

[53] Kaplan KB, Burds AA, Swedlow JR, et al. A role for the Adenomatous Polyposis Coli protein in chromosome segregation. Nat Cell Biol 2001;3:429–32.

[54] Tsushimi T, Noshima S, Oga A, et al. DNA amplification and chromosomal translocations are accompanied by chromosomal instability: analysis of seven human colon cancer cell lines by comparative genomic hybridization and spectral karyotyping. Cancer Genet Cytogenet 2001; 126:34–8.

[55] Buermeyer AB, Deschenes SM, Baker SM, et al. Mammalian DNA mismatch repair. Annu Rev Genet 1999;33:533–64.

[56] Kolodner RD, Marsischky GT. Eukaryotic DNA mismatch repair. Curr Opin Genet Dev 1999;9: 89–96.

[57] Marra G, Boland CR. DNA repair and colorectal cancer. Gastroenterol Clin North Am 1996;25: 755–72.

[58] Peltomaki P. Deficient DNA mismatch repair: a common etiologic factor for colon cancer. Hum Mol Genet 2001;10:735–40.

[59] Fishel R. Mismatch repair, molecular switches, and signal transduction. Genes Dev 1998;12: 2096–101.

[60] Parsons R, Myeroff LL, Liu B, et al. Microsatellite instability and mutations of the transforming growth factor beta type II receptor gene in colorectal cancer. Cancer Res 1995;55: 5548–50.

[61] Rampino N, Yamamoto H, Ionov Y, et al. Somatic frameshift mutations in the BAX gene in colon cancers of the microsatellite mutator phenotype. Science 1997;275:967–9.

[62] Ryan SV, Carrithers SL, Parkinson SJ, et al. Hypotensive mechanisms of amifostine. J Clin Pharmacol 1996;36:365–73.

[63] Baylin SB, Esteller M, Rountree MR, et al. Aberrant patterns of DNA methylation, chromatin formation and gene expression in cancer. Hum Mol Genet 2001;10:687–92.

[64] Baylin SB, Herman JG. DNA hypermethylation in tumorigenesis: epigenetics joins genetics. Trends Genet 2000;16:168–74.

[65] Tycko B. Epigenetic gene silencing in cancer. J Clin Invest 2000;105:401–7.

[66] Reik W, Dean W, Walter J. Epigenetic reprogramming in mammalian development. Science 2001;293:1089–93.

[67] Costello JF, Fruhwald MC, Smiraglia DJ, et al. Aberrant CpG-island methylation has nonrandom and tumour-type-specific patterns. Nat Genet 2000;24:132–8.

[68] Esteller M, Corn PG, Baylin SB, et al. A gene hypermethylation profile of human cancer. Cancer Res 2001;61:3225–9.

[69] Esteller M, Sparks A, Toyota M, et al. Analysis of adenomatous polyposis coli promoter hypermethylation in human cancer. Cancer Res 2000;60:4366–71.

[70] Esteller M, Toyota M, Sanchez-Cespedes M, et al. Inactivation of the DNA repair gene O6-methylguanine-DNA methyltransferase by promoter hypermethylation is associated with G to A mutations in K-ras in colorectal tumorigenesis. Cancer Res 2000;60:2368–71.

[71] Herman JG, Umar A, Polyak K, et al. Incidence and functional consequences of hMLH1 promoter hypermethylation in colorectal carcinoma. Proc Natl Acad Sci USA 1998;95: 6870–5.

[72] Veigl ML, Kasturi L, Olechnowicz J, et al. Biallelic inactivation of hMLH1 by epigenetic gene silencing, a novel mechanism causing human MSI cancers. Proc Natl Acad Sci USA 1998;95: 8698–702.

[73] Cui H, Horon IL, Ohlsson R, et al. Loss of imprinting in normal tissue of colorectal cancer patients with microsatellite instability. Nat Med 1998;4:1276–80.

[74] Nakagawa H, Chadwick RB, Peltomaki P, et al. Loss of imprinting of the insulin-like growth factor II gene occurs by biallelic methylation in a core region of H19-associated CTCF-binding sites in colorectal cancer. Proc Natl Acad Sci USA 2001;98:591–6.

[75] Takano Y, Shiota G, Kawasaki H. Analysis of genomic imprinting of insulin-like growth factor 2 in colorectal cancer. Oncology 2000;59:210–6.

[76] Toyota M, Ahuja N, Ohe-Toyota M, et al. CpG island methylator phenotype in colorectal cancer. Proc Natl Acad Sci USA 1999;96:8681–6.

[77] Toyota M, Ohe-Toyota M, Ahuja N, et al. Distinct genetic profiles in colorectal tumors with or without the CpG island methylator phenotype. Proc Natl Acad Sci USA 2000;97:710–5.

[78] Powell SM, Petersen GM, Krush AJ, et al. Molecular diagnosis of familial adenomatous polyposis. N Engl J Med 1993;329:1982–7.

[79] Barker N, Clevers H. Catenins, Wnt signaling and cancer. Bioessays 2000;22:961–5.

[80] Bienz M, Clevers H. Linking colorectal cancer to Wnt signaling. Cell 2000;103:311–20.

[81] Fearnhead NS, Britton MP, Bodmer WF. The ABC of APC. Hum Mol Genet 2001;10:721–33.

[82] Uthoff SM, Eichenberger MR, McAuliffe TL, et al. Wingless-type frizzled protein receptor signaling and its putative role in human colon cancer. Mol Carcinog 2001;31:56–62.

[83] Henderson BR. Nuclear-cytoplasmic shuttling of APC regulates beta-catenin subcellular localization and turnover. Nat Cell Biol 2000;2:653–60.

[84] Rosin-Arbesfeld R, Townsley F, Bienz M. The APC tumour suppressor has a nuclear export function. Nature 2000;406:1009–12.

[85] Ikeda S, Kishida M, Matsuura Y, et al. GSK-3beta-dependent phosphorylation of adenomatous polyposis coli gene product can be modulated by beta-catenin and protein phosphatase 2A complexed with Axin. Oncogene 2000;19:537–45.

[86] Yamamoto H, Kishida S, Kishida M, et al. Phosphorylation of axin, a Wnt signal negative regulator, by glycogen synthase kinase-3beta regulates its stability. J Biol Chem 1999;274: 10681–4.

[87] Peters JM, McKay RM, McKay JP, et al. Casein kinase I transduces Wnt signals. Nature 1999; 401:345–50.

[88] Willert K, Shibamoto S, Nusse R. Wnt-induced dephosphorylation of axin releases beta-catenin from the axin complex. Genes Dev 1999;13:1768–73.

[89] Hecht A, Kemler R. Curbing the nuclear activities of beta-catenin. Control over Wnt target gene expression. EMBO 2000;1:24–8.

[90] Hecht A, Vleminckx K, Stemmler MP, et al. The p300/CBP acetyltransferases function as transcriptional coactivators of beta-catenin in vertebrates. EMBO J 2000;19:1839–50.

[91] Polakis P. Wnt signaling and cancer. Genes Dev 2000;14:1837–51.

[92] Takemaru KI, Moon RT. The transcriptional coactivator CBP interacts with beta-catenin to activate gene expression. J Cell Biol 2000;149:249–54.

[93] Waltzer L, Bienz M. Drosophila CBP represses the transcription factor TCF to antagonize Wingless signalling. Nature 1998;395:521–5.

[94] Crawford HC, Fingleton BM, Rudolph-Owen LA, et al. The metalloproteinase matrilysin is a target of beta-catenin transactivation in intestinal tumors. Oncogene 1999;18:2883–91.

[95] He TC, Chan TA, Vogelstein B, et al. PPARdelta is an APC-regulated target of nonsteroidal anti-inflammatory drugs. Cell 1999;99:335–45.

[96] He TC, Sparks AB, Rago C, et al. Identification of c-MYC as a target of the APC pathway. Science 1998;281:1509–12.

[97] Howe LR, Subbaramaiah K, Chung WJ, et al. Transcriptional activation of cyclooxygenase-2 in Wnt-1-transformed mouse mammary epithelial cells. Cancer Res 1999;59:1572–7.

[98] Koh TJ, Bulitta CJ, Fleming JV, et al. Gastrin is a target of the beta-catenin/TCF-4 growth-signaling pathway in a model of intestinal polyposis. J Clin Invest 2000;106:533–9.

[99] Tetsu O, McCormick F. Beta-catenin regulates expression of cyclin D1 in colon carcinoma cells. Nature 1999;398:422–6.

[100] McCormick F. Signalling networks that cause cancer. Trends Cell Biol 1999;9:M53–6.

[101] Gottardi CJ, Wong E, Gumbiner BM. E-cadherin suppresses cellular transformation by inhibiting beta-catenin signaling in an adhesion-independent manner. J Cell Biol 2001;153: 1049–60.

[102] Orsulic S, Huber O, Aberle H, et al. E-cadherin binding prevents beta-catenin nuclear localization and beta-catenin/LEF-1-mediated transactivation. J Cell Sci 1999;112:1237–45.

[103] Palmer HG, Gonzalez-Sancho JM, Espada J, et al. Vitamin D(3) promotes the differentiation of colon carcinoma cells by the induction of E-cadherin and the inhibition of beta-catenin signaling. J Cell Biol 2001;154:369–87.

[104] Stockinger A, Eger A, Wolf J, et al. E-cadherin regulates cell growth by modulating proliferation-dependent beta-catenin transcriptional activity. J Cell Biol 2001;154:1185–96.

[105] Takaku K, Sonoshita M, Sasaki N, et al. Suppression of intestinal polyposis in Apc(delta 716) knockout mice by an additional mutation in the cytosolic phospholipase A(2) gene. J Biol Chem 2000;275:34013–6.

[106] Cormier RT, Hong KH, Halberg RB, et al. Secretory phospholipase Pla2g2a confers resistance to intestinal tumorigenesis. Nat Genet 1997;17:88–91.

[107] Wang SS, Esplin ED, Li JL, et al. Alterations of the PPP2R1B gene in human lung and colon cancer. Science 1998;282:284–7.

[108] Oshima M, Oshima H, Kitagawa K, et al. Loss of Apc heterozygosity and abnormal tissue building in nascent intestinal polyps in mice carrying a truncated Apc gene. Proc Natl Acad Sci USA 1995;92:4482–6.

[109] Su LK, Kinzler KW, Vogelstein B, et al. Multiple intestinal neoplasia caused by a mutation in the murine homolog of the APC gene. Science 1992;256:668–70.

[110] Spirio LN, Samowitz W, Robertson J, et al. Alleles of APC modulate the frequency and classes of mutations that lead to colon polyps. Nat Genet 1998;20:385–8.

[111] Korinek V, Barker N, Morin PJ, et al. Constitutive transcriptional activation by a beta-catenin-Tcf complex in APC −/− colon carcinoma. Science 1997;275:1784–7.

[112] Morin PJ, Sparks AB, Korinek V, et al. Activation of beta-catenin-Tcf signaling in colon cancer by mutations in beta-catenin or APC. Science 1997;275:1787–90.

[113] Huang J, Papadopoulos N, McKinley AJ, et al. APC mutations in colorectal tumors with mismatch repair deficiency. Proc Natl Acad Sci USA 1996;93:9049–54.

[114] Miyaki M, Iijima T, Kimura J, et al. Frequent mutation of beta-catenin and APC genes in primary colorectal tumors from patients with hereditary nonpolyposis colorectal cancer. Cancer Res 1999;59:4506–9.

[115] Smith KJ, Johnson KA, Bryan TM, et al. The APC gene product in normal and tumor cells. Proc Natl Acad Sci USA 1993;90:2846–50.

[116] Murata M, Iwao K, Miyoshi Y, et al. Activation of the beta-catenin gene by interstitial deletions involving exon 3 as an early event in colorectal tumorigenesis. Cancer Lett 2000;159:73–8.

[117] Rubinfeld B, Robbins P, El-Gamil M, et al. Stabilization of beta-catenin by genetic defects in melanoma cell lines. Science 1997;275:1790–2.

[118] Harada N, Tamai Y, Ishikawa T, et al. Intestinal polyposis in mice with a dominant stable mutation of the beta-catenin gene. EMBO J 1999;18:5931–42.

[119] Sparks AB, Morin PJ, Vogelstein B, et al. Mutational analysis of the APC/beta-catenin/Tcf pathway in colorectal cancer. Cancer Res 1998;58:1130–4.

[120] Samowitz WS, Powers MD, Spirio LN, et al. Beta-catenin mutations are more frequent in small colorectal adenomas than in larger adenomas and invasive carcinomas. Cancer Res 1999;59: 1442–4.

[121] Zhurinsky J, Shtutman M, Ben-Ze'ev A. Plakoglobin and beta-catenin: protein interactions, regulation and biological roles. J Cell Sci 2000;113:3127–39.

[122] Kolligs FT, Kolligs B, Hajra KM, et al. gamma-catenin is regulated by the APC tumor suppressor and its oncogenic activity is distinct from that of beta-catenin. Genes Dev 2000;14: 1319–31.

[123] Zhurinsky J, Shtutman M, Ben-Ze'ev A. Differential mechanisms of LEF/TCF family-dependent transcriptional activation by beta-catenin and plakoglobin. Mol Cell Biol 2000;20: 4238–52.

[124] Ratcliffe MJ, Itoh K, Sokol SY. A positive role for the PP2A catalytic subunit in Wnt signal transduction. J Biol Chem 2000;275:35680–3.

[125] Seeling JM, Miller JR, Gil R, et al. Regulation of beta-catenin signaling by the B56 subunit of protein phosphatase 2A. Science 1999;283:2089–91.

[126] Satoh S, Daigo Y, Furukawa Y, et al. AXIN1 mutations in hepatocellular carcinomas, and growth suppression in cancer cells by virus-mediated transfer of AXIN1. Nat Genet 2000;24:245–50.

[127] Korinek V, Barker N, Moerer P, et al. Depletion of epithelial stem-cell compartments in the small intestine of mice lacking Tcf-4. Nat Genet 1998;19:379–83.

[128] Mariadason JM, Bordonaro M, Aslam F, et al. Down-regulation of beta-catenin TCF signaling is linked to colonic epithelial cell differentiation. Cancer Res 2001;61:3465–71.

[129] Naishiro Y, Yamada T, Takaoka AS, et al. Restoration of epithelial cell polarity in a colorectal cancer cell line by suppression of beta-catenin/T-cell factor 4-mediated gene transactivation. Cancer Res 2001;61:2751–8.

[130] Hovanes K, Li TW, Munguia JE, et al. Beta-catenin-sensitive isoforms of lymphoid enhancer factor-1 are selectively expressed in colon cancer. Nat Genet 2001;28:53–7.

[131] Lewin B. DNA replication. In: Lewin B, editor. Genes VII. New York: Oxford University Press; 2000. p. 385–415.

[132] Lipkin SM, Wang V, Jacoby R, et al. MLH3: a DNA mismatch repair gene associated with mammalian microsatellite instability. Nat Genet 2000;24:27–35.

[133] Carrithers SL, Parkinson SJ, Goldstein SD, et al. Escherichia coli heat-stable enterotoxin receptors. A novel marker for colorectal tumors. Dis Colon Rectum 1996;39:171–81.

[134] Fishel R, Wilson T. MutS homologs in mammalian cells. Curr Opin Genet Dev 1997;7:105–13.

[135] Allen DJ, Makhov A, Grilley M, et al. MutS mediates heteroduplex loop formation by a translocation mechanism. EMBO J 1997;16:4467–76.

[136] Gradia S, Acharya S, Fishel R. The human mismatch recognition complex hMSH2-hMSH6 functions as a novel molecular switch. Cell 1997;91:995–1005.

[137] Bellacosa A, Cicchillitti L, Schepis F, et al. MED1, a novel human methyl-CpG-binding endonuclease, interacts with DNA mismatch repair protein MLH1. Proc Natl Acad Sci USA 1999;96:3969–74.

[138] Berry SE, Garces C, Hwang HS, et al. The mismatch repair protein, hMLH1, mediates 5-substituted halogenated thymidine analogue cytotoxicity, DNA incorporation, and radiosensitization in human colon cancer cells. Cancer Res 1999;59:1840–5.

[139] Duckett DR, Bronstein SM, Taya Y, et al. hMutSalpha- and hMutLalpha-dependent phosphorylation of p53 in response to DNA methylator damage. Proc Natl Acad Sci USA 1999;96: 12384–8.

[140] Hickman MJ, Samson LD. Role of DNA mismatch repair and p53 in signaling induction of apoptosis by alkylating agents. Proc Natl Acad Sci USA 1999;96:10764–9.

[141] Aebi S, Kurdi-Haidar B, Gordon R, et al. Loss of DNA mismatch repair in acquired resistance to cisplatin. Cancer Res 1996;56:3087–90.

[142] de Wind N, Dekker M, Berns A, et al. Inactivation of the mouse Msh2 gene results in mismatch repair deficiency, methylation tolerance, hyperrecombination, and predisposition to cancer. Cell 1995;82:321–30.

[143] Drummond JT, Anthoney A, Brown R, et al. Cisplatin and adriamycin resistance are associated with MutLalpha and mismatch repair deficiency in an ovarian tumor cell line. J Biol Chem 1996;271:19645–8.

[144] Vasen HF, Watson P, Mecklin JP, et al. New clinical criteria for hereditary nonpolyposis color-

ectal cancer (HNPCC, Lynch syndrome) proposed by the International Collaborative group on HNPCC. Gastroenterology 1999;116:1453–6.

[145] Vasen HF, Mecklin JP, Khan PM, et al. The International Collaborative Group on Hereditary Non-Polyposis Colorectal Cancer (ICG-HNPCC). Dis Colon Rectum 1991;34:424–5.

[146] Hamilton SR, Liu B, Parsons RE, et al. The molecular basis of Turcot's syndrome. N Engl J Med 1995;332:839–47.

[147] Kruse R, Rutten A, Lamberti C, et al. Muir-Torre phenotype has a frequency of DNA mismatch-repair-gene mutations similar to that in hereditary nonpolyposis colorectal cancer families defined by the Amsterdam criteria. Am J Hum Genet 1998;63:63–70.

[148] Boland CR, Thibodeau SN, Hamilton SR, et al. A National Cancer Institute workshop on microsatellite instability for cancer detection and familial predisposition: development of international criteria for the determination of microsatellite instability in colorectal cancer. Cancer Res 1998;58:5248–57.

[149] Liu B, Parsons R, Papadopoulos N, et al. Analysis of mismatch repair genes in hereditary nonpolyposis colorectal cancer patients. Nat Med 1996;2:169–74.

[150] Peltomaki P, Vasen HF. Mutations predisposing to hereditary nonpolyposis colorectal cancer: database and results of a collaborative study. The International Collaborative Group on Hereditary Nonpolyposis Colorectal Cancer. Gastroenterology 1997;113:1146–58.

[151] Akiyama Y, Sato H, Yamada T, et al. Germ-line mutation of the hMSH6/GTBP gene in an atypical hereditary nonpolyposis colorectal cancer kindred. Cancer Res 1997;57:3920–3.

[152] Huang J, Kuismanen SA, Liu T, et al. MSH6 and MSH3 are rarely involved in genetic predisposition to nonpolypotic colon cancer. Cancer Res 2001;61:1619–23.

[153] Kolodner RD, Tytell JD, Schmeits JL, et al. Germ-line msh6 mutations in colorectal cancer families. Cancer Res 1999;59:5068–74.

[154] Liu T, Yan H, Kuismanen S, et al. The role of hPMS1 and hPMS2 in predisposing to colorectal cancer. Cancer Res 2001;61:7798–802.

[155] Miyaki M, Konishi M, Tanaka K, et al. Germline mutation of MSH6 as the cause of hereditary nonpolyposis colorectal cancer. Nat Genet 1997;17:271–2.

[156] Wu Y, Berends MJ, Sijmons RH, et al. A role for MLH3 in hereditary nonpolyposis colorectal cancer. Nat Genet 2001;29:137–8.

[157] Wijnen J, de Leeuw W, Vasen H, et al. Familial endometrial cancer in female carriers of MSH6 germline mutations. Nat Genet 1999;23:142–4.

[158] Kane MF, Loda M, Gaida GM, et al. Methylation of the hMLH1 promoter correlates with lack of expression of hMLH1 in sporadic colon tumors and mismatch repair-defective human tumor cell lines. Cancer Res 1997;57:808–11.

[159] Das Gupta R, Kolodner RD. Novel dominant mutations in Saccharomyces cerevisiae MSH6. Nat Genet 2000;24:53–6.

[160] Nicolaides NC, Littman SJ, Modrich P, et al. A naturally occurring hPMS2 mutation can confer a dominant negative mutator phenotype. Mol Cell Biol 1998;18:1635–41.

[161] Heyer J, Yang K, Lipkin M, et al. Mouse models for colorectal cancer. Oncogene 1999;18:5325–33.

[162] Grady WM, Rajput A, Myeroff L, et al. Mutation of the type II transforming growth factor-beta receptor is coincident with the transformation of human colon adenomas to malignant carcinomas. Cancer Res 1998;58:3101–4.

[163] Souza RF, Appel R, Yin J, et al. Microsatellite instability in the insulin-like growth factor II receptor gene in gastrointestinal tumours. Nat Genet 1996;14:255–7.

[164] Losi L, Ponz de Leon M, Jiricny J, et al. K-ras and p53 mutations in hereditary non-polyposis colorectal cancers. Int J Cancer 1997;74:94–6.

[165] Samowitz WS, Holden JA, Curtin K, et al. Inverse relationship between microsatellite instability and K-ras and p53 gene alterations in colon cancer. Am J Pathol 2001;158:1517–24.

[166] Yagi OK, Akiyama Y, Nomizu T, et al. Proapoptotic gene BAX is frequently mutated in hereditary nonpolyposis colorectal cancers but not in adenomas. Gastroenterology 1998;114:268–74.

[167] Yamamoto H, Sawai H, Weber TK, et al. Somatic frameshift mutations in DNA mismatch

repair and proapoptosis genes in hereditary nonpolyposis colorectal cancer. Cancer Res 1998; 58:997–1003.

[168] Riccio A, Aaltonen LA, Godwin AK, et al. The DNA repair gene MBD4 (MED1) is mutated in human carcinomas with microsatellite instability. Nat Genet 1999;23:266–8.

[169] Ejima Y, Yang L, Sasaki MS. Aberrant splicing of the ATM gene associated with shortening of the intronic mononucleotide tract in human colon tumor cell lines: a novel mutation target of microsatellite instability. Int J Cancer 2000;86:262–8.

[170] Calin GA, Gafa R, Tibiletti MG, et al. Genetic progression in microsatellite instability high (MSI-H) colon cancers correlates with clinico-pathological parameters: a study of the TGRbetaRII, BAX, hMSH3, hMSH6, IGFIIR and BLM genes. Int J Cancer 2000;89: 230–5.

[171] Yoshitaka T, Matsubara N, Ikeda M, et al. Mutations of E2F−4 trinucleotide repeats in colorectal cancer with microsatellite instability. Biochem Biophys Res Commun 1996;227: 553–7.

[172] Duval A, Iacopetta B, Ranzani GN, et al. Variable mutation frequencies in coding repeats of TCF-4 and other target genes in colon, gastric and endometrial carcinoma showing microsatellite instability. Oncogene 1999;18:6806–9.

[173] Steele-Perkins G, Fang W, Yang XH, et al. Tumor formation and inactivation of RIZ1, an Rb-binding member of a nuclear protein-methyltransferase superfamily. Genes Dev 2001;15: 2250–62.

[174] Schwartz Jr. S, Yamamoto H, Navarro M, et al. Frameshift mutations at mononucleotide repeats in caspase-5 and other target genes in endometrial and gastrointestinal cancer of the microsatellite mutator phenotype. Cancer Res 1999;59:2995–3002.

[175] Ionov Y, Peinado MA, Malkhosyan S, et al. Ubiquitous somatic mutations in simple repeated sequences reveal a new mechanism for colonic carcinogenesis. Nature 1993;363: 558–61.

[176] Lothe RA, Peltomaki P, Meling GI, et al. Genomic instability in colorectal cancer: relationship to clinicopathological variables and family history. Cancer Res 1993;53:5849–52.

[177] Thibodeau SN, Bren G, Schaid D. Microsatellite instability in cancer of the proximal colon. Science 1993;260:816–9.

[178] Fujiwara T, Stolker JM, Watanabe T, et al. Accumulated clonal genetic alterations in familial and sporadic colorectal carcinomas with widespread instability in microsatellite sequences. Am J Pathol 1998;153:1063–78.

[179] Liu B, Nicolaides NC, Markowitz S, et al. Mismatch repair gene defects in sporadic colorectal cancers with microsatellite instability. Nat Genet 1995;9:48–55.

[180] Ma AH, Xia L, Littman SJ, et al. Somatic mutation of hPMS2 as a possible cause of sporadic human colon cancer with microsatellite instability. Oncogene 2000;19:2249–56.

[181] Kuismanen SA, Holmberg MT, Salovaara R, et al. Genetic and epigenetic modification of MLH1 accounts for a major share of microsatellite-unstable colorectal cancers. Am J Pathol 2000;156:1773–9.

[182] Wong SF, Lai LC. The role of TGFbeta in human cancers. Pathology 2001;33:85–92.

[183] Rooke HM, Crosier KE. The smad proteins and TGFbeta signalling: uncovering a pathway critical in cancer. Pathology 2001;33:73–84.

[184] de Caestecker MP, Piek E, Roberts AB. Role of transforming growth factor-beta signaling in cancer. J Natl Cancer Inst 2000;92:1388–402.

[185] Massague J, Blain SW, Lo RS. TGFbeta signaling in growth control, cancer, and heritable disorders. Cell 2000;103:295–309.

[186] Itoh S, Itoh F, Goumans MJ, et al. Signaling of transforming growth factor-beta family members through Smad proteins. Eur J Biochem 2000;267:6954–67.

[187] Massague J, Wotton D. Transcriptional control by the TGF-beta/Smad signaling system. EMBO J 2000;19:1745–54.

[188] Verrecchia F, Chu ML, Mauviel A. Identification of novel TGF-beta /Smad gene targets in dermal fibroblasts using a combined cDNA microarray/promoter transactivation approach. J Biol Chem 2001;276:17058–62.

[189] Chiao PJ, Hunt KK, Grau AM, et al. Tumor suppressor gene Smad4/DPC4, its downstream target genes, and regulation of cell cycle. Ann N Y Acad Sci 1999;880:31–7.

[190] Ulloa L, Doody J, Massague J. Inhibition of transforming growth factor-beta/SMAD signalling by the interferon-gamma/STAT pathway. Nature 1999;397:710–3.
[191] Kretzschmar M, Doody J, Timokhina I, et al. A mechanism of repression of TGFbeta/ Smad signaling by oncogenic Ras. Genes Dev 1999;13:804–16.
[192] Grady WM, Myeroff LL, Swinler SE, et al. Mutational inactivation of transforming growth factor beta receptor type II in microsatellite stable colon cancers. Cancer Res 1999;59:320–4.
[193] Markowitz S, Wang J, Myeroff L, et al. Inactivation of the type II TGF-beta receptor in colon cancer cells with microsatellite instability. Science 1995;268:1336–8.
[194] Togo G, Okamoto M, Shiratori Y, et al. Does mutation of transforming growth factor-beta type II receptor gene play an important role in colorectal polyps? Dig Dis Sci 1999;44: 1803–9.
[195] Wang J, Sun L, Myeroff L, et al. Demonstration that mutation of the type II transforming growth factor beta receptor inactivates its tumor suppressor activity in replication error-positive colon carcinoma cells. J Biol Chem 1995;270:22044–9.
[196] Hahn SA, Schutte M, Hoque AT, et al. DPC4, a candidate tumor suppressor gene at human chromosome 18q21.1. Science 1996;271:350–3.
[197] Thiagalingam S, Lengauer C, Leach FS, et al. Evaluation of candidate tumour suppressor genes on chromosome 18 in colorectal cancers. Nat Genet 1996;13:343–6.
[198] Eppert K, Scherer SW, Ozcelik H, et al. MADR2 maps to 18q21 and encodes a TGFbeta-regulated MAD-related protein that is functionally mutated in colorectal carcinoma. Cell 1996; 86:543–52.
[199] Riggins GJ, Thiagalingam S, Rozenblum E, et al. Mad-related genes in the human. Nat Genet 1996;13:347–9.
[200] Heyer J, Escalante-Alcalde D, Lia M, et al. Postgastrulation Smad2-deficient embryos show defects in embryo turning and anterior morphogenesis. Proc Natl Acad Sci USA 1999;96: 12595–600.
[201] Takaku K, Oshima M, Miyoshi H, et al. Intestinal tumorigenesis in compound mutant mice of both Dpc4 (Smad4) and Apc genes. Cell 1998;92:645–56.
[202] Riggins GJ, Kinzler KW, Vogelstein B, et al. Frequency of Smad gene mutations in human cancers. Cancer Res 1997;57:2578–80.
[203] Zhu Y, Richardson JA, Parada LF, et al. Smad3 mutant mice develop metastatic colorectal cancer. Cell 1998;94:703–14.
[204] Gold LI. The role for transforming growth factor-beta (TGF-beta) in human cancer. Crit Rev Oncog 1999;10:303–60.
[205] Matsushita M, Matsuzaki K, Date M, et al. Down-regulation of TGF-beta receptors in human colorectal cancer: implications for cancer development. Br J Cancer 1999;80:194–205.
[206] Oft M, Heider KH, Beug H. TGFbeta signaling is necessary for carcinoma cell invasiveness and metastasis. Curr Biol 1998;8:1243–52.
[207] Vogelstein B, Fearon ER, Hamilton SR, et al. Genetic alterations during colorectal-tumor development. N Engl J Med 1988;319:525–32.
[208] Daujat S, Neel H, Piette J. MDM2: life without p53. Trends Genet 2001;17:459–64.
[209] Ryan KM, Phillips AC, Vousden KH. Regulation and function of the p53 tumor suppressor protein. Curr Opin Cell Biol 2001;13:332–7.
[210] Soussi T. The p53 tumor suppressor gene: from molecular biology to clinical investigation. Ann NY Acad Sci 2000;910:121–37 [discussion 137–9].
[211] Woods DB, Vousden KH. Regulation of p53 function. Exp Cell Res 2001;264:56–66.
[212] el-Deiry WS. Regulation of p53 downstream genes. Semin Cancer Biol 1998;8:345–57.
[213] Donehower LA. The p53-deficient mouse: a model for basic and applied cancer studies. Semin Cancer Biol 1996;7:269–78.
[214] Donehower LA, Harvey M, Slagle BL, et al. Mice deficient for p53 are developmentally normal but susceptible to spontaneous tumours. Nature 1992;356:215–21.
[215] Srivastava S, Zou ZQ, Pirollo K, et al. Germ-line transmission of a mutated p53 gene in a cancer-prone family with Li-Fraumeni syndrome. Nature 1990;348:747–9.
[216] Lane DP. Cancer. p53, guardian of the genome. Nature 1992;358:15–6.

[217] Hussain SP, Amstad P, Raja K, et al. Increased p53 mutation load in noncancerous colon tissue from ulcerative colitis: a cancer-prone chronic inflammatory disease. Cancer Res 2000;60: 3333–7.

[218] Losi L, Roncucci L, di Gregorio C, et al. K-ras and p53 mutations in human colorectal aberrant crypt foci. J Pathol 1996;178:259–63.

[219] Baker SJ, Preisinger AC, Jessup JM, et al. p53 gene mutations occur in combination with 17p allelic deletions as late events in colorectal tumorigenesis. Cancer Res 1990;50: 7717–22.

[220] Kikuchi-Yanoshita R, Konishi M, Ito S, et al. Genetic changes of both p53 alleles associated with the conversion from colorectal adenoma to early carcinoma in familial adenomatous polyposis and non-familial adenomatous polyposis patients. Cancer Res 1992;52:3965–71.

[221] Bleeker WA, Hayes VM, Karrenbeld A, et al. Impact of KRAS and TP53 mutations on survival in patients with left- and right-sided Dukes' C colon cancer. Am J Gastroenterol 2000;95: 2953–7.

[222] Buglioni S, D'Agnano I, Cosimelli M, et al. Evaluation of multiple bio-pathological factors in colorectal adenocarcinomas: independent prognostic role of p53 and bcl-2. Int J Cancer 1999; 84:545–52.

[223] Nemunaitis J, Khuri F, Ganly I, et al. Phase II trial of intratumoral administration of ONYX-015, a replication-selective adenovirus, in patients with refractory head and neck cancer. J Clin Oncol 2001;19:289–98.

[224] Raj K, Ogston P, Beard P. Virus-mediated killing of cells that lack p53 activity. Nature 2001; 412:914–7.

[225] Offringa R, Vierboom MP, van der Burg SH, et al. p53: a potential target antigen for immunotherapy of cancer. Ann NY Acad Sci 2000;910:223–33 [discussion 233–6].

[226] Selivanova G, Iotsova V, Okan I, et al. Restoration of the growth suppression function of mutant p53 by a synthetic peptide derived from the p53 C-terminal domain. Nat Med 1997; 3:632–8.

[227] Watanabe T, Sullenger BA. Induction of wild-type p53 activity in human cancer cells by ribozymes that repair mutant p53 transcripts. Proc Natl Acad Sci USA 2000;97:8490–4.

[228] Carrithers SL, Taylor B, Cai WY, et al. Guanylyl cyclase-C receptor mRNA distribution along the rat nephron. Regul Pept 2000;95:65–74.

[229] Pruitt K, Der CJ. Ras and Rho regulation of the cell cycle and oncogenesis. Cancer Lett 2001; 171:1–10.

[230] Gallinger S, Vivona AA, Odze RD, et al. Somatic APC and K-ras codon 12 mutations in periampullary adenomas and carcinomas from familial adenomatous polyposis patients. Oncogene 1995;10:1875–8.

[231] Ichii S, Takeda S, Horii A, et al. Detailed analysis of genetic alterations in colorectal tumors from patients with and without familial adenomatous polyposis (FAP). Oncogene 1993;8: 2399–405.

[232] McMahon M, Woods D. Regulation of the p53 pathway by Ras, the plot thickens. Biochim Biophys Acta 2001;1471:M63–71.

[233] Irby RB, Mao W, Coppola D, et al. Activating SRC mutation in a subset of advanced human colon cancers. Nat Genet 1999;21:187–90.

[234] Herrlich P, Morrison H, Sleeman J, et al. CD44 acts both as a growth- and invasiveness-promoting molecule and as a tumor-suppressing cofactor. Ann NY Acad Sci 2000;910:106–18 [discussion 118–20].

[235] Park BH, Vogelstein B, Kinzler KW. Genetic disruption of PPARdelta decreases the tumorigenicity of human colon cancer cells. Proc Natl Acad Sci USA 2001;98:2598–603.

[236] Seed B. PPARgamma and colorectal carcinoma: conflicts in a nuclear family. Nat Med 1998; 4:1004–5.

[237] Carrithers SL, Barber MT, Biswas S, et al. Guanylyl cyclase C is a selective marker for metastatic colorectal tumors in human extraintestinal tissues. Proc Natl Acad Sci USA 1996;93: 14827–32.

HEMATOLOGY/
ONCOLOGY
CLINICS OF
NORTH AMERICA

Hematol Oncol Clin N Am
16 (2002) 811–840

Primary prevention: phytoprevention and chemoprevention of colorectal cancer

Marco E. Turini, PhD[a], Raymond N. DuBois, MD, PhD[b],*

[a]Department of Nutrition, Nestlé Research Center, Post Office Box 44,
CH-1000 Lausanne 26, Switzerland
[b]Departments of Medicine/Gastrointestinal and Cell Biology, MCN C-2104,
Vanderbilt University Medical Center, Nashville, TN 37232-2279, USA

Colorectal cancer (CRC) is a leading cause of mortality and morbidity in the United States and other Western countries. It is the third most common form of cancer in the United States. Estimated figures for 2002 are 148,000 new cases and more than 56,000 deaths (American Cancer Society, Cancer Facts and Figures 2002, http://www.cancer.org). The 5-year survival rate depends on the stage of disease, with a 90%, 65%, and 10% rates of survival for localized, regional, and distant cancers, respectively [1]. It has been reported that only 37% of cases are diagnosed at an early stage.

Poor prognosis associated with late-stage diagnosis and the possibility of modulating the course of carcinogenesis make phytoprevention and chemoprevention attractive approaches for the primary prevention of colorectal cancer. Primary prevention aims at decreasing the risk for cancer by inhibiting or reversing the tumorigenic process through environmental or dietary modifications and through pharmacologic or endoscopic interventions. As reviewed elsewhere, prophylactic endoscopic polypectomy and early detection of cancer decrease colorectal cancer incidence and death [2]. Persons at risk for colorectal cancer, such as those with familial adenomatous polyposis (FAP), may benefit most from prevention therapy. In this regard, inherited factors may account for up to 30% of colorectal cancer cases [2]. A long-term prevention approach to colon cancer for the overall population or an at-risk population may also be suitable using dietary modifications or diet-derived chemoprevention agents.

Genetic and environmental factors have been identified as causes of cancer. It has been estimated that 35% to 50% of colorectal cancers could be prevented by proper nutrition. In addition to agents such as nonsteroidal antiinflammatory drugs (NSAIDs), a number of micronutrients and dietary constituents with chemo-

---

* Corresponding author.
E-mail address: raymond.dubois@mcmail.vanderbilt.edu (R.N. DuBois).

prevention properties have been identified. These components include fibers and carotenoids such as lycopene, vitamins (A, C, D, E), folate, calcium, and selenium. Groups of phytochemicals associated with cancer prevention are, to cite a few, organosulfurs, phenols including flavonoids and isoflavones, glucosinolates, and saponins. A select number of agents with evidence of potential chemoprevention properties are presented in this review.

Phytoprevention versus chemoprevention

The term phytoprevention has been widely used, though differentiation between phytoprevention and chemoprevention is unclear and may in some ways be artificial. Phyt(o) comes from the Greek *phytum* for plant. Consequently, phytoprevention indicates prevention through the use of chemical compounds derived from plants, and the perception is that they are natural. On the other hand, the term chemoprevention may reflect the use of drugs and of a more aggressive therapeutic approach than that with phytochemicals. This is confusing, however, because many drugs were originally discovered as natural components of plants. In addition, preventive agents are difficult to classify in one of these categories (eg, calcium, vitamins). Keeping in mind the above considerations but to maintain the clarity of this review, sections on chemoprevention and phytoprevention have been distinguished.

Carcinogenesis

Carcinogenesis is a complex, multistep process involving initiation and promotion stages that are not necessarily discrete or well-defined events. During the initiation stage, mutations accumulate in protooncogenes and tumor-suppressor genes that are meditated by carcinogens and followed by subsequent loss of heterozygosity. It is estimated that 85% of colorectal cancers are associated with a mutation in the adenomatous polyposis carcinomatous (*APC*) gene. Mutations in other tumor-suppressor genes such as *MCC*, *DCC*, and *p53*, and in oncogenes such as K-*ras*, also can occur. During the promotion stage, cell proliferation increases and aberrant crypt foci and a preneoplastic structure develop that may lead to adenoma (benign neoplastic polyps) and potentially result in tumor formation (carcinoma). The adenoma-to-carcinoma sequence results from a series of mutations affecting cell growth, differentiation, and programmed cell death [3–6]. Colorectal neoplasms can also arise from another distinct genetic pathway in which the frequent loss of expression of one of the DNA mismatch repair enzymes, usually hMLH1 or hMSH2, results in microsatellite instability [7,8]. Hereditary nonpolyposis colon cancer is a form of cancer caused by defective mismatch repair enzymes [9,10].

Molecular, phenotypic, and histopathologic differences and variations in lesion distribution within the colon between these two groups of tumors have important implications for chemoprevention strategies. Whereas COX-2 expression is increased in 80% to 90% of adenocarcinomas, tumors with defective mismatch repair often exhibit low or no COX-2 staining [11]. Tumor type may be an important consideration when assessing the efficacy of chemoprevention agents such as COX-2 inhibitors [12]. Conversely, a chemoprevention agent must be chosen carefully and adequately according to the targeted tumor type and location. For instance, in one study, protection by NSAID use was most pronounced for right-sided lesions in a population-based retrospective cohort study [13]. Sulindac has been shown to prevent and treat colorectal adenomas, but some FAP patients acquired rectal cancer during the therapy, indicating an uncoupling between the inhibition of prostaglandin production and carcinogenesis in some patients [14,15]. Rats treated with azoxymethane (AOM) develop colon cancer and aberrant crypt foci (ACF); aspirin treatment reduced ACF, prostaglandin E_2 (PGE_2) levels, and mitosis at concentrations that did not prevent cancer, supporting an uncoupling between the inhibition of prostaglandin production and carcinogenesis under certain conditions [16]. Aspirin and sulindac also reduced microsatellite instability in colorectal cancer cells deficient in a subset of human mismatch repair genes (hMLH1, hMSH2, hMSH6). This effect was specific for nonapoptotic cells and independent of cell proliferation rate and COX activity.

Cancer chemoprevention strategies primarily target cell growth inhibition, differentiation, and apoptosis. The mechanisms for chemoprevention are numerous; some of these involve arachidonic metabolism, sphingomyelin synthesis, modulation of procarcinogen and carcinogen metabolism, and interference with growth signaling, cell division, and differentiation.

Genetics and biomarkers

The development and validation of biomarkers to identify persons at risk for colorectal cancer and to serve as surrogate end-points to assess therapeutic efficacy have gained much interest and have been critically reviewed [17–23]. Criteria for a useful biomarker to serve as a surrogate end-point include variability and expression between key phases of carcinogenesis, association with risk for cancer, modulation by bioactive molecules, easy-to-perform noninvasive assay, reproducibility, and reliability [23]. The use of surrogate biomarkers allows investigators to design shorter, smaller, and less expensive trials [24].

Numerous clinical and molecular measurements have been suggested as biomarkers for risk assessment and as surrogate end-points for colorectal cancer. Clinical assessments include adenomatous polyps, ACF, and mucosal proliferation. Epidemiologic and clinical studies indicate adenoma as a valid biomarker and intermediate end-point for colorectal cancer, whereas ACF holds promise [25]. Programmed cell death is negatively correlated with colon cancer, responds to chemoprevention agents in AOM-treated rats, and is considered seriously as a biomarker [16,26,27]. The polyamines spermidine and spermine and their precursor, putrescine, are required for the growth and proliferation of eukaryotic cells. Elevated polyamine levels and ornithine decarboxylase (ODC) activity have been associated with abnormal cell proliferation and tumor promotion but are also observed in apparently normal colorectal mucosa of FAP patients [28]. None of these parameters was significantly correlated with polyp history, number of prevalent polyps found at colonoscopy, or polyp size when measured in unaffected colorectal mucosa [29]. The latter study indicates that rectal mucosal proliferation may not be an adequate marker of risk. On the other hand, it has been suggested that the spermidine-to-spermine ratio may be used as an end-point marker of the consequence of polyamine synthesis inhibition in chemoprevention trials [29]. Others [30] reported an increase in polyamine levels in the colon mucosa of cancer patients; however, four to eight biopsy samples in the cancer patients were necessary for acceptable reliability. Other putative biomarkers include rectal mucosal PGE_2 [31,32] and blood lymphocyte–glutathione S-transferase [33] measurements. Variability in PGE_2 levels calls for a large number of subjects to be included in the study [32].

Genetic DNA markers such as K-*ras*, *p53*, and *APC* are becoming available for early detection of patients at risk for cancer, as a substitute end-point measurement, or both [23]. Identification of DNA mutations in stool, especially K-*ras*, is considered a sensitive, specific, and cost-effective approach for use in chemoprevention trials and screening protocols; however, problems with the assay must first be overcome [34]. Stool DNA assays appear encouraging as a potential screening tool [35]. DNA methylation [36] and DNA strand break [36,37] have been considered putative surrogate markers. Confounding factors seem to interfere, as indicated by a folate supplementation study of patients after polypectomy [36].

Molecular genetics, gene array, genomics, and proteomics provide tools for a better understanding of neoplastic events involved in inherited colorectal cancer syndromes and for the identification of new biomarkers and intermediate endpoints. As the precise molecular events leading to malignant tumors are unraveled, optimized strategies using natural or synthetic agents may be developed. At-risk patients may also benefit from screening for early detection, whereas population-based genetic screening may soon be available to identify at-risk populations [38,39]. In addition, it might be possible to evaluate chemoprevention efficacy by high-throughput microarray analyses of gene expression profiles [40].

Chemoprevention by drugs

Chemoprevention by NSAIDs and COX-2 selective inhibitors

Nonsteroidal antiinflammatory drugs (NSAIDs) have some promise as chemoprevention agents for colorectal cancer. Animal, epidemiological, and clinical studies indicate an inverse association between NSAID use and colorectal cancer risk [41–43]. Antineoplastic properties of various NSAIDs were demonstrated in animal models of colon cancer [44–47]. Multiple intestinal neoplasia (Min) mice (a model of familial adenomatous polyposis) develop intestinal adenomas caused by a germline mutation in the *APC* gene. Adenomas in these mice can be prevented or reduced by treatment with piroxicam [48], sulindac sulfide [49,50], or high-dose aspirin [51]. Waddell and Loughry [52] were the first to report a reduced number of polyps by sulindac in an uncontrolled small clinical study in patients with FAP. In a follow-up study, similar results were obtained, and cessation of the treatment resulted in the recurrence of polyp formation, whereas reinitiating the therapy led to the disappearance of these polyps [53]. Subsequent intervention in FAP patients resulted in a regression of colorectal polyps by sulindac [54–56]. Recently, sulindac (mean, 158 mg/day) was effective in the long-term treatment and prevention of FAP, as observed in 7 of 12 patients who had undergone ileorectal anastomosis and had rectal segments free of adenoma [14]. Further support for reduced colorectal cancer risk by aspirin and NSAID use was indicated by 22 of 24 case-control and cohort studies in patients with sporadic colorectal neoplasia [57].

Many studies implicate PGE_2 as a factor modulating cell proliferation, tumor growth, and immune function [58]. Cyclooxygenase enzymes catalyze the first step in the conversion of arachidonic acid to prostanoids, including PGE_2. Cyclooxygenase has two isoforms, COX-1 and COX-2. COX-1 is expressed constitutively in many tissues, and it is thought that COX-1 is involved in tissue homeostasis and repair. COX-2, an immediate/early growth response gene, is induced by various stimuli mediating inflammation and tumor promotion. COX-2 expression is elevated in colorectal tumors [59–64], and animal and human data support its role in neoplasia [65,66]. Excellent reviews provide further detailed information on the structural, cellular, and molecular biology of cyclooxygenases [67,68], the prostanoid receptors [69], and the role of prostanoids in the large intestine under normal and abnormal conditions [70,71].

Recently, a new class of COX-2 selective inhibitors (COXIBs) has been developed that provide the antiinflammatory benefits of traditional NSAIDs with reduced gastrointestinal toxicity. The possible involvement of COX-2 in tumors and the recognized beneficial effects of NSAIDs on colon cancer led to an evaluation of COXIBs for their chemoprevention potential [72,73]. Rat colon tumors induced by AOM were reduced by the administration of COXIBs, celecoxib [74], or NS-398 [75], as indicated by a lower preneoplastic or tumor incidence and multiplicity, respectively, compared with control AOM-treated rats. The dose-response effect of celecoxib, administered during the initiation and postinitiation stages of colon tumorigenesis, was further investigated in AOM-treated rats [76]. Celecoxib inhibited adenocarcinoma incidence, suggesting its potential as a chemoprevention agent for primary prevention. In addition, efficacy of the drug was demonstrated when treatment was initiated at the later stages of colon cancer, indicating that celecoxib may also be effective for the secondary prevention of colon cancer in patients with FAP and sporadic polyps. Celecoxib was effective in preventing and treating adenomas in the Min mouse model [77]. The latter finding was further substantiated by Oshima et al [78], who assessed the effect of a COXIB on the development of intestinal adenomas in ApcΔ716 mice (a model in which a targeted truncation deletion in the tumor-suppressor gene, *APC*, causes intestinal polyposis). Drug treatment dramatically reduced the number and size of polyps by 50% and 80%, respectively. Nimesulfide, another COXIB, reduced AOM-induced ACF in rats, colon carcinogenesis in mice, and intestinal polyp formation in Min mice [79]. In contrast to these studies, orally fed formulations of 5-ASA (free acid, sulfasalazine, Pentasa) at various dosages were without chemoprevention activity against the development of nascent intestinal adenomas in Min mice [80]. In a pilot study of patients with colorectal cancer, mesalazine, a compound derived from salicylic acid, selectively induced apoptosis of tumor cells but had no effect on cell proliferation of normal or malignant tissues [81].

The mechanisms by which NSAIDs reduce the risk for colon cancer are still unclear. It is thought that NSAIDs in part mediate the inhibition of colon carcinogenesis through the inhibition of prostaglandin production by the cyclo-oxygenase enzymes [82]. Additional prostaglandin-independent effects, including those on cell adhesion and apoptosis, have been documented [83]. To reconcile the current contradictions of COX-dependent and COX-independent inhibition of colon carcinogenesis by NSAIDs, Rigas and Shiff [84] proposed a model in which NSAIDs exert their effects on different steps of the multistage process of colon carcinogenesis or on different control mechanisms, resulting in the same outcome. Different views persist, however, on the mechanisms by which NSAIDs exert their potentially beneficial effects [85]. In this regard, gene knockout mouse models, such as COX-1 and COX-2, have been useful in demonstrating the specificity of the effects of a drug. Clearly, at high concentrations, COXIBs inhibit the growth of cultured cells in a cyclooxygen-ase-independent fashion [86].

It is recognized that NSAIDs may have a role in cancer prevention, but the optimal dose of NSAID and the duration and frequency of treatment have not been established. In addition, the long-term use of aspirin and classical NSAIDs is limited because of significant adverse effects [87]. An animal study using 1,2-dimethylhydrazine (DMH) as the carcinogen suggested that aspirin treatment through the entire carcinogenic period is required to gain a protective effect [88]. The latter is supported by a population-based study of the elderly indicating that duration of use, but not daily dose, of NSAIDs is important for chemoprevention [13]. Whether COXIBs offer an alternative to classical NSAIDs without the side effects is under investigation. Noteworthy is that NSAIDs have COX-independent effects that may be important for their antineoplastic effect. In addition, not all NSAIDs, including COXIBs, may have the same chemoprevention properties. The National Cancer Institute (NCI) is sponsoring a randomized clinical trial assessing the safety and efficacy of celecoxib for reducing the occurrence of new sporadic colorectal adenomatous polyps in patients who have undergone polyp-ectomy. Results from ongoing and future clinical trials should provide some answers before the development of NSAID and COXIB recommendations for gastrointestinal cancer.

Chemoprevention by α-difluoromethylornithine

An enzyme-activated irreversible inhibitor of ornithine decarboxylase, α-difluoromethylornithine (DFMO)—the first enzyme in polyamine synthesis catalyzing the conversion of ornithine to putrescine—was developed more than 2 decades ago as a drug for proliferative diseases; it is now being developed as a chemoprevention agent [89]. Polyamine depletion arrests the growth of untransformed (IEC-6) and p53-mutated (Caco-2) cells by different mechanisms [90]. The growth inhibition of normal small intestinal mucosa in DFMO-induced polyamine depletion occurred through increased p53 mRNA stability [91], whereas in tumorigenic cells the mechanism remains unknown [90]. Polyamine-mediated regulation of gap junctions, thought to be crucial for normal tissue function and during various steps of tumorigenesis, has also been demonstrated [92].

The chemoprevention efficacy of DFMO against colon tumors was shown in preclinical studies using various animal models [93]. In human rectal mucosa, DFMO mediated a dose-dependent decrease in polyamines [94–96], though 0.4 g/m^2/day was more efficacious in decreasing putrescine levels than 0.2 g/m^2/day. Higher dropout and discontinuation rates were observed in patients on the highest dose [96]. In a smaller randomized, placebo-controlled trial, rectal mucosal polyamines were also decreased at 3 and 12 months of treatment with 0.5 g/m^2/day DFMO [97]. Concerns regarding toxicity that results in loss of hearing have been addressed. Combining the data of two clinical studies, a dose-dependent shift in auditory thresholds by DFMO (0.5–3.0 g/m^2/day) was reported [98]. Similarly, 3 of 24 patients acquired clinically noticeable and audiologically demonstrated hearing loss, which was reversible and was attributed to 0.5 g/m^2/day DFMO treatment [97]. Lower doses of the drug resulted only in marginal auditory losses, leading to a recommendation of 0.2g/m^2/day dose in combination phase 2b or single-agent phase 3 chemoprevention trials [96]. A phase 2 randomized, double-blind study of low-grade superficial bladder cancer using DFMO is ongoing, as are evaluations of its effectiveness in the prevention of colorectal cancer.

Chemoprevention by micronutrients and fibers

Chemoprevention by folate

Metabolic defects in folate metabolism are associated with atherogenic diseases causing cerebral (spina bifida), coronary, or peripheral vascular disease and venous thrombotic diathesis [99,100]. The potential role of folate in neoplastic changes, especially in the colon, and the proposed mechanisms have been recently reviewed [101,102]. Evidence for low folate status in certain segments of the population was previously reported [103–105]. Insufficient intake of this vitamin by a large proportion of the American population was further substantiated by the average intake of 242 µg/day dietary folate, compared with the

Dietary Reference Intake (DRI) of 400 µg/day [106]. This is in agreement with the subclinical, biochemically evident folate deficiency reported for up to 30% of the healthy, ambulatory United States population [107]. It has important implications for the at-risk population because long-term mild deficiency of certain vitamins may be involved in the development of chronic diseases, including cancer [108].

Folic acid is involved in DNA synthesis and repair, DNA methylation, and modulation of cell proliferation. In immortalized human colonocytes, folate deficiency decreases DNA stability as indicated by increased strand breakage and uracil misincorporation [109]. Absence of folate resulted in DNA hypomethylation. On the other hand, feeding rats a diet deficient in methyl donor, including folate, primarily affected DNA stability in isolated colonocytes without affecting overall DNA methylation [109].

In a series of experiments, Kim et al [110,111] investigated the effects of dietary folate on DNA methylation and strand breaks. DMH treatment resulted in exon-specific p53 hypomethylation, an effect that was prevented by folic acid supplementation [110]. Exon-specific strand breaks in the p53 tumor-suppressor gene occur in the colon of rats fed a folate-deficient diet but was not observed in the *APC* and *β-actin* genes or at the genomic level. After dietary folate supplementation at 4 times the rat basal requirement, p53 integrity increased above the degree observed with a basal diet. Folic acid deficiency may lead to functional dysregulation of the p53 tumor-suppressor gene, promoting carcinogenesis; on the other hand, folate supplementation above required amounts may inhibit this pathologic process. In this regard, Lashner et al [112] studied a cohort of 95 patients with long-standing ulcerative colitis and reported that folic acid supplementation may prevent p53 mutation. An involvement of folate on K-*ras* protooncogene mutation has also been suggested [113,114]. Thus, folate deficiency results in DNA hypomethylation and genomic instability that may be prevented by folate supplementation. In addition, folic acid dose dependently reduced the proliferation of colon cancer cell lines (Caco-2, HCT-116) induced by transforming growth factor-α, an effect that may involve the regulation of epidermal growth factor receptor (EGFR) tyrosine kinase [115].

Case-control studies investigating the association between folate and risk for colorectal cancer, in which folate intake was assessed by a food frequency questionnaire, gave varying results. Only weak associations were found in these studies [116–118], whereas some nutrients (vitamin C, carotenoid, fiber) had a strong correlation with folate. The folate-protective effect was greatly decreased [117,118] or disappeared [116] when these nutritional factors were taken into account. In addition, a negative association was reported for rectal and colon cancer in one study [116], whereas such an association was only observed for rectal cancer in another study [117]. In these case-control trials, the possibility of systematic bias, including imprecise estimates of energy and nutrient intake obtained from food frequency questionnaires, is of concern.

The influence of folate on the risk for neoplasia has been investigated in large prospective cohort studies. Decreased relative risk to develop colorectal adenoma with high versus low intake of folate was reported for women (relative risk [RR] = 0.66; 95% confidence interval [CI] = 0.46–0.95) and men (RR = 0.63; 95% CI = 0.41–0.98) in the Nurses' Health study and the Health Professional follow-up study, respectively [119]. In a subsequent study selecting subjects who underwent endoscopic procedures, folate intake was negatively associated with hyperplastic polyps of the distal colon and rectum in women (RR = 0.45; 95% CI = 0.28–0.74), whereas only a trend was observed for men (RR = 0.74; 95% CI = 0.49–1.11) [120].

In the National Health and Nutrition Epidemiologic follow-up study, decreased colon cancer risk was found only in men (RR = 0.40; 95% CI = 0.18–0.88) who consumed more than 249 μg/day folate [121]. On the other hand, Giovannucci et al [122] reported a decreased risk for colon cancer with folate intake above 400 μg/day in women in the Nurses' Health study, independent of vitamins A, C, D, and E. Use of multivitamins by most participants in the study group suggests that folate derived from multivitamin supplements may account for part of the beneficial effect. In contrast, folate intake derived from food, but not from supplements, was marginally negatively associated with recurrence of large bowel adenoma [123]. Whether the source of folate influences the risk for adenoma and CRC is unclear; the effect may depend on whether the neoplasia is cancerous.

Patients with longstanding ulcerative colitis frequently exhibit the expansion of proliferating cells to the crypt surface. In these patients, 3-month folate supplementation (15 mg/day) resulted in a reduction of rectal cell proliferation [124].

A limited number of animal studies have been performed. DMH-treated rats fed a diet deficient in folic acid exhibited enhanced neoplasia [125,126]. Folic acid supplementation, up to 8 mg/kg of diet, progressively reduced the incidence and average number of macroscopic tumors per rat [126]. No further benefit was obtained by supplementation beyond 8 mg/kg diet, a dose equal to 4 times the basal requirement. Song et al investigated the chemoprevention effect of folate on intestinal tumorigenesis in the $apc^{+/-}$ Msh2 $^{-/-}$ [127] and Min [128] mice. In these studies, the chemoprevention effects of folate were dependent on the dose and timing of administration and on the intestinal site of the lesion.

Chemoprevention by dietary fiber

The greatest limitation in the field of fiber research is the reluctance to recognize that fibers represent a complex mixture of components. The presence of complex mixtures of varying compositions may account for many of the discrepancies in the fiber effects reported in the literature. To understand the unique physiological effects of individual components, a better characterization of the fiber components themselves is still required.

Since the hypothesis of Burkitt [129,130] that dietary fiber may protect from CRC, the effects of dietary fiber on carcinogenesis has been extensively studied. This topic will only be summarized here because the large body of literature has recently been reviewed [131,132]. Particular attention has been given to the potential protective effect of wheat bran [133–138], which appears to inhibit colon tumorigenesis more consistently than oat bran, corn bran, rice bran, or soy bran [131,138].

The definition of the word *fiber* varies, based on different criteria, and is still a matter of debate [132,139]. The physiological definition remains today as it was initially—"the remnants of plant components that are resistant to hydrolyses by human alimentary enzymes" [140]. It includes cellulose, hemicellulose, lignin, gums, modified celluloses, mucilages, oligosaccharides, pectin, and associated minor substances such as wax, cutin, and suberin. Thus, the word encompasses a mixture of components that vary in their physico-chemical properties and, as a consequence, that differ in their biological effects. Animal studies indicate that the nature, amount, and form of fiber influence the outcome of the study. For instance, a diet supplemented with fermentable fiber was more efficacious in protecting against colon tumorigenesis than one of nonfermentable fiber in DMH-treated rats [141]. A decreased rate of aberrant crypt foci in AOM-treated rats was only observed with butyrate-producing fibers, such as type 2 resistant starch and fructooligosaccharides [142]. Although not assessed, changes in the colonic ecosystem, in addition to the fermentation of fiber, may account for the effect. The main mechanisms by which dietary fiber may mediate a beneficial health effect include stool bulking with concomitant dilution of toxic compounds, increased intestinal transit time, changes in the intestinal microflora, modifications of the colonic physico-chemical environment, and production of short-chain fatty acids [143]. Some of these mechanisms are supported by human studies. Recently, a link between insulin resistance and CRC has been suggested [144–146] and is supported by a recent case-control study [147]. Fiber-mediated decreased insulin resistance [148] may be another mechanism by which fiber exerts a preventive effect on CRC.

Overall, results from case-control studies generally support the protective effect of fiber or fiber-rich foods on CRC [132]. Prospective and intervention studies have yielded conflicting results, but because of limitations definitive conclusions are difficult to make [132]. Burkitt [129] associated the rarity of CRC in African populations with their high intake of fiber and their low intake of refined carbohydrates. This hypothesis has recently been challenged by Keefe et al [149], who reported that the rarity of CRC in Africans is associated with low animal product consumption and not with dietary fiber content. In this regard, a number of prospective and intervention studies reported fiber as having marginal or no effect on CRC risk [150–154]. Two recent studies reported the effect of lack of fiber on the recurrence of colorectal adenomas in humans [155,156]. It must be acknowledged that long-term high-fiber, low-fat intake is necessary for a beneficial outcome on a disease that may develop over a 10- to 20-year period. In addition, soluble fibers may be better for cancer prevention than nonsoluble fibers.

Although wheat bran is rich in fiber, other nutrients and phytochemicals, including phytic acid and phenolic components, may also protect against cancer [134,157]. Phytic acid derived from wheat bran or added exogenously to a low-fiber diet increased cell apoptosis and differentiation and favorably affected colon morphogenesis in AOM-treated rats [158]. The latter study relied on biomarker measurements to assess the effect of phytic acid. In this regard, the impact of wheat bran fractions was investigated on carcinogenesis in the same rat model [159]. Wheat bran fractions included wheat bran (WB), dephynitized wheat bran (WB-P), defatted wheat bran (WB-F), and dephynitized and defatted wheat bran (WB-PF). Compared with WB, WB-PF resulted in increased tumorigenicity, whereas removal of either phytic acid or lipids had no effect. Specific antitumor properties of bran oil was suggested by the inhibition of tumorigenesis and the inhibition of tumor activities and expression of iNOS and COX-2 in rats receiving WB-PF fortified with bran oil. These effects were not shared or altered by phytic acid. In contrast, WB was less effective in limiting the number of ACFs than butyrogenic fibers, such as type 3 resistant starch and short-chain fructo-oligosaccharides in AOM-treated rats [142].

The protective role of fiber against CRC is under careful evaluation. Nevertheless, taken together, the data from epidemiological, animal, and intervention studies support an inverse relationship between dietary fiber and CRC risk. The American Gastroenterological Association, in its medical position statement on the impact of fiber on colon cancer occurrence, recommends 30 to 35 g/day fiber from all fiber sources, including vegetables, fruits, and whole-grain cereals [160]. This amount of dietary fiber represents 3 to 3.5 times the mean dietary fiber intake of the United States adult population [132]. These recommendations are higher than the dietary guidelines (20–30 g/day fiber) of the American Cancer Society and the NCI. Consequently, fiber may need to be considered in the context of the whole diet, and it efficacy may be best considered in combination with a low-fat diet [137,161]. A role for other components derived from fiber-rich foods cannot be excluded. The type and source of dietary fiber may be important; the use of mixtures of fibers selected for their demonstrated protective efficacy may deserve attention [142]. The potential to combine prebiotics (nonabsorbable carbohydrate including inulin and oligofructose) with probiotics to enhance the beneficial effects of butyrogenic fibers should not be overlooked. Noteworthy is that high-fiber diets should remain palatable and not too bulky to ensure long-term compliance.

Chemoprevention by calcium

The role of the source or form of calcium in mediating biological effects is poorly understood, which may be a key determinant for biological activity. It is recognized that intestinal calcium absorption depends on habitual intake. It has been suggested that the bioavailability of the calcium source plays a role at low but not at high calcium intake (higher than 800 mg/day) [162]. Under conditions of adequate or high calcium intake, passive absorption in jejunum and ileum is the major absorptive process. This passive absorption of calcium is highly dependent on the solubility of the calcium. It has been reported, however, that at adequate or high calcium intake, the calcium available for solubilization may be sufficient to meet dietary needs [163]. Nevertheless, the bioavailability of micellar calcium phosphopeptide complex was higher than that of whey calcium, an effect attributed in part to the difference in intestinal solubility between the two calcium sources [164]. In addition, the bioavailability of calcium from calcium-rich mineral waters is comparable or better than from dairy products [165,166]. Considering the potential for low calcium intake, especially in the elderly population, it is important to obtain a readily available calcium source. Interestingly, the availability of calcium is not dependent on the particle size of the calcium source [167].

For at least two decades, calcium has been the focus of much interest as a potential chemoprevention agent. A protective effect of calcium for colon cancer is supported by in vitro and animal studies [168,169]. Induction of colonic cell apoptosis after calcium supplementation in mice [170] and rats [171] was recently reported. Calcium-associated decreased cell proliferation was observed in rats but not in mice. Findings from clinical trials investigating the effects of calcium on colorectal epithelial cell proliferation have been inconclusive [172–174]. Overall, colorectal epithelial cell proliferation is marginally decreased by calcium supplementation, but the distribution of proliferating cells within colonic crypts may normalize [172]. Low-fat dairy foods have been associated with decreased colonic cell proliferation [175]. A pilot study also indicated that such foods may positively modulate cell differentiation biomarkers of colorectal cancer risk [176]. It should be recognized that food-related studies do not address specifically the effect of calcium and that other components may provide beneficial effects.

In randomized, double-blind, placebo-controlled clinical trials, calcium carbonate supplementation resulted in a modest reduction of recurrent polyp formation that was independent of initial dietary fat and calcium intake [177] and in a moderate decrease in fecal bile acids and deoxycholic acid [178]. The underlying mechanisms involved in decreased colon cancer risk associated with calcium are unclear. The ability of calcium to bind bile acids, preventing their proliferative and carcinogenic effects, has been hypothesized as a possible mechanism [179].

The clinical evidence for calcium as a putative chemoprevention agent primarily relies on colorectal epithelial cell proliferation measurement. Although difficult to perform, long-term clinical trials investigating the effect of calcium, alone or in combination with vitamin D, on more reliable surrogate end-points such as adenomas or ACF are lacking. Noteworthy is the necessity to monitor possible micronutrient imbalances during calcium supplementation (ie, Ca/P).

Chemoprevention by vitamins

There are conflicting results on the potential chemoprevention properties of antioxidant vitamins such as vitamins A, C, and E. Available data do not provide a coherent body of evidence to support antioxidant vitamins as reducing the risk for colorectal cancer [131,180–182]. In addition, a recent randomized, placebo-controlled study of patients (34 treated, 43 placebo) with resected colorectal cancer Dukes stage B–C—taking combinations of calcium plus vitamin A, C, and E—failed to show differences in the cell kinetics of normal colonic mucosa, as assessed by proliferating cell nuclear antigen [183]. Vitamins may have some cancer protective effects. What's more, they do appear to be good markers of fruit and vegetable intake.

Prevention by phytochemicals

Phytochemicals are biologically active molecules derived from plants. More than 40 promising diet-derived agents or agent combinations have been clinically evaluated for their chemoprevention role against major types of cancer, among them colon, breast, prostate, and lung cancer [184]. Plant extracts containing a mixture of bioactive molecules have been prepared and tested for their anti-carcinogenic activity. Identification and purification of the active phytoprevention agents and subsequent mechanistic and pharmacologic studies have been the focus of much research. With the growing interest in herbal medicine and the use of plant extracts, a science-based approach to their evaluation and development has been advocated by the NCI [184]. Food-derived products such as extracts and concentrates and purified active biomolecules should be subjected to the same scientific scrutiny as drugs if they are to be used as therapy. In addition, to evaluate the safety and efficacy of their use, the compositional and functional properties of the extracts or pure phytochemicals and the technology used for their preparation must be monitored to ensure reproducibility. Knowledge of comparative effects, potency, and toxicity between the whole extracts and the identified purified active agents may be an asset to determine their specific conditions of use (ie, general healthy population versus at-risk patients).

Phytoprevention by curcumin

Curcumin, a natural plant phenolic commonly used as a yellow coloring and flavoring agent in food, is a major component of the rhizomes of *Curcuma* species. The chemoprevention properties of curcumin are supported by in vitro and animal experiments. The pharmacodynamics and pharmacokinetics of curcumin have not been extensively studied. Systemic bioavailability of curcumin in humans and rodents is low [185–188], indicating that some of the biological effects are mediated by curcumin metabolites. In this regard, transformation of curcumin during absorption from the intestine has been demonstrated [189]. Curcumin was recovered in feces from patients with colorectal cancer who were taking a standardized Curcuma extract supplement [188]; the gastrointestinal tract may thus be a good target for unmetabolized curcumin. In the latter dose-escalation pilot study, dose-limiting toxicity was not observed during the 4-month supplementation, with daily doses of Curcuma extract corresponding to up to 180 mg curcumin [188].

Various effects may account for the chemoprevention properties of curcumin, including decreased cell growth and proliferation and increased apoptosis [190,191]. The mechanisms by which curcumin may exert its effects include antioxidation, inhibition of enzymes involved in the mitogenic transduction signal pathways (c-*jun*, c-*fos*, c-*myc*, AP-1), decreased iNOS and protein kinase C, and inhibition of arachidonic acid metabolism such as COX-mediated prostaglandin synthesis.

Curcumin preferentially inhibited COX-2 over COX-1 in various cancer cell lines, including colon cancer cells [192]. In this regard, curcumin may exert COX-2–specific inhibition through the blockage of nuclear factor κB activation at the level of the NIK/IKKα/β signaling complex [193]. In human colonic epithelial cells, curcumin prevented phorbol ester-induced PGE_2 production, whereas curcumin metabolites showed only weak PGE_2 inhibitory activity [185]. In rats, the AOM-induced iNOS and COX-2 activities in colonic mucosa were reduced by curcumin supplementation [194], as was PGE_2 production [195].

In C57BL/6J $^-$ Min/$^+$ mice, curcumin inhibited the tumor formation associated with increased enterocyte apoptosis and proliferation [196]. Suppressed APC-associated intestinal carcinogenesis may also be the result of decreased expression of the oncogenic β-catenin [196]. The increased enterocyte proliferation reported by Mahmoud et al [196] is in contrast to reports indicating curcumin-mediated inhibition of cell proliferation through cell-cycle arrest in G2-M phase [40,190,197]. Although results were similar for the two human cancer cell lines investigated (HT-29, HCT-15), differences in their ability to produce prostaglandins indicated that the inhibition of cell proliferation does occur independently of prostaglandin inhibition [197]. Noteworthy, curcumin induced apoptosis in immortalized and transformed cells [198]. Curcumin inhibited the incidence and multiplicity of adenomas in AOM-treated rats [195,199] and mice [200] in a dose-dependent manner [199]. In addition, tumor size was reduced after curcumin supplementation [195,200]. Colonic ACF formation was 45% lower in AOM-treated rats receiving curcumin supplement than in AOM-treated control rats [194]. In addition, the chemoprevention activity of curcumin is observed at all stages of tumorigenesis, as indicated in AOM-treated rats fed curcumin before, during, and after carcinogen treatment or only during the promotion/progression phase [201]. Supplementation with tetrahydrocurcumin, but not curcumin, of DMH-treated mice resulted in a decreased number of ACFs and aberrant crypts per mouse, which was paralleled by a decreased proliferation of colonic crypt epithelial cells [202]. Thus, the available preclinical data provide support for curcumin as a candidate for colon cancer chemoprevention. Human clinical trials are urgently needed to confirm results from in vitro and animal studies.

Phytoprevention by tea

Much interest has been focused on tea as a chemoprevention agent against cancer [203–206]. Green tea and black tea contain catechin polyphenol compounds. The major catechins in green tea are epigallocatechin gallate (EGCG), epigallocatechin (EGC), epicatechin gallate (ECG), and epicatechin (EC), with EGCG representing the most abundant catechin. Theaflavin (TF-1), theaflavin-3-monogallate (TF-2), and theaflavin-3,3′-digallate (TF-3) are major black tea polyphenols.

Population studies investigating tea consumption based on dietary questionnaire and risk for colorectal cancer showed varying results. In five Asian studies, the association between tea consumption and relative risk for colon cancer was reported to be negative in three and positive in one, whereas no association was found in another study [207]. For rectal cancers, the association was positive in two studies, negative in one study, and absent in one study [207]. No association between black tea consumption and risk for colorectal cancer was observed in the Netherlands Cohort Study on Diet and Cancer [208]. Similarly, Baron et al [209] found no association between the intake of tea and the risk for recurrent colorectal adenoma. A Finnish cohort clinical trial reported a positive association for colon cancer that depended on the numbers of cups of tea consumed; no such association was observed for rectal cancer [210]. On the other hand, decreased risk was reported for rectal cancer in a comparative case-control study [211]. The discrepancies among these reports reflect some of the limitations of epidemiologic studies using dietary surveys.

In vitro and animal studies have been performed to assess more precisely the effects and mechanisms of action of tea and its components revealing multiple mechanisms. Effects of the various tea catechins (EGCG, ECG, EGC, EC) on athymic Balb/c nude mice inoculated with HT29 human colon cancer cells were investigated [212]. EGCG treatment inhibited tumor growth, microvessel density, and tumor cell proliferation. Tumor and endothelial cell apoptosis were increased. In vitro studies with this cell line suggest that EGCG, but not the other catechins, may exert part of the anticancer effect through an inhibition of vascular endothelial growth factor-mediated angiogenesis [212]. EGCG and EGC inhibited the growth of cancerous human colonic cells (HT-29, HCT116, Lovo), whereas ECG and EC were less effective or had no effect [213–215]. Apoptosis was also induced in cells treated with EGCG or EGC [213]. EGCG inhibited Caco-2 colon cell growth, but only a marginal effect was observed on the normal cell counterpart [216]. Similar differential effects on cell growth were observed with TF-2, a polyphenol found primarily in black tea [217]. This effect was TF-2 specific because no such differential growth was observed with either TF-1 or TF-3.

In 2-amino-1-methyl-6-phenyimidazo[4,5b]pyridine (PhIP)–induced tumorigenesis in rats, green tea and black tea exhibited chemoprevention properties as indicated by the inhibition of PhIP-DNA adducts; however, the effects were site specific and time dependent [218]. Green tea and black tea also inhibited ACF formation in 2-amino-3-methylimidazo[4,5-f]quinoline (IQ)–induced ACFs and tumors [219]. Green tea catechins did not inhibit the incidence or multiplicity of colon tumors in carcinogen-treated rats [220]. Surprisingly, animals fed 0.1% green tea catechins exhibited decreased colon adenomas, but carcinomas were increased. In AOM-treated rats, green tea or black tea solutions provided before or during various stages of carcinogenesis did not result in beneficial outcomes for colon cancer [221,222]. An absence of effect was also observed with ECGC [221]. Under certain conditions, higher doses of tea solutions adversely affected the end-point measurements. Although tea may affect various metabolic sites, it is suggested that part of these results are accounted for by a lack of effect of tea on cytochrome P4502E1, an enzyme system required for metabolic activation of AOM [221,222]. In contrast, crude green tea extract, provided in the drinking water of AOM-treated rats after the initiation phase of colon carcinogenesis, resulted in a decrease in the number of aberrant crypts and crypt multiplicity relative to control animals [223]. COX-2 may be involved in this positive outcome, as indicated by the selective decrease in COX-2 but not COX-1 activity in colonic tissue. In this regard, TF-2 and, to a lesser extent, EGCG also selectively inhibited *COX-2* gene expression in cell culture studies [217]. A transiently decreased level of PGE_2 in rectal mucosa of healthy volunteers after the administration of a single dose of green tea was also reported [224]. In addition to COX-2 inhibition, catechins may act by inducing the expression of uridine-5'-diphosphate–glucuronyl transferase, inhibition of NADPH-cyto-chrome P450 reductase, or scavenging of reactive intermediates [219]. EGCG-induced H_2O_2 production may also mediate apoptosis [225].

Discrepancies in evaluating tea as a chemoprevention agent may be accounted for by differences in the experimental model and tea preparations used. In this regard, standardization for reporting the results with reference to polyphenol content of the various tea preparations used has been proposed by the Inter-national Life Science Institute. Profiles of bioactive molecule content between green and black teas and among tea extracts may vary greatly. Differences in catechin chemoprevention efficacy may also be partly accounted for by structural differences. Number and steric disposition of hydroxyl groups within poly-phenols may be important factors for biological activities such as the inhibition of matrix metalloproteinase, association with tumor invasion and metastasis, and induction of apoptosis [226].

Inconsistent and limited epidemiologic and clinical data on the relationship between tea and colorectal cancer, together with data derived from laboratory studies, suggest that purified tea components, alone or in combination, may be more suitable than tea or tea extracts as chemoprevention agents. In contrast to cases in which putative purified micronutrients did not support the chemo-prevention effect observed with whole food, much of the chemoprevention effects of green tea appear to be mediated by EGCG and, to a lesser extent, EGC. Preclinical and clinical trials are warranted to further assess the chemo-prevention potential of tea components, especially EGCG and EGC.

Other chemoprevention agents

There is a wide array of chemoprevention agents under evaluation; however, only a few have the potential for reaching clinical trial testing. In addition to those reviewed, bioactive molecules of interest for colon cancer prevention include lycopene, derived from tomato; rumenic acid (referred to conjugated linoleic acid) and butyrate, found in milk and dairy products; resveratrol, a potent antioxidant extracted from grapes; and soy and its components, such as genistein and daidzein.

Dietary intervention

It is well recognized that dietary habits have an important impact on cancer risk and incidence. It has been suggested that 35% to 50% of cancer could be prevented by proper nutrition. On the other hand, analyses of prospective studies suggest that the effect of fat on colorectal cancer may not be as important as previously thought; similarly, recent prospective studies indicate that the association with fruits and vegetables may have been overestimated [227]. Based on epidemiologic, clinical, and animal studies, a balanced diet rich in fruits and vegetables with an adequate supply of grain and cereals and a limited amount of meat, especially red meat, is generally recommended [228,229]. On an ingredient basis, this translates to decreased total and saturated fat intake and increased consumption of dietary fiber, together with vitamins and specific minerals. It also includes the nonnutrient phytochemicals. A number of studies using the pure, isolated bioactive molecules (beta-carotene, specific fibers) failed to demonstrate a beneficial clinical outcome, suggesting that the combination of active biomolecules within the whole diet and the complex interactions that may occur among them are important for the prevention of chronic disease. The general population may thus benefit from dietary intervention to decrease cancer risk, which in turn may significantly reduce healthcare costs.

Combination therapy

From the data available, it appears that the use of a single agent does not eradicate all tumors. Combination therapy is now considered a more efficient chemoprevention approach than monotherapy to modulate carcinogenesis through additive or synergistic effects. In this regard, the growth inhibition and apoptotic effects of sulindac in two human colon cancer cell lines, SW-480 and HT-29, were enhanced by the coadministration of S-allylmercaptocysteine, a water-soluble derivative of garlic [230]. Whereas sulindac inhibited cell-cycle progression from G1 to S, S-allylmercaptocysteine resulted in an accumulation of cells in G_2-M. Caco-2 cells and K-ras–transfected Caco-2 cells treated with sulindac sulfide or sulindac sulfone exhibited reduced viability through the induction of apoptosis [231]. An apoptosis-independent decrease in cell viability by DMFO occurred in K-ras oncogene-activated Caco-2 cells but not in parental cells. The sequential treatment of DMFO and either of the sulindac metabolites resulted in an additive effect on cell viability.

In azoxymethane-treated rats, the incidence (percentage of animals with tumors) and the multiplicity (number of tumors/rat) of colon adenocarcinoma were inhibited by piroxicam or DMFO in comparison with control animals [232,233].

An enhanced anticarcinogenic effect was obtained by the coadministration of piroxicam and DMFO than by either agent alone. Piroxicam or DMFO alone had no inhibitory effect on colon adenoma incidence and multiplicity, whereas colon adenomas were decreased by the combination of these compounds [233]. Similar effects were observed in the Min mouse model with a number of mice completely free of adenoma [77]. In vivo growth of human colonic adenocarcinoma cells (HT-29) in athymic mice was synergistically reduced by the intraperitoneal administration of all-*trans* retinoic acid plus oral DMFO treatment [234]. Two large clinical trials evaluating coronary events indicated that Lovastatin, a 3-hydroxy-3-methylglutary-coenzyme A (HMG-CoA) reductase inhibitor, reduced new cases of colon cancer. Subsequently, in AOM-treated rats, the inhibition of total number of ACFs by sulindac was enhanced by lovastatin [235].

Neoplasia of the colon, lung, and breast is frequently associated with dysregulation in the EGFR signaling pathway, suggesting inhibitors of EGFR-kinase as potential chemoprevention agents [236]. Recently, polyp formation in the APC$^{Min/+}$ mice, a murine model of human FAP, was inhibited more than 95% by the coadministration of an EGFR-kinase inhibitor and an NSAID, EKB-569 (20 mg/kg/mouse/day) and sulindac (5 mg/kg/mouse/day), respectively [237]. The effect of EKB-569 alone accounted for an 85% reduction in intestinal neoplasia compared with findings in control animals, whereas sulindac had no effect at the dose tested. Of interest is the absence of polyps in nearly half the mice receiving the combinatorial treatment. Convergence and interactions between the cyclooxygenases and EGFR signaling pathways in relation to the combinatorial approach to cancer prevention have been discussed elsewhere [238]. Although not yet tested, the combination of COX-2 and iNOS inhibitors may be an attractive strategy. As for COX-2, NOS is frequently overexpressed in colon cancers of humans and rats. AOM-induced ACF in rats was inhibited by the NOS inhibitor L-NG-nitroarginine methylester [79].

The NCI is sponsoring a phase 2b randomized placebo control clinical trial investigating the efficacy of combined sulindac and eflornithine (DMFO) on the prevention of colorectal cancer development in patients with previously resected colorectal adenoma. Unfortunately, the possible better efficacy of combination therapy will not be assessed because groups treated with either drug alone are not included. In vitro and animal study findings reported in this chapter support the concept of better efficacy of combination therapy through a mechanistic approach. A combinatorial strategy may provide for enhanced chemoprevention efficacy or may allow the administration of lower, less toxic doses of the respective drugs. The usefulness of this strategy must be confirmed in adequately designed clinical trials.

Summary

Considering the various stages of carcinogenesis and the numerous tumor types and available chemoprevention agents, knowledge of the etiology and the type of cancer to be treated, or possibly prevented, and understanding of the mechanisms by which agents exert their chemoprevention benefits may provide for improved strategy in designing therapeutic regimens. Because cancer usually develops over a 10- to 20-year period, it may be necessary for some agents to be provided before or early in the initiation steps of carcinogenesis to have beneficial effects. On the other hand, some agents may be more suitable for CRC prevention if provided at a later stage of carcinogenesis.

Gene array, genomics, and proteomics are useful tools in advancing our understanding of the molecular events involved in carcinogenesis and in identifying markers of risk and surrogate end-points for colorectal cancer progression. These techniques may also serve for screening, identifying, and providing treatment targets for high-risk patient populations. Treatment could be developed depending on a patient's individual needs and genomic tumor profile. Clinical markers and surrogate end-points should be considered, together with molecular measurements, to more accurately assess risk.

NSAIDs and COXIBs are clinically recognized as chemoprevention agents, and clinical trials evaluating their efficacy are ongoing. Treatment protocols, including dose and timing, remain to be determined, however. DFMO may best be used in combination with other chemoprevention agents. Dietary fiber and calcium supplements, as part of an overall low-fat diet, may decrease CRC risk. Long-term compliance with this regimen may be necessary to effect a beneficial outcome. Folate holds promise but needs further investigation, especially because its beneficial effects may depend on cancer type. Phytochemicals have been identified as strong candidates for use as agents to prevent colorectal cancer in cell culture and in rodent models of carcinogenesis. Their potential as chemoprevention agents must be demonstrated in clinical trials. In vitro and animal studies indicate that combination therapy may be a promising strategy over the monotherapy approach; clinical trials addressing the safety and efficacy of some combinations (DFMO/sulindac, fiber/calcium) are underway.

The gastrointestinal tract and other organs are constantly exposed to a mixture of potentially toxic compounds and molecules considered favorable to health. Homeostasis between stress-mediated by toxic compounds and defensive mechanisms, is key for the maintenance of health and the prevention of disease. Whereas aggressive pharmacologic treatment may be necessary for patients at high risk for cancer, dietary supplements may be useful for populations at normal risk. The message for cancer prevention in the general population may well remain: keep a balanced healthy diet, eating a variety from all food groups, as part of a healthy lifestyle that includes moderate exercise.

Acknowledgments

The authors thank Dr. E. Offord and Dr. Bruce German for their editing and valuable comments during the preparation of this manuscript.

References

[1] Crucitti F, Sofo L, Doglietto GB, et al. Prognostic factors in colorectal cancer: current status and new trends. J Surg Oncol 1991;2:76–82.
[2] Dove-Edwin I, Thomas HJ. Review article: the prevention of colorectal cancer. Aliment Pharmacol Ther 2001;15:323–36.
[3] Bedi A, Pasricha PJ, Akhtar AJ, et al. Inhibition of apoptosis during development of colorectal cancer. Cancer Res 1995;55:1811–6.
[4] Boland CR. The biology of colorectal cancer: implications for pretreatment and follow-up management. Cancer 1993;71:4180–6.
[5] Fearon ER. Molecular genetic studies of the adenoma-carcinoma sequence. Adv Intern Med 1994;39:123–47.
[6] Rustgi AK. Molecular genetics and colorectal cancer. Gastroenterology 1993;104:1223–5.
[7] Eshleman JR, Markowitz SD. Microsatellite instability in inherited and sporadic neoplasms. Curr Opin Oncol 1995;7:83–9.
[8] Thibodeau SN, Bren G, Schaid D. Microsatellite instability in cancer of the proximal colon. Science 1993;260:816–9.
[9] Marra G, Boland CR. Hereditary nonpolyposis colorectal cancer: the syndrome, the genes, and historical perspectives. J Natl Cancer Inst 1995;87:1114–25.
[10] Peltomaki P, Vasen HF. Mutations predisposing to hereditary nonpolyposis colorectal cancer: database and results of a collaborative study. The International Collaborative Group on Hereditary Nonpolyposis Colorectal Cancer. Gastroenterology 1997;113:1146–58.
[11] Karnes WE Jr, Shattuck-Brandt R, Burgart LJ, et al. Reduced COX-2 protein in colorectal cancer with defective mismatch repair. Cancer Res 1998;58:5473–7.
[12] Karnes WE Jr. Implications of low COX-2 expression in colorectal neoplasms with defective DNA mismatch repair. J Cell Biochem 2000;34:S23–7.
[13] Smalley W, Ray WA, Daugherty J, et al. Use of nonsteroidal anti-inflammatory drugs and incidence of colorectal cancer: a population-based study. Arch Intern Med 1999;159:161–6.
[14] Cruz-Correa MR, Hylind LM, Romans KE, et al. Long-term treatment with sulindac in familial adenomatous polyposis: a prospective cohort study. In: Programs and Abstracts of the Digestive Disease Week Conference, Atlanta GA: DDW Abstracts—Sanders; 2001. p. 265–6.
[15] Giardiello FM, Spannhake EW, DuBois RN, et al. Prostaglandin levels in human colorectal mucosa: effects of sulindac in patients with familial adenomatous polyposis. Dig Dis Sci 1998;43:311–6.
[16] Li H, Schut HA, Conran P, et al. Prevention by aspirin and its combination with alpha-difluoromethylornithine of azoxymethane-induced tumors, aberrant crypt foci and prostaglandin E_2 levels in rat colon. Carcinogenesis 1999;20:425–30.
[17] Baron JA. Intermediate effect markers for colorectal cancer. IARC Sci Publ 2001;154:113–29.
[18] Einspahr JG, Alberts DS, Gapstur SM, et al. Surrogate end-point biomarkers as measures of colon cancer risk and their use in cancer chemoprevention trials. Cancer Epidemiol Biomarkers Prev 1997;6:37–48.
[19] Hill MJ. Molecular and clinical risk markers in colon cancer trials. Eur J Cancer 2000;36:1288–91.
[20] Kelloff GJ, Boone CW, Crowell JA, et al. Risk biomarkers and current strategies for cancer chemoprevention. J Cell Biochem 1996;25:1–14.
[21] Lipkin M. Summary of recommendations for colonic biomarker studies of candidate chemopreventive compounds in phase II clinical trials. J Cell Biochem 1994;19(suppl):94–8.
[22] Schatzkin A, Freedman LS, Dorgan J, et al. Surrogate end points in cancer research: a critique. Cancer Epidemiol Biomarkers Prev 1996;5:947–53.
[23] Syngal S, Clarke G, Bandipalliam P. Potential roles of genetic biomarkers in colorectal cancer chemoprevention. J Cell Biochem 2000;34:28–34.
[24] Lippman SM, Lee JJ, Sabichi AL. Cancer chemoprevention: progress and promise. J Natl Cancer Inst 1998;90:1514–28.

[25] Wargovich MJ, Chen CD, Jimenez A, et al. Aberrant crypts as a biomarker for colon cancer: evaluation of potential chemopreventive agents in the rat. Cancer Epidemiol Biomarkers Prev 1996;5:355–60.
[26] Pereira MA. Prevention of colon cancer and modulation of aberrant crypt foci, cell proliferation, and apoptosis by retinoids and NSAIDs. Adv Exp Med Biol 1999;470:55–63.
[27] Samaha HS, Kelloff GJ, Steele V, et al. Modulation of apoptosis by sulindac, curcumin, phenylethyl-3-methylcaffeate, and 6-phenylhexyl isothiocyanate: apoptotic index as a biomarker in colon cancer chemoprevention and promotion. Cancer Res 1997;57:1301–5.
[28] Giardiello FM, Hamilton SR, Hylind LM, et al. Ornithine decarboxylase and polyamines in familial adenomatous polyposis. Cancer Res 1997;57:199–201.
[29] Hixson LJ, Emerson SS, Shassetz LR, et al. Sources of variability in estimating ornithine decarboxylase activity and polyamine contents in human colorectal mucosa. Cancer Epidemiol Biomarkers Prev 1994;3:317–23.
[30] Wang W, Liu LQ, Higuchi CM. Mucosal polyamine measurements and colorectal cancer risk. J Cell Biochem 1996;63:252–7.
[31] Barnes CJ, Hamby-Mason RL, Hardman WE, et al. Effect of aspirin on prostaglandin E_2 formation and transforming growth factor alpha expression in human rectal mucosa from individuals with a history of adenomatous polyps of the colon. Cancer Epidemiol Biomarkers Prev 1999;8:311–5.
[32] Chow HH, Earnest DL, Clark D, et al. Effect of subacute ibuprofen dosing on rectal mucosal prostaglandin E_2 levels in healthy subjects with a history of resected polyps. Cancer Epidemiol Biomarkers Prev 2000;9:351–6.
[33] Szarka CE, Pfeiffer GR, Hum ST, et al. Glutathione S-transferase activity and glutathione S-transferase mu expression in subjects with risk for colorectal cancer. Cancer Res 1995;55:2789–93.
[34] Lev Z, Kislitsin D, Rennert G, et al. Utilization of K-ras mutations identified in stool DNA for the early detection of colorectal cancer. J Cell Biochem 2000;34:35–9.
[35] Traverso G, Shuber A, Levin B, et al. Detection of APC mutations in fecal DNA from patients with colorectal tumors. N Engl J Med 2002;346:311–20.
[36] Kim YI, Baik HW, Fawaz K, et al. Effects of folate supplementation on two provisional molecular markers of colon cancer: a prospective, randomized trial. Am J Gastroenterol 2001;96:184–95.
[37] Pool-Zobel BL, Abrahamse SL, Collins AR, et al. Analysis of DNA strand breaks, oxidized bases, and glutathione S-transferase P1 in human colon cells from biopsies. Cancer Epidemiol Biomarkers Prev 1999;8:609–14.
[38] Cunningham C, Dunlop MG. Genetics of colorectal cancer. Br Med Bull 1994;50:640–55.
[39] Lynch HT, Lynch JF. Genetics of colonic cancer. Digestion 1998;59:481–92.
[40] Mariadason JM, Corner GA, Augenlicht LH. Genetic reprogramming in pathways of colonic cell maturation induced by short chain fatty acids: comparison with trichostatin A, sulindac, and curcumin and implications for chemoprevention of colon cancer. Cancer Res 2000;60:4561–72.
[41] Arber N, DuBois RN. Nonsteroidal anti-inflammatory drugs and prevention of colorectal cancer. Curr Gastroenterol Rep 1999;1:441–8.
[42] DuBois RN, Giardiello FM, Smalley WE. Nonsteroidal anti-inflammatory drugs, eicosanoids, and colorectal cancer prevention. Gastroenterol Clin North Am 1996;25:773–91.
[43] Reddy BS. The Fourth DeWitt S. Goodman lecture: novel approaches to the prevention of colon cancer by nutritional manipulation and chemoprevention. Cancer Epidemiol Biomarkers Prev 2000;9:239–47.
[44] Kudo T, Narisawa T, Abo S. Antitumor activity of indomethacin on methylazoxymethanol-induced large bowel tumors in rats. Gann 1980;71:260–4.
[45] Narisawa T, Sato M, Sano M, et al. Inhibition of development of methylnitrosourea-induced rat colonic tumors by peroral administration of indomethacin. Gann 1982;73:377–81.
[46] Pollard M, Luckert PH. Treatment of chemically-induced intestinal cancers with indomethacin. Proc Soc Exp Biol Med 1981;167:161–4.

[47] Pollard M, Luckert PH. Effect of piroxicam on primary intestinal tumors induced in rats by N-methylnitrosourea. Cancer Lett 1984;25:117–21.

[48] Jacoby RF, Marshall DJ, Newton MA, et al. Chemoprevention of spontaneous intestinal adenomas in the Apc Min mouse model by the nonsteroidal anti-inflammatory drug piroxicam. Cancer Res 1996;56:710–4.

[49] Beazer-Barclay Y, Levy DB, Moser AR, et al. Sulindac suppresses tumorigenesis in the Min mouse. Carcinogenesis 1996;17:1757–60.

[50] Boolbol SK, Dannenberg AJ, Chadburn A, et al. Cyclooxygenase-2 overexpression and tumor formation are blocked by sulindac in a murine model of familial adenomatous polyposis. Cancer Res 1996;56:2556–60.

[51] Barnes CJ, Lee M. Chemoprevention of spontaneous intestinal adenomas in the adenomatous polyposis coli Min mouse model with aspirin. Gastroenterology 1998;114:873–7.

[52] Waddell WR, Loughry RW. Sulindac for polyposis of the colon. J Surg Oncol 1983;24:83–7.

[53] Waddell WR, Ganser GF, Cerise EJ, et al. Sulindac for polyposis of the colon. Am J Surg 1989; 157:175–9.

[54] Giardiello FM, Hamilton SR, Krush AJ, et al. Treatment of colonic and rectal adenomas with sulindac in familial adenomatous polyposis. N Engl J Med 1993;328:1313–6.

[55] Labayle D, Fischer D, Vielh P, et al. Sulindac causes regression of rectal polyps in familial adenomatous polyposis. Gastroenterology 1991;101:635–9.

[56] Nugent KP, Farmer KC, Spigelman AD, et al. Randomized controlled trial of the effect of sulindac on duodenal and rectal polyposis and cell proliferation in patients with familial adenomatous polyposis. Br J Surg 1993;80:1618–9.

[57] Strul H, Arber N. Non-steroidal anti-inflammatory drugs and selective apoptotic anti-neoplastic drugs in the prevention of colorectal cancer: the role of super aspirins. Isr Med Assoc J 2000;2: 695–702.

[58] Marnett LJ. Aspirin and the potential role of prostaglandins in colon cancer. Cancer Res 1992; 52:5575–89.

[59] Chapple KS, Cartwright EJ, Hawcroft G, et al. Localization of cyclooxygenase-2 in human sporadic colorectal adenomas. Am J Pathol 2000;156:545–53.

[60] Eberhart CE, Coffey RJ, Radhika A, et al. Up-regulation of cyclooxygenase 2 gene expression in human colorectal adenomas and adenocarcinomas. Gastroenterology 1994;107:1183–8.

[61] Kargman SL, Neill GP, Vickers PJ, et al. Expression of prostaglandin G/H synthase-1 and -2 protein in human colon cancer. Cancer Res 1995;55:2556–9.

[62] Kutchera W, Jones DA, Matsunami N, et al. Prostaglandin H synthase 2 is expressed abnormally in human colon cancer: evidence for a transcriptional effect. Proc Natl Acad Sci U S A 1996;93:4816–20.

[63] Sano H, Kawahito Y, Wilder RL, et al. Expression of cyclooxygenase-1 and -2 in human colorectal cancer. Cancer Res 1995;55:3785–9.

[64] Shao J, Sheng H, Aramandla R, et al. Coordinate regulation of cyclooxygenase-2 and TGF-β1 in replication error-positive colon cancer and azoxymethane-induced rat colonic tumors. Carcinogenesis 1999;20:185–91.

[65] Agoff SN, Brentnall TA, Crispin DA, et al. The role of cyclooxygenase 2 in ulcerative colitis-associated neoplasia. Am J Pathol 2000;157:737–45.

[66] Shattuck-Brandt RL, Varilek GW, Radhika A, et al. Cyclooxygenase 2 expression is increased in the stroma of colon carcinomas from IL-10(−/−) mice. Gastroenterology 2000;118: 337–45.

[67] Katori M, Majima M. Cyclooxygenase-2: its rich diversity of roles and possible application of its selective inhibitors. Inflamm Res 2000;49:367–92.

[68] Smith W, Elmer PJ, Tharp TM, et al. Increasing vegetable and fruit intake: randomized intervention and monitoring in an at-risk population. Cancer Epidemiol Biomarkers Prev 2000;9: 307–17.

[69] Narumiya S, Sugimoto Y, Ushikubi F. Prostanoid receptors: structures, properties, and functions. Physiol Rev 1999;79:1193–226.

[70] Gupta R, DuBois RN. Colorectal cancer prevention and treatment by inhibition of cyclooxy-genase-2. Nature Rev Cancer 2001;1:11–21.

[71] Krause W, DuBois RN. Eicosanoids and the large intestine. Prostaglandins Other Lipid Mediat 2000;61:145–61.

[72] Dempke W, Rie C, Grothey A, et al. Cyclooxygenase-2: a novel target for cancer chemo-therapy? J Cancer Res Clin Oncol 2001;127:411–7.

[73] Turini ME, DuBois RN. Cyclooxygenase-2: a therapeutic target. Annu Rev Med 2002;53:35–57.

[74] Kawamori T, Rao CV, Seibert K, et al. Chemopreventive activity of celecoxib, a specific cyclooxygenase-2 inhibitor, against colon carcinogenesis. Cancer Res 1998;58:409–12.

[75] Yoshimi N, Shimizu M, Matsunaga K, et al. Chemopreventive effect of N- (2-cyclohexyloxy-4-nitrophenyl)methane sulfonamide (NS-398), a selective cyclooxygenase-2 inhibitor, in rat colon carcinogenesis induced by azoxymethane. Jpn J Cancer Res 1999;90:406–12.

[76] Reddy BS, Hirose Y, Lubet R, et al. Chemoprevention of colon cancer by specific cyclo-oxygenase-2 inhibitor, celecoxib, administered during different stages of carcinogenesis. Can-cer Res 2000;60:293–7.

[77] Jacoby RF, Cole CE, Tutsch K, et al. Chemopreventive efficacy of combined piroxicam and difluoromethylornithine treatment of Apc mutant Min mouse adenomas, and selective toxicity against Apc mutant embryos. Cancer Res 2000;60:1864–70.

[78] Oshima M, Murai N, Kargman S, et al. Chemoprevention of intestinal polyposis in the Apcdelta716 mouse by rofecoxib, a specific cyclooxygenase-2 inhibitor. Cancer Res 2001; 61:1733–40.

[79] Watanabe K, Kawamori T, Nakatsugi S, et al. COX-2 and iNOS, good targets for chemo-prevention of colon cancer. Biofactors 2000;12:129–33.

[80] Ritland SR, Leighton JA, Hirsch RE, et al. Evaluation of 5-aminosalicylic acid (5-ASA) for cancer chemoprevention: lack of efficacy against nascent adenomatous polyps in the Apc(Min) mouse. Clin Cancer Res 1999;5:855–63.

[81] Bus PJ, Nagtegaal ID, Verspaget HW, et al. Mesalazine-induced apoptosis of colorectal cancer: on the verge of a new chemopreventive era? Aliment Pharmacol Ther 1999;13:1397–402.

[82] Williams CS, Smalley W, DuBois RN. Aspirin use and potential mechanisms for colorectal cancer prevention. J Clin Invest 1997;100:1325–9.

[83] Chan TA, Morin PJ, Vogelstein B, et al. Mechanisms underlying nonsteroidal antiinflammatory drug-mediated apoptosis. Proc Natl Acad Sci U S A 1998;95:681–6.

[84] Rigas B, Shiff SJ. Is inhibition of cyclooxygenase required for the chemopreventive effect of NSAIDs in colon cancer? A model reconciling the current contradiction. Med Hypotheses 2000;54:210–5.

[85] Marx J. Cancer research: anti-inflammatories inhibit cancer growth–but how? Science 2001; 291:581–2.

[86] Williams CS, Watson AJ, Sheng H, et al. Celecoxib prevents tumor growth *in vivo* without toxicity to normal gut: lack of correlation between *in vitro* and *in vivo* models. Cancer Res 2000; 60:6045–51.

[87] Singh AK, Trotman BW. Use and safety of aspirin in the chemoprevention of colorectal cancer. J Assoc Acad Minor Phys 1998;9:40–4.

[88] Barnes CJ, Lee M. Determination of an optimal dosing regimen for aspirin chemoprevention of 1,2-dimethylhydrazine-induced colon tumours in rats. Br J Cancer 1999;79:1646–50.

[89] Meyskens FL, Gerner EW. Development of difluoromethylornithine (DFMO) as a chemopre-vention agent. Clin Cancer Res 1999;5:945–51.

[90] Ray RM, McCormack SA, Johnson LR. Polyamine depletion arrests growth of IEC-6 and Caco-2 cells by different mechanisms. Am J Physiol 2001;281:G37–43.

[91] Li L, Rao JN, Guo X, et al. Polyamine depletion stabilizes p53 resulting in inhibition of normal intestinal epithelial cell proliferation. Am J Physiol 2001;281:C941–53.

[92] Shore L, McLean P, Gilmour SK, et al. Polyamines regulate gap junction communication in connexin 43-expressing cells. Biochem J 2001;357:489–95.

[93] Steele VE, Moon RC, Lubet RA, et al. Preclinical efficacy evaluation of potential chemo-

preventive agents in animal carcinogenesis models: methods and results from the NCI Chemo-prevention Drug Development Program. J Cell Biochem 1994;20:32–54.

[94] La V, Negri E, Franceschi S, et al. Tea consumption and cancer risk. Nutr Cancer 1992;17:27–31.

[95] Meyskens FL, Emerson SS, Pelot D, et al. Dose de-escalation chemoprevention trial of alpha-difluoromethylornithine in patients with colon polyps. J Natl Cancer Inst 1994;86: 1122–30.

[96] Meyskens FL, Gerner EW, Emerson S, et al. Effect of alpha-difluoromethylornithine on rectal mucosal levels of polyamines in a randomized, double-blinded trial for colon cancer prevention. J Natl Cancer Inst 1998;90:1212–8.

[97] Love RR, Jacoby R, Newton MA, et al. A randomized, placebo-controlled trial of low-dose alpha-difluoromethylornithine in individuals at risk for colorectal cancer. Cancer Epidemiol Biomarkers Prev 1998;7:989–92.

[98] Pasic TR, Heisey D, Love RR. Alpha-difluoromethylornithine ototoxicity. Chemoprevention clinical trial results. Arch Otolaryngol Head Neck Surg 1997;123:1281–6.

[99] Selhub J, D'Angelo A. Relationship between homocysteine and thrombotic disease. Am J Med Sci 1998;316:129–41.

[100] Shields DC, Kirke PN, Mills JL, et al. The "thermolabile" variant of methylenetetrahydrofolate reductase and neural tube defects: an evaluation of genetic risk and the relative importance of the genotypes of the embryo and the mother. Am J Hum Genet 1999;64:1045–55.

[101] Kim Y. Folate and carcinogenesis: evidence, mechanisms, and implications. J Nutr Biochem 1999;10:66–88.

[102] Ryan BM, Weir DG. Relevance of folate metabolism in the pathogenesis of colorectal cancer. J Lab Clin Med 2001;138:164–76.

[103] Bailey LB, Mahan CS, Dimperio D. Folacin and iron status in low-income pregnant adolescents and mature women. Am J Clin Nutr 1980;33:1997–2001.

[104] Bailey LB, Wagner PA, Christakis GJ, et al. Folacin and iron status and hematological findings in predominately black elderly persons from urban low-income households. Am J Clin Nutr 1979;32:2346–53.

[105] Bailey LB, Wagner PA, Davis CG, et al. Food frequency related to folacin status in adolescents. J Am Diet Assoc 1984;84:801–4.

[106] Subar AF, Block G, James LD. Folate intake and food sources in the U.S. population. Am J Clin Nutr 1989;50:508–16.

[107] Selhub J, Jacques PF, Wilson PW, et al. Vitamin status and intake as primary determinants of homocysteinemia in an elderly population. JAMA 1993;270:2693–8.

[108] Ames BN. DNA damage from micronutrient deficiencies is likely to be a major cause of cancer. Mutat Res 2001;475:7–20.

[109] Duthie SJ, Narayanan S, Blum S, et al. Folate deficiency *in vitro* induces uracil misincorpora-tion and DNA hypomethylation and inhibits DNA excision repair in immortalized normal human colon epithelial cells. Nutr Cancer 2000;37:245–51.

[110] Kim YI, Pogribny IP, Salomon RN, et al. Exon-specific DNA hypomethylation of the p53 gene of rat colon induced by dimethylhydrazine: modulation by dietary folate. Am J Pathol 1996; 149:1129–37.

[111] Kim YI, Shirwadkar S, Choi SW, et al. Effects of dietary folate on DNA strand breaks within mutation-prone exons of the p53 gene in rat colon. Gastroenterology 2000;119:151–61.

[112] Lashner BA, Shapiro BD, Husain A, et al. Evaluation of the usefulness of testing for p53 mutations in colorectal cancer surveillance for ulcerative colitis. Am J Gastroenterol 1999;94: 456–62.

[113] Martinez ME, Maltzman T, Marshall JR, et al. Risk factors for Ki-ras protooncogene mutation in sporadic colorectal adenomas. Cancer Res 1999;59:5181–5.

[114] Slattery ML, Curtin K, Anderson K, et al. Associations between dietary intake and Ki-ras mutations in colon tumors: a population-based study. Cancer Res 2000;60:6935–41.

[115] Jaszewski R, Khan A, Sarkar FH, et al. Folic acid inhibition of EGFR-mediated proliferation in human colon cancer cell lines. Am J Physiol 1999;277:C1142–8.

[116] Ferraroni M, La V, Avanzo B, et al. Selected micronutrient intake and the risk for colorectal cancer. Br J Cancer 1994;70:1150–5.

[117] Freudenheim JL, Graham S, Marshall JR, et al. Folate intake and carcinogenesis of the colon and rectum. Int J Epidemiol 1991;20:368–74.

[118] Meyer F, White E. Alcohol and nutrients in relation to colon cancer in middle-aged adults. Am J Epidemiol 1993;138:225–36.

[119] Giovannucci E, Stampfer MJ, Colditz GA, et al. Folate, methionine, and alcohol intake and risk for colorectal adenoma. J Natl Cancer Inst 1993;85:875–84.

[120] Kearney J, Giovannucci E, Rimm EB, et al. Diet, alcohol, and smoking and the occurrence of hyperplastic polyps of the colon and rectum (United States). Cancer Causes Control 1995; 6:45–56.

[121] Su LJ, Arab L. Nutritional status of folate and colon cancer risk: evidence from NHANES I epidemiologic follow-up study. Ann Epidemiol 2001;11:65–72.

[122] Giovannucci E, Stampfer MJ, Colditz GA, et al. Multivitamin use, folate, and colon cancer in women in the Nurses' Health Study. Ann Intern Med 1998;129:517–24.

[123] Baron JA, Sandler RS, Haile RW, et al. Folate intake, alcohol consumption,95% CIgarette smoking, and risk for colorectal adenomas. J Natl Cancer Inst 1998;90:57–62.

[124] Biasco G, Zannoni U, Paganelli GM, et al. Folic acid supplementation and cell kinetics of rectal mucosa in patients with ulcerative colitis. Cancer Epidemiol Biomarkers Prev 1997;6:469–71.

[125] Cravo ML, Mason JB, Dayal Y, et al. Folate deficiency enhances the development of colonic neoplasia in dimethylhydrazine-treated rats. Cancer Res 1992;52:5002–6.

[126] Kim YI, Salomon RN, Graeme C, et al. Dietary folate protects against the development of macroscopic colonic neoplasia in a dose responsive manner in rats. Gut 1996;39:732–40.

[127] Song J, Sohn KJ, Medline A, et al. Chemopreventive effects of dietary folate on intestinal polyps in Apc+/−Msh2−/− mice. Cancer Res 2000;60:3191–9.

[128] Song J, Medline A, Mason JB, et al. Effects of dietary folate on intestinal tumorigenesis in the apcMin mouse. Cancer Res 2000;60:5434–40.

[129] Burkitt DP. Epidemiology of cancer of the colon and rectum. Cancer 1971;28:3–13.

[130] Burkitt DP. Some neglected leads to cancer causation. J Natl Cancer Inst 1971;47:913–9.

[131] Faivre J, Bonithon-Kopp C. Chemoprevention of colorectal cancer. Recent Results Cancer Res 1999;151:122–33.

[132] Kim YI. AGA technical review: impact of dietary fiber on colon cancer occurrence. Gastroenterology 2000;118:1235–57.

[133] Earnest DL, Einspahr JG, Alberts DS. Protective role of wheat bran fiber: data from marker trials. Am J Med 1999;106:S32–7.

[134] Ferguson LR, Harris PJ. Protection against cancer by wheat bran: role of dietary fibre and phytochemicals. Eur J Cancer Prev 1999;8:17–25.

[135] Kritchevsky D. Protective role of wheat bran fiber: preclinical data. Am J Med 1999;106: S28–31.

[136] Lupton JR, Turner ND. Potential protective mechanisms of wheat bran fiber. Am J Med 1999;106:S24–S27.

[137] Macrae F. Wheat bran fiber and development of adenomatous polyps: evidence from randomized, controlled clinical trials. Am J Med 1999;106:S38–42.

[138] Reddy BS. Role of dietary fiber in colon cancer: an overview. Am J Med 1999;106:16S–9S.

[139] DeVries JW, Prosky L, Li B, et al. A historical perspective on defining dietary fiber. St. Paul: American Association of Cereal Chemists; 1999

[140] Trowell H. Definitions of fibre [editorial]. Lancet 1974;1:503.

[141] Wijnands MV, Appel MJ, Hollanders VM, et al. A comparison of the effects of dietary cellulose and fermentable galacto-oligosaccharide, in a rat model of colorectal carcinogenesis: fermentable fibre confers greater protection than non-fermentable fibre in both high and low fat backgrounds. Carcinogenesis 1999;20:651–6.

[142] Perrin P, Pierre F, Patry Y, et al. Only fibres promoting a stable butyrate producing colonic ecosystem decrease the rate of aberrant crypt foci in rats. Gut 2001;48:53–61.

[143] Russo GL, Della P, Mercurio C, et al. Protective effects of butyric acid in colon cancer. Adv Exp Med Biol 1999;472:131–47.

[144] Bruce WR, Wolever TM, Giacca A. Mechanisms linking diet and colorectal cancer: the possible role of insulin resistance. Nutr Cancer 2000;37:19–26.

[145] Giovannucci E. Insulin and colon cancer. Cancer Causes Control 1995;6:164–79.

[146] Zhuo XG, Watanabe S. Factor analysis of digestive cancer mortality and food consumption in 65 Chinese counties. J Epidemiol 1999;9:275–84.

[147] Franceschi S, Dal M, Augustin L, et al. Dietary glycemic load and colorectal cancer risk. Ann Oncol 2001;12:173–8.

[148] Hu FB. van D, Liu S. Diet and risk for type II diabetes: the role of types of fat and carbohydrate. Diabetologia 2001;44:805–17.

[149] Keefe SJ, Kidd M, Espitalier N, et al. Rarity of colon cancer in Africans is associated with low animal product consumption, not fiber. Am J Gastroenterol 1999;94:1373–80.

[150] Fuchs CS, Giovannucci EL, Colditz GA, et al. Dietary fiber and the risk for colorectal cancer and adenoma in women. N Engl J Med 1999;340:169–76.

[151] Giovannucci E, Rimm EB, Stampfer MJ, et al. Intake of fat, meat, and fiber in relation to risk for colon cancer in men. Cancer Res 1994;54:2390–7.

[152] MacLennan R, Macrae F, Bain C, et al. Randomized trial of intake of fat, fiber, and beta carotene to prevent colorectal adenomas: the Australian Polyp Prevention Project. J Natl Cancer Inst 1995;87:1760–6.

[153] McKeown-Eyssen GE, Bright See E, Bruce WR et al: A randomized trial of a low fat high fibre diet in the recurrence of colorectal polyps: Toronto Polyp Prevention Group. J Clin Epidemiol 1994;47:525–36.

[154] Steinmetz KA, Kushi LH, Bostick RM, et al. Vegetables, fruit, and colon cancer in the Iowa Women's Health Study. Am J Epidemiol 1994;139:1–15.

[155] Alberts DS, Martinez ME, Roe DJ, et al. Lack of effect of a high-fiber cereal supplement on the recurrence of colorectal adenomas: Phoenix Colon Cancer Prevention Physicians' Network. N Engl J Med 2000;342:1156–62.

[156] Schatzkin A, Lanza E, Corle D, et al. Lack of effect of a low-fat, high-fiber diet on the recurrence of colorectal adenomas: Polyp Prevention Trial Study Group. N Engl J Med 2000; 342:1149–55.

[157] Slavin JL, Martini MC, Jacobs DR, et al. Plausible mechanisms for the protectiveness of whole grains. Am J Clin Nutr 1999;70:S459–63.

[158] Jenab M, Thompson LU. Phytic acid in wheat bran affects colon morphology, cell differentiation and apoptosis. Carcinogenesis 2000;21:1547–52.

[159] Reddy BS, Hirose Y, Cohen LA, et al. Preventive potential of wheat bran fractions against experimental colon carcinogenesis: implications for human colon cancer prevention. Cancer Res 2000;60:4792–7.

[160] American Gastroenterological Association. Impact of dietary fiber on colon cancer occurrence: American College of Gastroenterology medical position statement. Gastroenterology 2000; 118:1233–4.

[161] Faivre J, Giacosa A. Primary prevention of colorectal cancer through fibre supplementation. Eur J Cancer Prev 1998;7(suppl 2):S29–32.

[162] Bronner F, Pansu D. Nutritional aspects of calcium absorption. J Nutr 1999;129:9–12.

[163] Duflos C, Bellaton C, Pansu D, et al. Calcium solubility, intestinal sojourn time and paracellular permeability codetermine passive calcium absorption in rats. J Nutr 1995;125: 2348–55.

[164] Toba Y, Kato K, Takada Y, et al. Bioavailability of milk micellar calcium phosphate-phosphopeptide complex in rats. J Nutr Sci Vitaminol (Tokyo) 1999;45:311–23.

[165] Bohmer H, Muller H, Resch KL. Calcium supplementation with calcium-rich mineral waters: a systematic review and meta-analysis of its bioavailability. Osteoporos Int 2000;11:938–43.

[166] Wynckel A, Hanrotel C, Wuillai A, et al. Intestinal calcium absorption from mineral water. Miner Electrolyte Metab 1997;23:88–92.

[167] Ross RD, Cromwell GL, Stahly TS. Effects of source and particle size on the biological availability of calcium in calcium supplements for growing pigs. J Anim Sci 1984;59:125–34.

[168] Kleibeuker JH, van der Meer R, de Vries E. Calcium and vitamin D: possible protective agents against colorectal cancer? Eur J Cancer 1995;31A:1081–4.

[169] Lipkin M. Preclinical and early human studies of calcium and colon cancer prevention. Ann N Y Acad Sci 1999;889:120–7.

[170] Penman ID, Liang QL, Bode J, et al. Dietary calcium supplementation increases apoptosis in the distal murine colonic epithelium. J Clin Pathol 2000;53:302–7.

[171] Liu Z, Tomotake H, Wan G, et al. Combined effect of dietary calcium and iron on colonic aberrant crypt foci, cell proliferation and apoptosis, and fecal bile acids in 1,2-dimethylhydrazine-treated rats. Oncol Rep 2001;8:893–7.

[172] Bostick RM. Human studies of calcium supplementation and colorectal epithelial cell proliferation. Cancer Epidemiol Biomarkers Prev 1997;6:971–80.

[173] Martinez ME, McPherson RS, Levin B, et al. A case-control study of dietary intake and other lifestyle risk factors for hyperplastic polyps. Gastroenterology 1997;113:423–9.

[174] Mobarhan S. Calcium and the colon: recent findings. Nutr Rev 1999;57:124–6.

[175] Holt PR. Dairy foods and prevention of colon cancer: human studies. J Am Coll Nutr 1999; 18:S379–91.

[176] Holt PR, Atillasoy EO, Gilman J, et al. Modulation of abnormal colonic epithelial cell proliferation and differentiation by low-fat dairy foods: a randomized controlled trial. JAMA 1998; 280:1074–9.

[177] Baron JA, Beach M, Mandel JS, et al. Calcium supplements for the prevention of colorectal adenomas: Calcium Polyp Prevention Study Group. N Engl J Med 1999;340:101–7.

[178] Alberts DS, Ritenbaugh C, Story JA, et al. Randomized, double-blinded, placebo-controlled study of effect of wheat bran fiber and calcium on fecal bile acids in patients with resected adenomatous colon polyps. J Natl Cancer Inst 1996;88:81–92.

[179] Newmark HL, Wargovich MJ, Bruce WR. Colon cancer and dietary fat, phosphate, and calcium: a hypothesis. J Natl Cancer Inst 1984;72:1323–5.

[180] Giacosa A, Filiberti R, Hill MJ, et al. Vitamins and cancer chemoprevention. Eur J Cancer Prev 1997;6(suppl 1):47S–54S.

[181] Langman M, Boyle P. Chemoprevention of colorectal cancer [review]. Gut 1998;43:578–85.

[182] Van Poppel G, van den Berg H. Vitamins and cancer. Cancer Lett 1997;114:195–202.

[183] Cascinu S, Ligi M, Del Ferro E, et al. Effects of calcium and vitamin supplementation on colon cell proliferation in colorectal cancer. Cancer Invest 2000;18:411–6.

[184] Kelloff GJ, Crowell JA, Steele VE, et al. Progress in cancer chemoprevention: development of diet-derived chemopreventive agents. J Nutr 2000;130:467S–71S.

[185] Ireson C, Orr S, Jones DJ, et al. Characterization of metabolites of the chemopreventive agent curcumin in human and rat hepatocytes and in the rat *in vivo*, and evaluation of their ability to inhibit phorbol ester-induced prostaglandin E_2 production. Cancer Res 2001;61:1058–64.

[186] Pan MH, Huang TM, Lin JK. Biotransformation of curcumin through reduction and glucuronidation in mice. Drug Metab Dispos 1999;27:486–94.

[187] Ravindranath V, Chandrasekhara N. Absorption and tissue distribution of curcumin in rats. Toxicology 1980;16:259–65.

[188] Sharma RA, McLelland HR, Hill KA, et al. Pharmacodynamic and pharmacokinetic study of oral curcuma extract in patients with colorectal cancer. Clin Cancer Res 2001;7:1894–900.

[189] Ravindranath V, Chandrasekhara N. *In vitro* studies on the intestinal absorption of curcumin in rats. Toxicology 1981;20:251–7.

[190] Moragoda L, Jaszewski R, Majumdar AP. Curcumin induced modulation of cell cycle and apoptosis in gastric and colon cancer cells. Anticancer Res 2001;21:873–8.

[191] Li JK, Lin-Shia SY. Mechanisms of cancer chemoprevention by curcumin. Proc Natl Sci Counc Repub China B 2001;25:59–66.

[192] Ramsewak RS, DeWitt DL, Nair MG. Cytotoxicity, antioxidant and anti-inflammatory activities of curcumins I–III from Curcuma longa. Phytomedicine 2000;7:303–8.

[193] Plummer SM, Holloway KA, Manson MM, et al. Inhibition of cyclo-oxygenase 2 expression in colon cells by the chemopreventive agent curcumin involves inhibition of NF-κB activation via the NIK/IKK signalling complex. Oncogene 1999;18:6013–20.

[194] Rao CV, Kawamori T, Hamid R, et al. Chemoprevention of colonic aberrant crypt foci by an inducible nitric oxide synthase-selective inhibitor. Carcinogenesis 1999;20:641–4.

[195] Rao CV, Rivenson A, Simi B, et al. Chemoprevention of colon carcinogenesis by dietary curcumin, a naturally occurring plant phenolic compound. Cancer Res 1995;55:259–66.

[196] Mahmoud NN, Carothers AM, Grunberger D, et al. Plant phenolics decrease intestinal tumors in an animal model of familial adenomatous polyposis. Carcinogenesis 2000;21: 921–7.

[197] Hanif R, Qiao L, Shiff SJ, et al. Curcumin, a natural plant phenolic food additive, inhibits cell proliferation and induces cell cycle changes in colon adenocarcinoma cell lines by a prosta-glandin-independent pathway. J Lab Clin Med 1997;130:576–84.

[198] Jiang MC, Yang Y, Yen JJ, et al. Curcumin induces apoptosis in immortalized NIH 3T3 and malignant cancer cell lines. Nutr Cancer 1996;26:111–20.

[199] Pereira MA, Grubbs CJ, Barnes LH, et al. Effects of the phytochemicals, curcumin and quer-cetin, upon azoxymethane-induced colon cancer and 7,12-dimethylbenz[a]anthracene-induced mammary cancer in rats. Carcinogenesis 1996;17:1305–11.

[200] Huang MT, Lou YR, Ma W, et al. Inhibitory effects of dietary curcumin on forestomach, duodenal, and colon carcinogenesis in mice. Cancer Res 1994;54:5841–7.

[201] Kawamori T, Lubet R, Steele VE, et al. Chemopreventive effect of curcumin, a naturally occurring anti-inflammatory agent, during the promotion/progression stages of colon cancer. Cancer Res 1999;59:597–601.

[202] Kim JM, Araki S, Kim DJ, et al. Chemopreventive effects of carotenoids and curcumins on mouse colon carcinogenesis after 1,2-dimethylhydrazine initiation. Carcinogenesis 1998;19: 81–5.

[203] Conney AH, Lou YR, Xie JG, et al. Some perspectives on dietary inhibition of carcinogenesis: studies with curcumin and tea. Proc Soc Exp Biol Med 1997;216:234–45.

[204] Katiyar SK, Mukhtar H. Tea antioxidants in cancer chemoprevention. J Cell Biochem 1997; 27:59–67.

[205] Kohlmeier L, Weterings KG, Steck S, et al. Tea and cancer prevention: an evaluation of the epidemiologic literature. Nutr Cancer 1997;27:1–13.

[206] Mukhtar H, Ahmad N. Tea polyphenols: prevention of cancer and optimizing health. Am J Clin Nutr 2000;71:1698S–702S.

[207] Bushman JL. Green tea and cancer in humans: a review of the literature. Nutr Cancer 1998;31: 151–9.

[208] Goldbohm RA, Hertog MG, Brants HA, et al. Consumption of black tea and cancer risk: a prospective cohort study. J Natl Cancer Inst 1996;88:93–100.

[209] Baron JA, Greenberg ER, Haile R, et al. Coffee and tea and the risk for recurrent colorectal adenomas. Cancer Epidemiol Biomarkers Prev 1997;6:7–10.

[210] Hartman TJ, Tangrea JA, Pietinen P, et al. Tea and coffee consumption and risk for colon and rectal cancer in middle-aged Finnish men. Nutr Cancer 1998;31:41–8.

[211] Inoue M, Tajima K, Hirose K, et al. Tea and coffee consumption and the risk for digestive tract cancers: data from a comparative case-referent study in Japan. Cancer Causes Control 1998; 9:209–16.

[212] Jung YD, Kim MS, Shin BA, et al. EGCG, a major component of green tea, inhibits tumour growth by inhibiting VEGF induction in human colon carcinoma cells. Br J Cancer 2001;84: 844–50.

[213] Tan X, Hu D, Li S, et al. Differences of four catechins in cell cycle arrest and induction of apoptosis in LoVo cells. Cancer Lett 2000;158:1–6.

[214] Uesato S, Kitagawa Y, Kamishimoto M, et al. Inhibition of green tea catechins against the growth of cancerous human colon and hepatic epithelial cells. Cancer Lett 2001;170:41–4.

[215] Valcic S, Timmermann BN, Alberts DS, et al. Inhibitory effect of six green tea catechins and

caffeine on the growth of four selected human tumor cell lines. Anticancer Drugs 1996;7: 461–8.

[216] Chen ZP, Schell JB, Ho CT, et al. Green tea epigallocatechin gallate shows a pronounced growth inhibitory effect on cancerous cells but not on their normal counterparts. Cancer Lett 1998;129:173–9.

[217] Lu J, Ho CT, Ghai G, et al. Differential effects of theaflavin monogallates on cell growth, apoptosis, and Cox-2 gene expression in cancerous versus normal cells. Cancer Res 2000;60: 6465–71.

[218] Schut HA, Yao R. Tea as a potential chemopreventive agent in PhIP carcinogenesis: effects of green tea and black tea on PhIP-DNA adduct formation in female F-344 rats. Nutr Cancer 2000;36:52–8.

[219] Xu M, Dashwood RH. Chemoprevention studies of heterocyclic amine-induced colon carcino-genesis. Cancer Lett 1999;143:179–83.

[220] Hirose M, Hoshiya T, Mizoguchi Y, et al. Green tea catechins enhance tumor development in the colon without effects in the lung or thyroid after pretreatment with 1,2-Dimethylhy-drazine or 2,2′-dihydroxy-di-n-propylnitrosamine in male F344 rats. Cancer Lett 2001;168: 23–9.

[221] Weisburger JH, Rivenson A, Aliaga C, et al. Effect of tea extracts, polyphenols, and epigallo-catechin gallate on azoxymethane-induced colon cancer. Proc Soc Exp Biol Med 1998;217: 104–8.

[222] Weisburger JH, Rivenson A, Reinhardt J, et al. Effect of black tea on azoxymethane-induced colon cancer. Carcinogenesis 1998;19:229–32.

[223] Metz N, Lobstein A, Schneider Y, et al. Suppression of azoxymethane-induced preneoplastic lesions and inhibition of cyclooxygenase-2 activity in the colonic mucosa of rats drinking a crude green tea extract. Nutr Cancer 2000;38:60–4.

[224] August DA, Landau J, Caputo D, et al. Ingestion of green tea rapidly decreases prostaglandin E_2 levels in rectal mucosa in humans. Cancer Epidemiol Biomarkers Prev 1999;8:709–13.

[225] Yang GY, Liao J, Kim K, et al. Inhibition of growth and induction of apoptosis in human cancer cell lines by tea polyphenols. Carcinogenesis 1998;19:611–6.

[226] Isemura M, Saeki K, Kimura T, et al. Tea catechins and related polyphenols as anti-cancer agents. Biofactors 2000;13:81–5.

[227] Willett WC. Diet and cancer: one view at the start of the millennium. Cancer Epidemiol Biomarkers Prev 2001;10:3–8.

[228] Levi F, Pasche C, La V, et al. Food groups and colorectal cancer risk. Br J Cancer 1999;79: 1283–7.

[229] Steinmetz KA, Potter JD. Vegetables, fruit, and cancer prevention: a review. J Am Diet Assoc 1996;96:1027–39.

[230] Shirin H, Pinto JT, Kawabata Y, et al. Antiproliferative effects of S-allylmercaptocysteine on colon cancer cells when tested alone or in combination with sulindac sulfide. Cancer Res 2001; 61:725–31.

[231] Lawson KR, Ignatenko NA, Piazza GA, et al. Influence of K-ras activation on the survival responses of Caco-2 cells to the chemopreventive agents sulindac and difluoromethylornithine. Cancer Epidemiol Biomarkers Prev 2000;9:1155–62.

[232] Rao CV, Tokumo K, Rigotty J, et al. Chemoprevention of colon carcinogenesis by dietary administration of piroxicam, alpha-difluoromethylornithine, 16 alpha-fluoro-5-androsten-17-one, and ellagic acid individually and in combination. Cancer Res 1991;51:4528–34.

[233] Reddy BS, Nayini J, Tokumo K, et al. Chemoprevention of colon carcinogenesis by con-current administration of piroxicam, a nonsteroidal antiinflammatory drug with D,L-alpha-difluoromethylornithine, an ornithine decarboxylase inhibitor, in diet. Cancer Res 1990;50: 2562–8.

[234] Paulsen JE, Lutzow H. *In vivo* growth inhibition of human colon carcinoma cells (HT-29) by all-trans-retinoic acid, difluoromethylornithine, and colon mitosis inhibitor, individually and in combination. Anticancer Res 2000;20:3485–9.

[235] Agarwal B, Rao CV, Bhendwal S, et al. Lovastatin augments sulindac-induced apoptosis in colon cancer cells and potentiates chemopreventive effects of sulindac. Gastroenterology 1999; 117:838–47.

[236] Kelloff GJ, Fay JR, Steele VE, et al. Epidermal growth factor receptor tyrosine kinase inhibitors as potential cancer chemopreventives. Cancer Epidemiol Biomarkers Prev 1996;5:657–66.

[237] Gupta RA, DuBois RN. Combinations for cancer prevention. Nat Med 2000;6:974–5.

[238] Torrance CJ, Jackson PE, Montgomery E, et al. Combinatorial chemoprevention of intestinal neoplasia. Nat Med 2000;6:1024–8.

HEMATOLOGY/
ONCOLOGY
CLINICS OF
NORTH AMERICA

Hematol Oncol Clin N Am
16 (2002) 841–865

Secondary prevention: screening and surveillance of persons at average and high risk for colorectal cancer

Kathryn A. Peterson, MD[a], James A. DiSario, MD[b],*

[a]Division of Gastroenterology, University of Utah Health Sciences Center, 50 North Medical Drive,
4R118, Salt Lake City, UT 84132, USA
[b]Huntsman Cancer Center, University of Utah Health Sciences Center, 50 North Medical Drive,
4R118, Salt Lake City, UT 84132, USA

Colorectal cancer is the third most common cancer, accounting for 9% of all new cancer diagnoses and affecting men and women alike. It was estimated that in 2001 there would be 138,900 new cases of colorectal cancer with 57,200 deaths, making this the second most common cause of cancer-related death after lung cancer. The average American experiences approximately a 6% lifetime risk for colorectal cancer [1]. Risk factors for colorectal cancer include country of birth, age, family history, rare syndromes, inflammatory bowel disease, and diet and lifestyle. Three fourths of all colon cancers, however, develop within those without risk factors other than country of birth and age greater than 50 years [2].

Colorectal cancer is treatable and has a good prognosis when it is discovered at an early stage. Adenomatous polyps are precursors to cancer, and the progression generally takes 5 to 10 years [3–5]. The development from early-stage malignancy to metastatic spread requires approximately 1 to 2 years. Therefore, there is ample time to diagnose and treat curable lesions. The overall 5-year survival rate is approximately 62%; however at diagnosis, only about 45% of patients have disease contained in the bowel, 25% have regional nodal spread, and 30% have distant metastases [1,2].

Colorectal cancers have long been staged using Duke classification with Astler-Coller modification. Currently, the American Joint Commission on Cancer and the Union Internationale Contre le Cancer tumor, node, metastasis (TNM) classification is preferred [6]. Table 1 shows these classification systems, and

Resources and support provided by the Huntsman Foundation, the Huntsman General Clinical Research Center (NIH M01 RR00064), and the National Cancer Institute (R01 CA80852).
* Corresponding author.
E-mail address: James.Disario@hsc.utah.edu (J.A. DiSario).

Table 1
Tumor stage

TNM	Duke/Aster-Coller	Tumor
Tumor		
Tx	—	Cannot be assessed
T0	—	No cancer in specimen, ie, post-polypectomy
Tis	Carcinoma in situ	High-grade dysplasia limited to epithelium
T1	A	Submucosal invasion
T2	B1	Muscularis propria invasion
T3	B2	Serosa or perirectal tissue invasion
T4	B3	Adjacent organs invaded/peritoneum perforated
Regional Lymph nodes		
Nx	—	Not assessed
N0	—	None
N1	—	1–3 involved
N2	—	4 or more
N3	—	Atypical nodes or nodes along vascular trunk
Distant Metastases		
Mx	—	Not assessed
M0	—	None
M1	—	Distant metastases

TNM, tumor, node, metastases; American Joint Commission on Cancer and Union Internationale Contre le Canceur Staging Classification.
Data from Handbook for staging of cancer: manual for staging of cancer. 4th edition. Philadelphia: JB Lippincott; 1993.

Table 2 shows survival by tumor stage. Only 10% to 15% of patients have symptoms before metastases occur.

Advances in endoscopic and diagnostic imaging and genetic technology are having a meaningful impact on the early diagnosis and prevention of colorectal malignancy. Controlled trials conducted in the last decade demonstrate a strong correlation between cancer screening using fecal occult blood testing (FOBT) and

Table 2
Survival by tumor stage

Stage	TNM	Duke/Aster-Coller	5-year survival (%)
I	T1,N0,Mo	A	90–100
	T2, N0,M0	B1	
II	T3, N0,M0	B2	80–85
	T4, N0,M0	B3	
III	T2, N1/2,M0	C1	50–70
	T3, N1/2,M0	C2	
	T4, N1/2,M0	C3	
IV	M1	D	5–15

TNM, tumor, node, metastases.
Data from Handbook for staging of cancer: manual for staging of cancer. 4th edition. Philadelphia: JB Lippincott; 1993.

flexible sigmoidoscopy and a reduction in deaths from colorectal cancer. Recent studies show that full colonoscopic screening may more adequately reduce risk. Genetic testing of germline mutations in persons from high-risk families holds strong promise for early detection of colorectal malignancy, as do somatic mutations from fecal cellular debris. Additionally, newer, imaging studies, often termed virtual colonoscopy (CT and MRI colonography), have the potential for a significant role in cancer screening in the near future.

Screening, surveillance, and prevention

Screening refers to testing asymptomatic persons at average risk, whereas surveillance implies examining persons at increased risk. Primary prevention entails altering diet and lifestyle and using chemopreventive medications to avoid the occurrence of cancer. Secondary prevention is intervention to treat premalignant lesions, thereby precluding cancer development. Strategies for primary and secondary colorectal cancer prevention are evolving.

Colorectal polyps

Adenomas are the most common polyps and occur in 25% to 50% of the population older than 50 years [4,5,7–9]. They are precursors to most colorectal cancers and are of greatest significance in colorectal cancer prevention. Detection and removal of adenomatous polyps is the foundation of secondary colorectal cancer prevention. Cancer risk is associated with adenoma size, degree of villous architecture, and grade of dysplasia. Adenomatous polyps larger than 1 cm, with villous architecture or moderate to high-grade dysplasia, are termed advanced and are of most importance in cancer prevention. Most adenomas are small and have tubular architecture and mild dysplasia. Multiplicity of adenomatous polyps is also associated with increased risk for advanced adenomas and cancer [3–5,7].

Adenomatous polyps occur throughout the colon and rectum and have a distal predominance. The older literature described a distal predominance of cancer, making flexible sigmoidoscopy a more reasonable screening tool. Recent literature, however, demonstrates a proximal shift in neoplasms. This may represent a shift in cancer demographics or in diagnostic accuracy. Multiple (synchronous) polyps often occur within a single person. Fifty percent of patients with a distal adenoma harbor more proximal lesions [4,5,7–9], and 3% to 6% of patients with newly diagnosed colorectal cancer have synchronous cancers [10]. Metachronous lesions are those that develop subsequent to the detection of the index lesion.

Gross morphology of polyps may be pedunculated or sessile. Pedunculated polyps result from forces of the fecal stream propelling the polyp downstream and causing the development of a stalk of normal mucosa, as shown in Fig. 1A. Sessile polyps are flat to protuberant and do not have stalks.

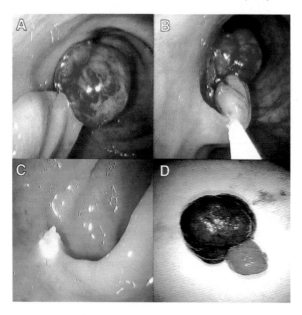

Fig. 1. (A) Pedunculated polyp within the colon. (B) Snare catheter to serve as a tourniquet and to cut and cauterize the stalk. (C) Coagulum on the colonic mucosa after removal of polyp. (D) Resected polyp ex vivo.

The malignant potential of an adenoma relates proportionally to its size, degree of dysplasia, and villous architecture. The presence of dysplasia defines neoplasia. By definition, adenomas are neoplasms; therefore, some degree of dysplasia is present in all adenomas. Adenomas that are larger than 1 cm in diameter, are predominantly villous, or have high-grade dysplasia are at high-risk for subsequent development of carcinoma [5,7,9].

Tubular adenomas comprise approximately 80% of all adenomas and have the minimal malignant potential. Grossly, these polyps appear darker or more erythematous than the surrounding mucosa and often have smooth surfaces. They have enlarged hyperchromatic nuclei with loss of polarity, as demonstrated in Fig. 2. Villous adenomas comprise approximately 5% of colorectal adenomas and occur more frequently in older persons. They are often large, flat, sessile polyps with abundant mucus production. By definition, the histologic architecture is at least 75% villous with infolding, proliferation, and branching of epithelial cells (Fig. 2). Thirty percent to 50% of villous adenomas contain foci of carcinoma. Tubulovillous adenomas comprise the remainder of adenomas. Histopathologic findings are at least 25% villous and 25% tubular. The risk for harboring carcinoma is intermediate [5,7].

Adenomatous polyps typically develop in the fifth or sixth decade of life and colorectal cancer in the sixth decade, supporting a 10-year adenoma-to-carcinoma interval. Numerous genetic mutations accumulate during the development of neoplasia and subsequent carcinogenesis. Sporadically occurring adenomatous

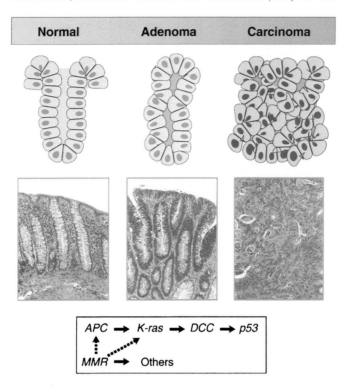

Fig. 2. Adenoma–carcinoma sequence. The progression from normal colonic mucosa to carcinoma involves an accumulating sequence of genetic mutations. Eighty-percent of adenomas are initiated from somatic mutations in the *APC* gene. The remaining 20% arise from mutations of the mismatch repair genes.

polyps arise from clonal cellular expansions initiated by a somatic mutation of the adenomatous polyposis coli (APC) gene in 80% of patients. The other 20% of adenomas appear to begin with mutations of the mismatch repair (MMR) genes (*HmSH2*, *HmLH1*, *HpMS1*, *HpMS2*). Interestingly, when inherited as germline mutations, APC leads to familial adenomatous polyposis (FAP) and MMR genes to hereditary nonpolyposis colorectal cancer (HNPCC). Subsequent mutations of oncogenes (k-*ras*), repair genes (*p53*), and tumor-suppressor genes (*DCC*) accumulate and eventually result in malignant degeneration, as is schematically demonstrated in Fig. 2.

Other types of colorectal polyps include hyperplastic, hamartomatous, and lymphoid nodules. There is controversy about the significance of hyperplastic polyps. These lesions are often small (smaller than 5 mm) and are usually located distally in the sigmoid colon and rectum. Histopathology consists of increased cellular proliferation within the basal third of the crypt, with increased epithelial enhancement and infolding. There may be an association with neoplasms in older men and in persons with multiple hyperplastic polyps [8,11]. Hamartomas may entail malignant degeneration in inherited syndromes, including Peutz-Jeghers and juvenile polyposis. Juvenile polyps are also known as retention polyps because, on histopathologic examination, they contain mucin-filled cystic glands and an edematous lamina propria, and they are hypervascular. They tend to be single, round, and red, and they are usually found in children younger than 10 years. Bleeding is common with juvenile polyps. Lymphoid nodules have no clinical significance relating to colorectal cancer.

Colonoscopic polypectomy

Several studies demonstrate the efficacy of polypectomy in the prevention of cancer [12,13]. Polypectomy includes the identification of a mucosal excrescences during endoscopy and the subsequent removal with a forceps or snare (see Fig. 1). Depending on the size and morphology of the polyp, injection with saline to separate the involved mucosa from the submucosal or electrocautery are used to facilitate removal. Morbidity after colonoscopic polypectomy is uncommon and usually mild. The most common serious complication is bleeding, which occurs in 1.4% of polypectomies and usually starts 7 days after the procedure. Perforation occurs in up to 0.3% of patients, and postpolypectomy serosal burns—manifest by abdominal pain, fever, and leukocytosis—develop in 0.3% of patients [14].

Several studies demonstrate the efficacy of colonoscopic polypectomy in reducing the incidence and mortality of colorectal cancer [13,15,16]. The National Polyp study showed a 76% to 90% decrease in colon cancer deaths compared to reference death rates after polypectomy, as demonstrated in Fig. 3 [13]. Postpolypectomy surveillance recommendations are outlined in Table 3 and depend

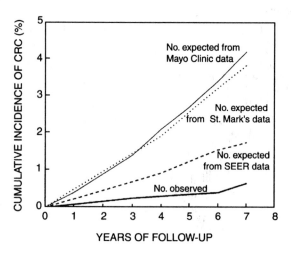

Fig. 3. Cumulative incidence of colorectal cancer deaths from the National Polyp Study. Observed incidence after polypectomy is less than the expected incidence from the three reference groups. (*From* Winauer SJ, Zauber AG, Ho MN, et al. Prevention of colorectal cancer by colonoscopic polypectomy. N Engl J Med 1993;329:1977-81; with permission of the Massachusetts Medical Society; Copyright © 1993, all rights reserved.)

Table 3
Post-polypectomy surveillance

Finding	Colonoscopy intervals
Single tubular adenoma < 1 cm	5 years
Single tubular adenoma and family history	3 years
Several adenomas, villous elements, or high-grade dysplasia completely resected	3 years
Numerous adenomas	1 year
Large sessile adenomas	2–6 months
Negative follow-up examination findings	5 years

on the findings at colonoscopy and the histopathologic characteristics of the removed lesions [12,16,17].

Average-risk colon cancer screening

Colorectal cancer screening entails the regular use of endoscopic, radiographic, or laboratory techniques to evaluate asymptomatic persons at average risk for adenomatous polyps or colorectal cancer. Death rates from colorectal cancer have declined by approximately 2% per year since 1984 [1]. This is attributed to enhanced screening with the removal of adenomatous polyps and the treatment of early-stage cancers. If the tumor is found at a localized stage, patients with colorectal cancer have a 94% probability of survival at 5 years [18].

Controlled studies from the 1990s provide sufficient evidence to recommend some form of colorectal cancer screening in all persons beginning at 50 years of age [1,3]. Table 3 outlines several recommended postpolypectomy surveillance strategies, and the box below illustrates several accepted screening strategies for persons of average risk. Such recommendations have been developed by several organizations, including the United States Preventive Services Task Force, the Federal Agency for Health Care Policy and Research, the American Society for Gastrointestinal Endoscopy, the American College of Gastroenterology, and the American Cancer Society [9,19–22]. All organizations recommend at least flexible sigmoidoscopy every 5 years or FOBT every year, preferably combined or supplanted by more sensitive methods. Currently recommended options for screening are outlined in the following box.

Risk factors

Each person in the United States has a 5.6% lifetime risk for colorectal cancer [1]. Family and personal history may confer increased risk. The risk for colon cancer increases with age; calculated risk ranges from 0.06% for those younger than 40 to 3.5% for those between 60 and 79 years of age [1]. Approximately 75% of all colorectal cancers occur in persons who are at average risk but are

---

Colorectal cancer screening recommendations for average risk

Begin at age 50

 Annual fecal occult blood test *or*
 Flexible sigmoidoscopy every 5 years *or*
 Annual fecal occult blood test and flexible sigmoidoscopy every
5 years *or*
 Colonoscopy every 10 years *or*
 Double-contrast barium enema every 5–10 years (less sensitive,
untested)

---

older than 50. The other 25% of these cancers generally occur in people with genetic or familial susceptibility [2,3,18].

In addition to age, a personal history of colorectal neoplasms increases the risk for colorectal malignancy. Prior diagnosis of advanced adenomas increases the risk by threefold [15]. Up to 50% of patients given diagnoses of colorectal adenomas have synchronous lesions and a 10% risk for metachronous neoplasms [5,10,23]. Cancer risk is increased fourfold for those with histories of colorectal malignancy [2,3]. Table 4 shows that a family history of early-onset cancer signifies increased risk to first-degree relatives.

Persons with certain genetic syndromes, such as FAP and hereditary nonpolyposis colorectal cancer (HPNCC), have a 100% and an 80% risk for colorectal malignancy, respectively, and require genetic and endoscopic surveillance. Inflammatory bowel disease increases the risk for colorectal cancer to up to 18-fold in persons with extensive ulcerative colitis or Crohn disease [24]. Surveillance strategies are empiric and include annual or biannual colonoscopy after 8 to 10 years of pan-colitis or 15 years of more localized disease [25].

Table 4
Familial risk for colorectal neoplasia

Familial setting	Approximate lifetime risk
General population	6%
One first-degree relative with CRC	2–3-fold increased
Two first-degree relatives with CRC	3–4-fold increased
First-degree relative with CRC younger than 50	3–4-fold increased
One second- or third-degree relative with CRC	1.5-fold increased
Two second-degree relatives with CRC	2–3-fold increased
One first-degree relative with an adenoma	2–3-fold increased

CRC, colorectal cancer.
Modified from Burt RW. Colon cancer screening. Gastroenterology 2000;119:837–53; with permission.

Fecal occult blood test

FOBT is based on the concept that two thirds of colorectal cancers bleed within the course of one week and that advanced adenomas bleed more than normal mucosa [26]. Hemoglobin has peroxidase activity that is detected using the guaiac test. Gum guaiac is a colorless indicator oxidized to a pigmented quinone in the presence of peroxidase and hydrogen peroxide. The pseudoperoxidase activity of blood turns guaiac from colorless to blue 30 to 60 seconds after hydrogen peroxide is applied. The recommended FOBT protocol involves taking two separated specimens from three consecutive stools. The test may be performed on a specimen obtained during digital rectal examination or in a person on low-dose aspirin [27]. Patients should be advised to eat a high-fiber diet beginning 2 days before collection. They should avoid eating peroxidase-containing foods (broccoli, cauliflower) to preclude false-negative results and red meat cooked rare, again to minimize false-positive findings. Antioxidants, such as vitamin C, interfere with the peroxidase reaction and may result in false-negative results. Hydration of specimens before the application of peroxide increases sensitivity but decreases specificity. Hydration has been shown to increase the rate of positive results by up to fourfold [26]. Visualization of the entire colon, preferably with colonoscopy, is recommended if there is any positive result, even from a single specimen. The sensitivity of FOBT ranges from 30% to 90% [28,29]. FOBT has been shown to decrease cancer deaths in three large-scale randomized, controlled trials when positive results were followed by endoscopic polypectomy or surgery. Annual FOBT with rehydration and subsequent colonoscopy for all positive results lead to a 15% to 33% reduction in deaths [26,28–31]. Increasing the frequency of testing does not appear to add any advantage because biennial FOBT yielded only a 21% decrease in deaths [32]. A nonrandomized study comparing sigmoidoscopy alone to sigmoidoscopy plus FOBT showed improvement with the addition of FOBT [33]. Another case-control study demonstrated a 31% decrease in cancer-related deaths in patients screened with FOBT [34].

Sigmoidoscopy

Flexible sigmoidoscopy offers advantages over FOBT. Sigmoidoscopy enables direct visualization of the bowel and the ability to biopsy lesions. Sensitivity is reported to be 92%, with a specificity of 85% for left-sided cancer [35]. Rigid sigmoidoscopy resulted in a 59% reduction in deaths from colorectal cancer in a well-conducted case-controlled study [36]. This significant decrease in deaths, however, was seen only in patients whose tumors could be examined with the sigmoidoscope, not in those with proximal cancer. The protection afforded by endoscopy persisted for as long as 10 years beyond the date of the procedure. Muller and Sonnenberg [37] demonstrated a 60% reduction in the development of colorectal cancer when sigmoidoscopic examination was performed at regular intervals. The protection afforded by flexible sigmoidoscopy screening lasted from 6 to 10 years [37]. Five-year intervals appear to be appropriate because progression from adenoma to carcinoma appears to require 5 to 10 years [38].

Combined FOBT and sigmoidoscopy

Accepted guidelines recommend screening with sigmoidoscopy and FOBT. Sigmoidoscopy accurately detects polyps and cancers within the left colon but does not visualize the right colon. Only 50% to 60% of all colon cancers arise from the left colon [5,23]. Combined FOBT and sigmoidoscopy resulted in a 20% improvement in survival from colorectal cancer over sigmoidoscopy alone [33]. Recently, a large prospective cohort study of colonoscopy and FOBT determined that combined FOBT and sigmoidoscopy would detect 76% of all advanced neoplasias within the population at average risk; this was increased from 70% detection with sigmoidoscopy alone [39]. Yet, even with the current screening recommendations, 24% of all advanced neoplasms are not detected within the study populations. Practical considerations are compliance difficulties, demonstrated by only 50% compliance in study settings [40].

Barium enema

No studies to date have evaluated the efficacy of barium enema for colorectal cancer screening. Appealing qualities are its relatively low cost and ability to examine the entire colon. Double-contrast barium enema (DCBE) is less effective than colonoscopy in detecting polyps and cancer [41,42]. The reported sensitivity of DCBE for detection of polyps is 55% to 80% [42]. In the National Polyp Study, barium enema did not detect 50% of polyps larger than 1 cm, which are considered to be high risk [16]. The American College of Gastroenterology (ACG) currently does not endorse the use of barium enema as a primary screening tool [9]. DCBE is also less accurate than colonoscopy for postpolypectomy surveillance; it detects only 35% of polyps seen at colonoscopy [43]. Barium enema seems appropriate for the detection of colorectal cancer only if colonoscopy cannot completed.

Colonoscopy

Colonoscopy is considered the most effective screening tool for colorectal cancer. In a retrospective study of 2193 patients with colorectal cancer in whom colonoscopy and barium enema were performed, colonoscopy had significantly higher sensitivity than barium enema (95% versus 83%, respectively) [42]. Additionally, after adjusting for the skill and training of the endoscopist, the sensitivity of colonoscopy in detecting colorectal cancer may be even greater (97% within those performed by a gastroenterologist versus 87% within those performed by other practitioners) [42]. Recent studies have focused attention on the need for full evaluation of the proximal colon [8,44]. In these well-designed studies, 26% of patients who had only trivial left-sided polyps had proximal neoplasms. These lesions would have been missed with traditional FOBT and flexible sigmoidoscopic screening. Despite the thorough examination and therapeutic capabilities, there are concerns over the risk and cost-effectiveness of screening colonoscopy [40,45]. Recently, Medicare approved reimbursement for colonoscopic colorectal cancer screening at 10-year intervals in persons at average risk.

Cost-effectiveness

Several analyses demonstrate that cost-effectiveness among the various methods of screening is similar. Twenty thousand dollars per year of life saved is generally considered to be the standard for cost-effectiveness [19]. A model developed in 1996 estimated the cost-effectiveness of the various screening strategies, and it appears to be approximately $25,000 per year of life saved [19,45].

Screening recommendations

The earlier box shows recommended colorectal cancer screening strategies. Guidelines for colorectal cancer screening continue to change as newer data become available. In 1996, the United States Preventive Task Force developed new guidelines that recommend FOBT every year, sigmoidoscopy every 5 years, or a combination of the two, because the data were felt to be inadequate to determine which modality was superior. No recommendations were made regarding digital rectal examination, barium enema, or colonoscopy [19].

The most comprehensive screening review was performed in 1997 by the American Gastroenterological Association and the Federal Agency for Health Care Policy and Research [20]. Recommendations for asymptomatic persons aged 50 or older and at average risk are as follows: annual FOBT or flexible sigmoidoscopy every 5 years, based on strong evidence; annual FOBT and flexible sigmoidoscopy every 5 years on the basis of theoretical findings; DCBE every 5 to 10 years or colonoscopy every 10 years, based on strong rationale [2,20].

The American Cancer Society developed a third set of recommendations in 1997 for asymptomatic, average risk persons starting at 50 years that includes annual FOBT and sigmoidoscopy every 5 years [22]. In 2000, The American Society for Gastrointestinal Endoscopy sanctioned the recommendations listed above with the caveat that DCBE is inferior to colonoscopy [21]. The ACG preferentially recommended colonoscopy every 10 years but also endorsed annual FOBT and flexible sigmoidoscopy every 5 years [9].

Familial risk and colon cancer

Familial clustering of colorectal cancer is common but derives from known inherited syndromes in only 1% to 3% of patients. Fig. 4 shows the proportion of

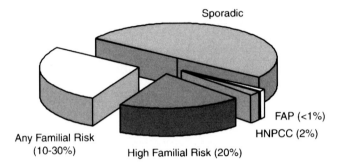

Fig. 4. Familial clustering of colorectal cancer. (*From* Burt RW. Colon cancer screening. Gastro-enterology 2000;119:837–53.)

colorectal cancers attributable to familial clustering, and Table 4 shows the magnitude of risk in various situations. Colorectal cancer risk is equivalent between a 40-year-old person with an affected first-degree relative and a 50-year-old person without a family history [46–49]. Additionally, persons with a family history of adenomas in a first-degree relative are at increased risk for colorectal malignancy [47]. The corollary also holds true in that persons with a first-degree relative with colorectal cancer are at greater risk for adenomas than the general population [47–49].

Certain factors increase the risk for cancer within first-degree relatives of affected probands. The younger the diagnosis of cancer in the proband, the greater the risk in the first-degree relative. In addition, the greater the number of relatives, the greater the risk. Second-degree relatives of patients with colorectal cancer are also at greater risk for colorectal cancer. All sites within the colon confer similar risk to relatives [50].

Adenomatous polyps also cluster in families [47,51]. The National Polyp Study demonstrated almost a twofold-increased risk in first-degree relatives of a proband with adenomas. The relative risk increased to 2.6 if diagnosis was made when the proband was younger than 60 years of age [51]. Another study found an odds ratio of 2.6 for high-risk adenomas in first-degree relatives of affected probands [52].

Etiology of familial risk

Familial risk for colorectal cancer likely stems from genetic determinants that increase susceptibility to environmental factors. Spouses of persons at increased familial risk for colorectal neoplasms are not at increased risk [4,53]. It appears that 10% to 30% of colorectal cancers result from an inherited predisposition [54]. A number of genes and chromosomal loci appear to be involved in inherited predisposition. Attenuated adenomatous polyposis coli (AAPC) and the I1307K APC mutation in the Ashkenazi Jewish population are mutations of the APC gene. Mutations in AAPC lead to a milder form of colorectal cancer predisposition than in classical FAP and may have a phenotype similar to that of sporadic colorectal cancers [54–57]. The Ashkenazi phenotype designated by this genetic mutation is no different from that of sporadic colorectal cancer.

Mutations of the *MSH6 MMR* gene have been found in 7% of patients with a family history of colon cancer [54,58]. MMR genes are responsible for a significant fraction of familial colon cancers that develop in older persons. Type I transforming growth factor receptor allele (TBR-I [6A]) is associated with colon cancer susceptibility. Higher percentages of homozygotes and heterozygotes with this allele are found in colon cancer patients than in controls [58,59].

Surveillance recommendations for persons at increased familial risk

Having a high-risk family history is defined as having a first-degree relative with cancer or adenoma diagnosed when the relative was younger than 60 or having two first-degree relatives diagnosed with colorectal cancer at any age. All current surveillance recommendations are empiric. Persons with a single first-degree relative with colorectal cancer diagnosed after the age of 50 should undergo the same surveillance as persons at average risk, but they should begin at 40 rather than 50 years of age [48,60]. This is because the risk in such a person is increased to a magnitude similar to that for an average-risk person at 50, as shown in Fig. 5 [49].

The American Cancer Society recommends full colonoscopy for persons with first-degree relatives who had adenomas or cancer diagnosed before they were 60 and for those with 2 or more first-degree relatives with colorectal cancer [22]. This screening should start at the age of 40 years or at 10 years younger

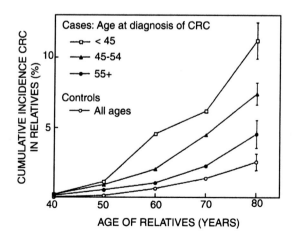

Fig. 5. Cumulative incidence of colorectal cancer in first-degree relatives by age at diagnosis in probands and control patients. CRC, colorectal cancer. (*From* St John JB, McDermott FT, Hopper JL, et al. Cancer risk in relatives of patients with common colorectal cancer. Ann Intern Med 1993;118:785–90; with permission).

Table 5
Colorectal cancer screening recommendations for people with familial risk

Familial risk	Recommendation
Second- or third- degree relatives with colon cancer	Same as average risk
First-degree relative with colon cancer or adenomatous polyps diagnosed at older than 59 years	Same as average risk but begin at age 40 years
Two or more first-degree relatives with colon cancer or adenomatous polyps diagnosed at age younger than 60 years	Colonoscopy every 5 years beginning at age 40 years or 10 years younger than the earliest diagnosis in the family, whichever comes first

From Burt RW. Colon cancer screening. Gastroenterology 2000;119:837–53.

than the age at diagnosis of the youngest affected relative. Full colonoscopic examination is advised every 5 years after that if no neoplasms are found. Table 5 outlines colorectal cancer surveillance recommendations in people with increased familial risk.

Inherited syndromes and screening

Familial adenomatous polyposis

FAP is characterized by the development of multiple adenomas within the colon at a young age. This syndrome accounts for only 0.5% of colorectal carcinomas. Colorectal cancer occurs in all affected persons if colectomy is not performed. Familial adenomatous polyposis arises from germline mutations of the APC gene and is inherited in an autosomal dominant fashion. The mean age for polyp development is 16 years, and for colorectal cancer diagnosis it is 39 years [61,62]. Other gastrointestinal manifestations of FAP include multiple gastric fundic gland polyps (hamartomas) and duodenal and ampulla of Vater neoplasms [10,62]. Upper endoscopy is recommended every 1 to 3 years starting at age 20 to 25 years [54].

Variants of FAP include Gardner syndrome, which includes gastrointestinal polyps and extraintestinal tumors, among them osteomas, epidermoid cysts, fibromas, and desmoid tumors [62]. Various subtypes of Gardner syndrome include congenital hypertrophy of the retinal pigment epithelium. Two thirds of the occurrences of Turcot syndrome arise from APC mutations and have the FAP phenotype with CNS malignancies [63]. Finally, there is AAPC, a milder form of FAP with fewer polyps, later onset, and decreased risk for colorectal malignancy than classical FAP [54,64].

Colorectal cancer surveillance for these syndromes is performed with genetic tests and interval endoscopies. APC gene mutations are detected in 80% to 90% of affected patients [61]. Once a mutation is detected in a proband, protein truncation genetic testing of family members can be performed with virtually 100% accuracy [54,63,64]. Genetic testing should be considered in anyone with 100 or more synchronous colorectal adenomatous polyps, anyone with 20 or more metachronous colorectal adenomas, and anyone who is a first-degree relative of a patient with known FAP or AAPC and who is 10 years of age or older [54,63,64]. It should be emphasized that negative findings on a protein truncation test of the first tested family member does not rule out the disease. Professional genetic counseling with informed consent is imperative before genetic testing. Patients and physicians must be able to understand how to appropriately use genetic testing and to better understand its advantages and risks.

Once affected patients have been identified, sigmoidoscopic surveillance should be initiated at approximately the age of 10 years [64–66]. Sigmoidoscopy is adequate for screening in classical FAP because the numerous adenomas are evenly distributed throughout the colon and rectum. Persons with, or at risk for, AAPC should have annual colonoscopy beginning in the second to third decades of life, depending on the age at which their family members have historically expressed the polyps [64–66]. Colonoscopy is indicated because of a proximal predilection for adenomas.

These guidelines for FAP surveillance are empiric and are based on autosomal dominant inheritance, clinical characteristics, and extreme risk for colorectal cancer. Sigmoidoscopy or colonoscopy is used primarily to recognize the emergence of colonic adenomas so that appropriately timed colectomy may be performed. Prophylactic colectomy is indicated for classical FAP sometime between the diagnosis in childhood and early adulthood and in AAPC, when numerous polyps are detected. Table 6 outlines surveillance guidelines for inherited syndromes.

Hereditary nonpolyposis colorectal cancer

HNPCC, also termed Lynch syndrome, is characterized by multiple family members with colorectal and other cancers. This syndrome accounts for 1% to 3% of all colorectal malignancies. HNPCC encompasses Muir Torre syndrome and approximately one third of cases of Turcot syndrome [67,68]. HNPCC

Table 6
Colorectal cancer surveillance guidelines for inherited syndromes

Syndrome	Recommendation
FAP gene carrier	Sigmoidoscopy annually
	Begin at age 10–12 years
AAPC	Colonoscopy annually
	Begin in late teens or early 20s
HNPCC, gene carrier	Colonoscopy every 1–2 years
	Begin at age 20–25 years or 10 years earlier than youngest affected relative
Peutz-Jeghers	Colonoscopy every 3 years or less
	Begin with symptoms or in the late teens
Juvenile polyposis	Colonoscopy every 3 years or less
	Begin with symptoms or in early teens
Cowden syndrome	No recommendations

FAP, familial adenomatous polyposis; AAPC, attenuated adenomatous polyposis coli; HNPCC, hereditary nonpolyposis colorectal cancer.
From Burt RW. Colon cancer screening. Gastroenterology 2000;119:837–53.

Table 7
Screening recommendations for extracolonic cancers in hereditary nonpolyposis colorectal cancer

Cancer	Recommendation
Endometrial and ovarian cancer	Pelvic examination, transvaginal ultrasound, endometrial aspirate
	Every 1–2 years starting at 25–35 years old
Gastric cancer	Upper gastrointestinal endoscopy
	Every 1–2 years starting at 25–35 years old
Urinary tract and renal cell cancer	Ultrasound and urinalysis
	Every 1–2 years starting at 30–35 years old
Biliary tract cancer	No recommendations
Central nervous system cancer	No recommendations
Small bowel cancer	No recommendations

From Burt RW. Colon cancer screening. Gastroenterology 2000;119:837–53.

derives from mutations of MMR genes, of which 6 are known. Two specific genes (*hMLH1* and *hMSH2*) appear to be responsible for more than 95% of these cases [69]. This condition is primarily transmitted by autosomal dominant inheritance and confers an 80% lifetime risk for colorectal cancer [70]. The average patient age for colorectal cancer diagnosis is 44 years. These neoplasms favor a proximal distribution and often occur with synchronous or metachronous lesions. Other types of cancer are common within these families, among them endometrial, ovarian, gastric, biliary, urinary tract, small bowel, pancreatic, and occasionally others [67]. Recommendations for screening for these extracolonic cancers are found in Table 7.

The clinical diagnosis of HNPCC remains controversial, and the Amsterdam criteria and its revisions are commonly used, as shown in following box. The 3-2-1 rule of diagnostic criteria should be considered: 3 relatives with colon cancer, 2 of whom are first-degree relatives of the third; at least 2 generations affected; and at least one person must be affected before the age of 50 [71].

Genetic testing also is available as a surveillance modality for this syndrome. Testing should be performed early in the second decade of life preferentially on the youngest person most likely to be carrying the gene [68,72]. Nevertheless, if all the Amsterdam criteria are present, the mutation is identified in only 50% of cases and in merely 8% if all the criteria are not met [73]. If no mutation is identified, all relatives must undergo periodic cancer surveillance, as described in Tables 6 and 7.

Prescreening with microsatellite instability (MSI) in a tumor specimen from a family member may be helpful. When an MMR gene is damaged, a replication error may occur during mitosis, and it accumulates throughout the involved tissue. These somatic mutations are easily identified as repeated DNA sequences throughout the genome called microsatellites. The tumor expresses MSI as these errors accumulate, and this can be easily and economically tested. MSI is present in only 15% of sporadic colorectal cancers in almost all such cancers

---

Amsterdam criteria for hereditary nonpolyposis colorectal cancer

Amsterdam I criteria

Three or more relatives with colorectal cancer and all the following:

One person must be a first-degree relative of the other two
At least two successive generations affected
At least one colorectal cancer diagnosed before the age of 50
Familial adenomatous polyposis excluded
Tumors verified by pathologic examination

Amsterdam II criteria

Three or more relatives with hereditary nonpolyposis colorectal cancer-associated and all the following:

One person must be a first-degree relative of the other two
At least two successive generations affected
At least one cancer diagnosed before the age of 50
Familial adenomatous polyposis excluded in patients with colorectal cancer
Tumors verified by pathologic examination

* Colon, rectum, stomach, small bowel, endometrium, ovary, urinary tract
Modified from Vasen HF, Watson P, Mecklin JP, Lynch HT. New clinical criteria for hereditary nonpolyposis colorectal cancer (HPNCC, Lynch syndrome) proposed by the International Collaborative Group on HPNCC. Gastroenterology 1999;116:1453–6; with permission.

---

associated with HNPCC [74]. Genetic testing may be performed on patients with a high family risk even if they do not meet all the Amsterdam criteria. If MSI is present in a tumor, the familial risk for HNPCC is much higher, and germline MMR gene testing is justified [75,76]. MSI testing is suggested for persons who have two first-degree relatives with colorectal cancer or one relative diagnosed before the age of 50, probands with colorectal cancer who have a family history of endometrial or colorectal cancer, and patients with multiple endometrial or colorectal cancers. A recently developed assay uses MSI testing on exfoliated tumor cells in the stool to detect adenomas and cancer. Sensitivity of this assay in the detection of cancer appears to approach 91%, with a specificity of 93%, whereas sensitivity for polyps larger than 1 cm approaches 82% [77].

The Bethesda criteria provide guidelines for genetic testing for HNPCC and recommend indicators for MSI testing, as shown in the following box [78]. Germline MMR gene testing should be performed in a patient who meets the Amsterdam criteria, harbors MSI in colorectal cancer tissue, is a member of a family meeting the first three Bethesda criteria or whose tumor tissue is unavailable for MSI testing, or is a first-degree relative of a person with a known mutation of one of the MMR genes.

Modified Bethesda criteria for hereditary nonpolyposis colorectal cancer

Patients with cancer in families that meet the Amsterdam criteria
Patients with two synchronous or metachronous HNPCC-related criteria
Patients with colorectal cancer *and*
A first-degree relative with colorectal cancer or HNPCC-related extracolonic cancer*, or colorectal adenoma *and*
   A cancer diagnosed before age 50
   An adenoma diagnosed before age 40
Patients with colorectal or endometrial cancer diagnosed before age 45
Patients with right-sided undifferentiated colon cancer diagnosed before age 45
Patients with signet-ring cell type colorectal cancer diagnosed before age 45
Patients with adenomas diagnosed before the age of 40

* Colon, rectum, stomach, small bowel, endometrium, ovary, ureter, and others
Data from Rodriquez-Bigas MA, Boland CR, Hamilton, SR, et al. A National Cancer Institute workshop on hereditary nonpolyposis colorectal cancer syndrome: meeting highlights and Bethesda guidelines. J Natl Cancer Inst 1997;89:1758–62.

Endoscopic surveillance guidelines are based on inheritance and characteristics of the disease. One study demonstrated decreased colorectal cancer incidence and mortality with colonoscopy every 3 years. The age to begin surveillance has been empirically determined based on the finding that most patients with HNPCC acquire colorectal cancer at an average age of 44 years. It should be emphasized that genetic testing is not recommended for all incidences of colorectal cancer because sporadic cases are significantly more frequent than HPNCC [79].

Hamartomatous polyposis syndromes

Peutz-Jeghers syndrome, juvenile polyposis, and Cowden syndrome are autosomal dominant transmitted syndromes manifest by hamartomatous polyps. These syndromes were formerly thought to be benign, but it has been determined they have malignant potential and known germline genetic mutations that can be tested [80–84]. The role of genetic testing in these syndromes is undefined, and the optimal age to begin testing is not established. Colorectal cancer surveillance recommendations for these syndromes are outlined in Table 6.

Peutz-Jeghers syndrome results from a mutation of the *STK11* gene. It has a phenotype of perioral-pigmented spots and multiple hamartomatous small bowel polyps. These polyps may cause benign conditions, such as intussusception, bleeding, and obstruction, in the earlier decades of life. Malignancy becomes a greater concern after the third decade of life, with a 2% to 13% risk for gastrointestinal cancer [54,81]. Extraintestinal malignancies are more common than colorectal cancer and include stomach, duodenum, small bowel, breast, ovary, uterus, pancreas, and testes [81,82]. Surveillance is recommended beginning at age of 10 years, with annual hemoglobin and testicular examination through ultrasound, and for signs of feminization. Biannual upper gastrointestinal endoscopy and small bowel radiographic series should also be performed. At the age of 20 years, annual pelvic examination with Papanicolaou smear and ultrasound are indicated. Annual breast examinations and mammography should be conducted every 2 to 3 years beginning at age 25, and endoscopic or trans-abdominal ultrasound of the pancreas should be performed every 1 to 2 years beginning at age 30 [54].

Juvenile polyposis is diagnosed when a young patient has 10 or more hamartomatous gastrointestinal polyps. These lesions are commonly found within the colon but may develop anywhere within the gastrointestinal tract. Often, the polyps are diagnosed after investigation for rectal bleeding or anemia early in life. Mutations of *SMAD4/DPC4* and *PTEN* genes are present in this condition. Colon cancer develops in up to 50% of affected persons and may arise from these hamartomatous polyps in those as young as 34 [83]. Gastric and duodenal cancers rarely occur, and surveillance with upper gastrointestinal endoscopy beginning in the teenage years is recommended, largely to avoid the complications of benign polyps [54].

Cowden syndrome includes juvenile and other hamartomatous polyps within the colon and throughout the gastrointestinal tract and mucous membranes. It results from a mutation of the *PTEN* gene. Trichilemmomas occur on the face and extremities. Cancers develop in extraintestinal organs, including thyroid in 10%, breast in 50%, and skin, uterus, and ovaries less frequently. Surveillance is recommended, with annual thyroid examination beginning in the second decade of life, annual breast examination beginning at 25 years of age, and annual mammography starting at 30 years [54]. Gastrointestinal malignancy is not established as a major risk in this syndrome, and no specific surveillance is recommended [81,84].

Future directions

Efforts are ongoing to increase public awareness about the benefits of colorectal cancer screening and surveillance. New and improved screening methodologies are also being developed. Present trends are aimed at improving the sensitivity of different FOBTs, genetic-based fecal screening tests, and improved noninvasive colonic imaging.

Fecal occult blood tests

FOBTs with increased sensitivity and specificity are being developed. One criticism in the past has been that the FOBT has low sensitivity and specificity for colorectal cancer. Hemoccult II (Beckman Coulter, Fullerton, CA) is widely used but has only 37% sensitivity (CI, 19.7–54.6%) [85]. A large study recently found Hemoccult II Sensa (Beckman Coulter), a more sensitive, guaiac-based test, to have a 79% sensitivity for cancer (95% CI, 63.0–94.5%). Specificity, however, was greater in Hemoccult II than Hemoccult II Sensa—98% and 87%, respectively [86]. The role of these tests in the era of screening colonoscopy requires careful consideration.

Genetic tests of cellular fecal debris

Genetic tests have a significant role in early screening for colorectal cancer. It has been well established that normal colonic mucosa undergoes a variety of mutations before it becomes malignant tissue. Neoplastic tissues have high turnover rates and thus shed tissue quickly; these exfoliated cells may be detected within the stool. One study examined stool debris for k-*ras*, *p53*, and *APC* mutations in 40 patients, including 21 with colon cancer, 9 with large adenomatous polyps, and 10 controls. All the adenoma patients had negative FOBT findings. Mutations were identified in 16 of 21 colon cancer patients and 7 of 9 adenoma patients. No mutations were identified in the control patients. Therefore, these mutation tests have a sensitivity of 83% and a specificity of 93% for adenomas larger than 1 cm. They provide enhanced detection for carcinomas compared with traditional FOBT [77].

Virtual colonoscopy

Virtual colonoscopy, also termed CT colonography, holds promise for future colorectal cancer screening. Potential advantages are improved patient acceptance, superior safety, possible avoidance of a bowel purge, no need for sedation and analgesia, and rapid performance. Applicability at present is limited by poor sensitivity for small polyps, inability of some patients to maintain a breath hold,

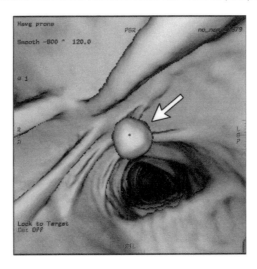

Fig. 6. Virtual colonoscopy (CT olonography) rendered in a 3-dimensional view. The arrow points to a polyp.

high cost, inadequate numbers of trained personnel, and lack of data in a screening setting. There are also issues concerning the significance and outcomes of evaluation for incidentally found extracolonic lesions. This could lead to costly and potentially morbid evaluations for findings of uncertain significance [87]. Patients come to the radiology suite after a bowel purge. Air is insufflated into the rectum, and imaging is performed during a 20- to 30-second breath hold in the supine and prone positions. Thin-sectioned, helical CT uses high-resolution, two-dimensional axial colonic images to reconstruct three-dimensional images that resemble a colonoscopic view (Fig. 6). Time requirements for software processing and interpretation may be lengthy. Most radiologists prefer the two-dimensional view.

Virtual colonoscopy offers a way to visualize the large intestine in the 5% to 10% of patients who are unable to undergo complete conventional colonoscopy [88]. When compared in a masked fashion with colonoscopy in 100 patients at high risk, virtual colonoscopy detected all cancers and 20 of 22 polyps larger than 1 cm, for a sensitivity and specificity of 96% [88]. Another recent study in high-risk patients demonstrated a 90% sensitivity of virtual colonoscopy for the detection of any polyp within the colon [89]. Patient tolerance of the procedure was good. Other studies have produced mixed results, with sensitivities for the detection of large adenomas varying from less than 50% to greater than 90% with variable patient satisfaction [90–92]. In follow-up interviews, many patients express either no preference or preference for conventional endoscopic colonoscopy [92,93].

New techniques include tagging the stool in vivo to eliminate the need for a bowel purge and developing electronic methods to detect lesions to minimize the interpretation time and expense required for this examination. Early results for magnetic resonance colonography appear promising [93].

Summary

Secondary prevention of colorectal cancer with FOBT and endoscopy with polypectomy decreases cancer deaths. Other available modalities include genetic tests and imaging studies, but outcomes data are not yet available. Issues remain concerning the most appropriate test, the optimal intervals, and cost-efficacy. Patients may be stratified by personal and family risk, and specific strategies may be used. Newer developments in genetic tests and imaging, including virtual colonoscopy, hold promise for the future. The most important issue at present is to have people screened or surveilled by any of the recommended modalities.

References

[1] Greenlee RT, Hill-Harmon MB, Murray T, et al. Cancer statistics, 2001. CA Cancer J Clin 2001;51:15–36.
[2] Winawer SJ, Fletcher RH, Miller L, et al. Colorectal cancer screening: clinical guidelines and rationale. Gastroenterology. 1997;112:594–642.
[3] Winawer SJ. Natural history of colorectal cancer. Am J Med 1999;10(1A):3S-6S,50S-57S.
[4] Cannon-Albright L, Bishop DT, Samowitz WS, et al. Colorectal polyps in an unselected population: prevalence, characteristics, and associations. Am J Gastroenterol 1994;89:827–31.
[5] DiSario JA, Foutch PG, Mai HD, et al. Prevalence and malignant potential of colorectal polyps in asymptomatic, average risk men. Am J Gastroenterol 1991;86:941–5.
[6] Beahrs OH. Handbook for staging of cancer. Manual for staging of cancer. 4th edition. Philadelphia: JB Lippincott; 1993.
[7] O'Brien MJ, Winawer SJ. Patient and polyp characteristics associated with high-grade dysplasia in colorectal adenomas. Gastroenterology 1990;98:371–9.
[8] Lieberman DA, Weiss DG, Bond J, et al. Use of colonoscopy to screen asymptomatic adults for colorectal cancer. N Engl J Med 2000;343:162–9.
[9] Rex DK, Johnson DA, Lieberman DA, et al. Colorectal cancer prevention 2000: screening recommendations of the American College of Gastroenterology. Am J Gastroenterol 2000;95: 868–77.
[10] Chu DZT, Giacco G, Martin RG, et al. The significance of synchronous carcinoma and polyps in colorectal cancer. Cancer 1986;59:445–51.
[11] Foutch PG, DiSario JA, Pardy K, Mai HD. The sentinel hyperplastic polyp – a marker for synchronous neoplasia in the proximal colon. Am J Gastroenterol 1991;86:1482–5.
[12] Khullar SK, DiSario JA. Colon cancer screening: sigmoidoscopy or colonoscopy. Gastrointest Endosc Clin North Am 1997;7:365–86.
[13] Winawer SJ, Zauber AG, Ho MN, et al. Prevention of colorectal cancer by colonoscopic polypectomy. N Engl J Med 1993;329:1977–81.
[14] Wexner SD, Garbus JE, Singh JJ. A prospective analysis of 13,580 colonoscopies. Surg Endosc 2001;15:251–61.
[15] Atkin WS, Morson BC, Cunak J. Long-term risk of colorectal cancer after excision of rectosigmoid adenomas. N Engl J Med 1992;326:658–62.
[16] Winawer SJ, Zauber AG, O'Brien MJ, et al. Randomized comparison of surveillance intervals after colonoscopic removal of newly diagnosed adenomatous polyps. N Engl J Med 1993;238: 901–6.

[17] Rex DK, Lehman GM, Ulbright TM, et al. The yield of second screening flexible sigmoidoscopy in average risk persons after one negative examination. Gastroenterology 1994;106:593–5.
[18] Ries LAG, Kosary CL, Hankey BF, Miller BA, Edwards NK. editors. SEER Cancer Statistics, 1973–1995. Bethesda: National Cancer Institute; 1998.
[19] US Preventive Services Task Force. Guide to clinical preventative. 2nd edition. Baltimore: Williams & Wilkins; 1996.
[20] Agency for Health Care Policy and Research. Colorectal cancer screening: technical review 1. Rockville, MD: AHCPR Publication 98–0033; May 1998.
[21] American Society for Gastrointestinal Endoscopy. Guidelines for Colorectal Cancer Screening and Surveillance. Gastrointest Endosc 2000;51:777–82.
[22] Smith RA, Mettlin CJ, Davis KJ, et al. American Cancer Society guidelines for the early detection of cancer. CA Cancer J Clin 2000;50:34–49.
[23] Muto T, Bussey HJR, Morson BC. The evolution of cancer of the colon and rectum. Cancer 1975; 36:2251–70.
[24] Gillen CD, Walmsley RS, Prior P, et al. Ulcerative colitis and Crohn's disease: a compilation of colorectal cancer risk in extensive colitis. Gut 1994;35:1590–2.
[25] Lewis JD, Deren JJ, Lichenstein GR. Cancer risk in patients with IBD. Gastroenterology Clin North Am 1999;28:459–71.
[26] Mandel JS, Bond JH, Church TR, et al. Reducing mortality from colorectal cancer by screening for fecal occult blood. N Engl J Med 1993;328:1365–71.
[27] Greenber PD, Cello JP, Rockey DC. Relationship of low-dose aspirin to GI injury and occult bleeding: a pilot study. Gastrointest Endosc 1999;50:618–22.
[28] Ransohoff DF, Lang CA. Screening for colorectal cancer with fecal occult blood test; a background paper. Ann Intern Med 1997;126:811–22.
[29] Church TR, Ederer F, Mandel JS. Fecal occult blood screening in the Minnesota study: sensitivity of the screening test. J Natl Cancer Inst 1997;89:1440–8.
[30] Hardcastle JD, Chamberalin JO, Robinson MHE, et al. Randomized controlled trial of fecal occult blood screening for colorectal cancer. Lancet 1996;348:1472–7.
[31] Kronborg O, Fenger C, Olsen J, et al. Randomized study of screening for colorectal cancer with fecal occult blood test. Lancet 1996;348:1467–71.
[32] Mandel JS, Church TR, Ederer F, Bond J. Colorectal cancer mortality: effectiveness of biennial screening for fecal occult blood. J Natl Cancer Inst 1999;91:434–7.
[33] Winawer SJ, Flehinger BH, Schottenfeld D, et al. Screening for colorectal cancer with fecal occult blood testing and sigmoidoscopy. J Natl Cancer Inst 1993;85:1311–8.
[34] Selby JV, Friedman GD, Quesenberry CP, et al. Effect of fecal occult blood testing on mortality from colorectal cancer: a case-control study. Ann Int Med 1993;118:1–6.
[35] Newcomb PA, Norfleet RG, Storer BE, et al. Screening sigmoidoscopy and colorectal cancer mortality. J Natl Cancer Inst. 1992;84:1572–5.
[36] Selby J, Friedman GD, Quesenberry CP, et al. A case-control study of screening sigmoidoscopy and mortality from colorectal cancer. N Engl J Med 1992;326:653–7.
[37] Muller AD, Sonnenberg A. Prevention of colorectal cancer by flexible endoscopy and polypectomy: a case-control study of 32,702 veterans. Ann Intern Med 1995;123:904–10.
[38] Stryker SJ, Wolff BG, Culp CE, et al. Natural history of untreated colonic polyps. Gastroenterology 1987;93:1009–13.
[39] Lieberman DA, Weiss DG. One time screening for colorectal cancer with combined fecal occult-blood testing and examination of the distal colon. N Engl J Med 2001;345:555–60.
[40] Vijan S, Hwang EW, Hofer TP, et al. Which colon cancer screening test? a comparison of costs, effectiveness, and compliance. Am J Med 2001;111:593–601.
[41] Schrock TR. Colonscopy versus barium enema for the diagnosis of colorectal cancer and polyps. Gastrointest Endosc Clin North Am 1993;3:585–610.
[42] Rex DK, Rahmani EY, Haseman JH, et al. Relative sensitivity of colonoscopy and barium enema for detection of colorectal cancer in clinical practice. Gastroenterology. 1997;112: 117–23.

[43] Winawer SJ, Stewart ET, Zauber AG, et al. A comparison of colonoscopy and double contrast barium enema for surveillance after polypectomy. N Engl J Med 2000;324:1766–72.
[44] Imperiale TF, Wagner DR, Lin CY, et al. Risk of advanced proximal neoplasms in asymptomatic adults according to the distal colorectal finding. N Engl J Med 2000;343:169–74.
[45] Lieberman DA. Cost-effectiveness of colon cancer screening. Gastroenterology 1995;109: 1781–90.
[46] Fuchs CS, Giovannucci EL, Colditz G, et al. A prospective study of family history and risk of colorectal cancer. N Engl J Med 1994;331:1669–74.
[47] Ahsan H, Neugut AI, Garbowski GC, et al. Family history of colorectal adenomatous polyps and increased frisk for colorectal cancer. Ann Intern Med 1998;128:900–5.
[48] Burt RW. Screening of patients with a positive family history of colorectal cancer. Gastrointest Endosc Clin North Am 1997;7:65–79.
[49] St John JB, McDermott FT, Hopper JL, et al. Cancer risk in relatives of patients with common colorectal cancer. Ann Intern Med 1993;118:785–90.
[50] Kune GA, Kune S, Watson LA. The Melbourne colorectal cancer study: characterization of patients with a family history of colorectal cancer. Dis Colon Rectum 1987;30:600–6.
[51] Winawer SJ, Zauber AG, Gerdes H. Risk of colorectal cancer in families of patients with adenomatous polyps. N Engl J Med 1996;334:82–7.
[52] Pariente A, Milan C, Lafor J, et al. Colon screening in first-degree relatives of patients with sporadic colorectal cancer: a case-control study. Gastroenterology 1998;115:7–12.
[53] Jensen OM, Sigtryggsson P, Nguyen-Dinh X, et al. Large bowel cancer in married couples in Sweden: a follow-up study. Lancet 1988;2:1161–3.
[54] Burt RW. Colon cancer screening. Gastroenterology 2000;119:837–53.
[55] Spirio L, Olschwang S, Groden J, et al. Alleles of the APC gene: an attenuated form of familial polyposis. Cell 1993;75:951–7.
[56] Soravia C, Berk T, Madlensky L, et al. Genotype-phenotype correlations in attenuated polyposis coli. Am J Hum Genet 1998;62:1290–301.
[57] Laken SJ, Peterson GM, Gruber SB, et al. Familial colorectal cancer in Ashkenazi due to a hypermutable tract in APC. Nat Genet 1997;17:79–83.
[58] Kolodner RD, Tytell JD, Schmeits JL, et al. Germ-line MSH6 mutations in colorectal cancer families. Cancer Res 1999;59:5068–74.
[59] Pasche B, Kolachana P, Nafa K, et al. TBR-1 is a candidate tumor susceptibility allele. Cancer Res 1999;59:5678–82.
[60] American Society for Gastrointestinal Endoscopy. Colonoscopy in the screening and surveillance of individuals at increased risk for colorectal cancer. Gastrointest Endosc 1998;48:676–8.
[61] King JE, Dozois RR, Lindor NM, et al. Care of patients and their families with familial adenomatous polyposis. Mayo Clin Proc 2000;75:57–67.
[62] Guillem JG, Smith AJ, Culle J, Ruo L. Gastrointestinal polyposis syndromes. Curr Prob Surg 1999;36:219–23.
[63] Hamilton SR, Liu B, Parsons RE, et al. The molecular basis of Turcot's syndrome. N Engl J Med 1995;332:839–47.
[64] Powell SM, Peterson GM, Krush AJ, et al. Molecular diagnosis of familial adenomatous polyposis. N Engl J Med 1993;329:1982–7.
[65] Giardiello FM, Brensinger JD, Petersen GM, et al. The use and interpretation of commercial APC gene testing for familial adenomatous polyposis. N Engl J Med 1997;336:823–7.
[66] Giardiello FM. Genetic testing in hereditary colorectal cancer. JAMA 1997;278:1278–81.
[67] Lynch HT, Smyrk T. Hereditary nonpolyposis colorectal cancer (Lynch syndrome): an updated review. Cancer 1996;78:1149–67.
[68] Giardiello FM, Brensinger JD, Peterson GM. American Gastroenterological Association technical review: hereditary colorectal cancer and genetic testing. Gastroenterology 2001;121:198–213.
[69] Lynch HT, Smyrk TC, Watson P, et al. Genetics, natural history, tumor spectrum, and pathology of hereditary nonpolyposis colorectal cancer: an updated review. Gastroenterology 1993;104: 1535–49.

[70] Marra G, Boland CR. Hereditary nonpolyposis colorectal cancer: the syndrome, the genes, and historical perspective. J Natl Cancer Inst 1995;87:1114–25.

[71] Vasen HF, Watson P, Mecklin JP, Lyncj HT. New clinical criteria for hereditary nonpolyposis colorectal cancer (HPNCC, Lynch syndrome) proposed by the International Collaborative group on HPNCC. Gastroenterology 1999;116:1453–6.

[72] Burke W, Petersen G, Lynch P, et al. Recommendations for follow up of individuals with an inherited predisposition to cancer, I: hereditary nonpolyposis colon cancer. JAMA 1997;277: 915–19.

[73] Winjen JT, Vasen HFA, Khan M, et al. Clinical findings with implications for genetic testing in families with clustering of colorectal cancer. N Engl J Med 1998;229:511–8.

[74] Thibodeau SN, French AJ, Cunningham JM, et al. Microsatellite instability in colorectal cancer: different mutator phenotypes and the principal involvement of hMLH1. Cancer Res 1998;58: 1713–8.

[75] Aaltonen LA, Salovaara R, Kristo P, et al. Incidence of hereditary nonpolyposis colorectal cancer and feasibility of molecular screening for the disease. N Engl J Med 1998;338:1481–7.

[76] Loukola A, de la Chapelle A, Aaltonen LA. Strategies for screening for hereditary nonpolyposis colorectal cancer. J Med Genet 1999;36:819–22.

[77] Ahlquist DA, Skoletsky JE, Boynton KA, et al. Colorectal cancer screening by detection of altered human DNA in stool: feasibility of a multi-target assay system. Gastroenterology 2000; 119:1219–27.

[78] Rodriquez-Bigas MA, Boland CR, Hamilton SR, et al. A National Cancer Institute workshop on hereditary nonpolyposis colorectal cancer syndrome: meeting highlights and Bethesda guidelines. J Natl Cancer Inst 1997;89:1758–62.

[79] Samowitz W, Slattery M, Kerber RA. Microsatellite instability in human colonic cancer is not a useful clinical indicator of familial colorectal cancer. Gastroenterology 1995;109:1765–71.

[80] Entius MM, Westerman AM, van Velthuysen ML, et al. Molecular and phenotypic markers of hamartomatous polyposis syndromes in the gastrointestinal tract. Hepatogastroenterology 1999; 46:661–6.

[81] McGarrity TJ, Kulin HE, Zaino RJ. Peutz-Jeghers Syndrome. Am J Gastroenterol 2000;95: 596–604.

[82] Tomlinson IPM, Houlston RS. Peutz-Jeghers syndrome. J Med Genet 1997;34:1007–11.

[83] Desai DC, Murday V, Phillips RKS, et al. A survey of phenotypic features in juvenile polyposis. J Med Genet 1998;35:476–81.

[84] Eng C. Cowden syndrome. J Genet Counsel 1997;6:181–92.

[85] Greenberg PD, Bertario L, Gnauck R, et al. A prospective multicenter evaluation of new fecal occult blood tests in patients undergoing colonoscopy. Gastroenterology 2000;95:1331–8.

[86] Allison JE, Tekawa IS, Ransom LJ, et al. A comparison of fecal occult blood tests for colorectal cancer surveillance. N Engl J Med 1996;234:155–59.

[87] Edwards JT, Wood CJ, Mendelson RM, et al. Extracolonic findings at virtual colonoscopy: implications for screening programs. Am J Gastroenterol 2001;96:3009–12.

[88] Fenlon HM, Nunes DP, Schroy PC III, et al. A comparison of virtual and conventional colonoscopy for the detection of colorectal polyps. N Engl J Med 1999;341:1496–503.

[89] Yee J, Akerkar GA, Hung RK, et al. Colorectal neoplasia: performance characteristics of CT colography for detection in 300 patients. Radiology 2001;219:685–92.

[90] Rex D. Virtual colonoscopy: time for some tough questions for radiologists and gastroenterologists. Endoscopy 2000;32:260–3.

[91] Johnson CD, Dachman AH. CT colography: the next colon screening examination. Radiology 2000;216:331–41.

[92] Kay CL, Kulling D, Hawes RH, et al. Virtual endoscopy: comparison with colonoscopy in the detection of space-occupying lesions within the colon. Endoscopy 2000;32:226–32.

[93] Forbes GM, Mendelson RM. Patient acceptance of virtual endoscopy. Endoscopy 2000;32: 274–5.

Hematol Oncol Clin N Am
16 (2002) 867–874

HEMATOLOGY/
ONCOLOGY
CLINICS OF
NORTH AMERICA

Colonoscopy and polypectomy

Douglas Nelson, MD*

Department of Gastroenterology, Veterans Affairs Medical Center, Minneapolis, MN 55417, USA
Department of Medicine, University of Minnesota, Minneapolis, MN 55417, USA

Flexible fiberoptic endoscopy of the colon was first described in 1968 [1]. Since that time, endoscopic technology has advanced considerably. The most commonly used instruments for colonoscopy rely on video chip technology, which has allowed a tremendous increase in the quality and resolution of the image. Colonoscopy is now widely accepted, and millions of procedures are performed annually in the United States. The purpose of the present review is to familiarize the non-endoscopist with the basic principles involved with colonoscopy.

Role of colonoscopy in colorectal cancer

Before discussing the technical aspects of colonoscopy, the role of colonoscopy in the treatment of colorectal cancer is reviewed. That role can be loosely divided into four areas:

1. Diagnostic study for patients with symptoms or signs suggestive of colorectal cancer. The highest yield is found for symptoms/signs related to bleeding, such as hematochezia, melena after an upper gastrointestinal source has been excluded, or unexplained iron-deficiency anemia. The lowest yield is found when colonoscopy is performed for abdominal symptoms (without evidence of bleeding) such as abdominal pain, altered bowel habits, or weight loss, and it is similar to the background prevalence of disease in an asymptomatic population [2].
2. Evaluation of a positive finding on a screening test (fecal occult blood testing [FOBT], flexible sigmoidoscopy, or double-contrast barium enema.)
3. Periodic surveillance for adenomas, dysplasia, or cancers in patient populations at high risk (eg, personal or family history of polyps or colorectal

---

* Department of Gastroenterology, Veterans Affairs Medical Center (111D), One Veterans Drive, Minneapolis, MN 55417, USA.

E-mail address: nelso195@tc.umn.edu (D. Nelson).

cancer, hereditary non-polyposis colorectal cancer syndrome, chronic inflammatory bowel disease).
4. Direct screening of asymptomatic persons for colorectal cancer [3].

The latter two indications are the subject of the article by Drs. DiSario and
Peterson in this issue.

The colonoscope

The colonoscope is a complex medical device that supplies images of the
colon to the endoscopist with the aid of two technologies. The fiberoptic
colonoscope uses glass fiber bundles to transmit images of the colon from the
objective lens at the tip of the instrument to an ocular lens viewed by the
endoscopist, much like a telescope. This instrument has largely been supplanted
by the video colonoscope, which incorporates a charge-coupled device at the tip
of the instrument to electronically transmit images to a video monitor. Both types
of endoscopes use fiberoptic bundles to transmit cold light from the base unit or
light source to the tip of the instrument to illuminate the visual field.

From a basic mechanical standpoint, both types of endoscope are similar. Each
consists of an insertion tube, a control section or handpiece, and an umbilical
section that connects the instrument to a cold light source/base unit. The insertion
tube is approximately 170 cm long and is composed of helical metal bands
sheathed by a waterproof plastic cover. The insertion tube contains an air/water
channel to allow the endoscopist to insufflate air into the colon or to spray water
across the lens to clear the visual field of adherent debris and a larger suction
channel to remove air or liquid from the colon, which also serves as the channel
to allow the passage of endoscopic accessories (such as a biopsy forceps or
polypectomy snare) into the lumen of the colon. The control section resembles a
pistol-grip that contains buttons or valves to activate the air/water or suction
features of the colonoscope and control dials that deflect the distal tip of the
instrument (up/down, right/left) to direct the instrument. The umbilical segment
connects the control section to the light source, which also provides pressurized
air and water, and it contains a port to which a suction line is attached.

Preparation for the procedure

The diagnostic accuracy of colonoscopy depends on the quality of mucosal
visualization after cleansing of the colon. This requires that the lumen of the
bowel be evacuated of all solid and liquid contents before the procedure.
Although there is no standard regimen for bowel preparation for colonoscopy,
the two most commonly used methods include polyethylene glycol (PEG) or
sodium phosphate solutions. PEG solutions are osmotically balanced, nonabsorbable electrolyte solutions that cleanse the bowel by simple lavage, without

significant fluid or electrolyte shifts. However, the use of a PEG solution requires patients to drink a large volume of the purgative (usually 4 L), which can be uncomfortable for some patients [4]. Sodium phosphate solutions (or tablets) are hyperosmotic preparations that promote fluid secretion into the bowel lumen to promote evacuation. Although these agents may offer great tolerability [5], they have the potential to alter serum electrolyte levels and to cause intravascular volume depletion; thus, they are contraindicated for patients with renal failure, ischemic heart disease, congestive heart failure, or ascites [6,7]. PEG and sodium phosphate preparations can be accompanied by a plethora of adjunctive agents (eg, magnesium citrate, bisacodyl, senna, metaclopramide) to enhance bowel evacuation. Patients are instructed to discontinue all iron-containing medications approximately 1 week before the procedure because an iron-containing residue coating the wall of the colon can make adequate visualization impossible.

Routine preprocedural laboratory testing is generally not recommended [8]. In the absence of a bleeding disorder, it is unnecessary for the patient to discontinue taking aspirin or other nonsteroidal antiinflammatory agents (NSAIDs) before colonoscopy (though there are no guidelines regarding the newer antiplatelet agents, such as clopidogrel). Anticoagulation therapy with warfarin should be discontinued 3 to 5 days before colonoscopy if polypectomy is anticipated; guidelines for the management of these patients are available [9].

Colonoscopy and polypectomy

After informed consent has been obtained by the endoscopist, which has included a discussion of the risks and benefits of the procedure and alternatives to it, the patient is placed in the left lateral decubitus position on the examination table. Although colonoscopy can be performed without sedation in motivated patients, premedication is almost always administered, most commonly with an opioid (meperidine or fentanyl), a benzodiazepine (diazepam or midazolam), or both. After a digital rectal examination is performed, which also serves to lubricate the anal canal, the instrument is inserted into the rectum. It is beyond the scope of the present text to describe in detail the numerous maneuvers required to advance the insertion tube to the cecum, though a recurrent technique is repeated advancement and withdrawal of the instrument to straighten and foreshorten the colon, in effect "pleating" or "telescoping" the bowel onto the colonoscope. Once the cecum has been reached and carefully inspected, the endoscopist withdraws the instrument. Although some evaluation of the colon does occur during insertion, the most thorough examination occurs as the instrument is withdrawn.

Polyps are generally classified as sessile (broad-based) or pedunculated (attached to the wall of the colon by a stalk of normal mucosa). Once a polyp has been identified, removal is performed using an electrocautery snare. As an electrosurgical generator delivers current, heat is generated in the tissue encircled by the snare, which cuts and coagulates the target tissue. The snare is gradually tightened, and the polyp base is transected. The degree of thermal damage created during polypectomy must balance the need for adequate coagulation of the blood supply feeding the polyp (to prevent bleeding) while avoiding damage to the underlying colon wall that might result in perforation. Retrieval of all resected tissue is attempted for subsequent histologic analysis. Most patients in whom adenomas are resected should undergo surveillance colonoscopy in 3 years; however, patients with large sessile adenomas should undergo repeat colonoscopy in 3 to 6 months to confirm complete resection of all adenomatous tissue [10,11].

The probability of an adenomatous polyp harboring invasive carcinoma is directly related to polyp size and degree of villous component [12]. Invasive carcinomas (cancer cells penetrating the muscularis mucosa) that are contained within the body of a resected polyp are considered malignant polyps. If the cancer is not poorly differentiated, has no evidence of vascular or lymphatic invasion, and contains a free margin of resection, the probability of residual disease is approximately 0.3% for pedunculated polyps and 1.5% for sessile polyps. This must be weighed against the risk for death from elective colonic resection, which ranges from 0.2% in young, healthy patients to more than 5% in elderly patients. Although the risks and benefits must be considered individually for each patient, in general surgical resection of the bowel is not recommended if patients meet the favorable prognostic criteria listed above. The patient should, however, undergo repeat colonoscopy in 1 to 3 months to assess the polypectomy site, especially if the polyp was sessile [10,11,13].

If a suspected carcinoma is identified during colonoscopy, every attempt should be made to complete the examination and to clear the remainder of the colon of other lesions. Approximately 2% to 5% of colorectal carcinomas entail a synchronous malignancy [2,14,15] that would obviously alter the surgical treatment of the patient. Histologic confirmation of the carcinoma is made through endoscopic biopsy of the lesion, which has a reported sensitivity ranging from 57% to 86% [16]. Thus it is clear that if histologic evidence of cancer is not present in a clinically suspicious lesion and tissue diagnosis is needed, the procedure should be repeated and the lesion should undergo another biopsy.

Efficacy

Numerous studies demonstrate the efficacy of screening for colorectal cancer. The final common pathway for indirect colorectal cancer screening strategies, whether FOBT, flexible sigmoidoscopy, or double-contrast barium enema, is colonoscopy. Case-control studies have suggested that FOBT screening, followed by colonoscopy for positive results, reduces mortality from colorectal cancer [17–21]. Stronger evidence is provided by three prospective randomized trials that have demonstrated reductions in mortality using FOBT to screen for colorectal cancer [22–24]. Similarly, case-control studies of sigmoidoscopy also point to a reduction in mortality [25,26]. Although these studies have shown that colorectal cancer screening results in a shift of diagnosed cancers to an earlier and, thus, more curable stage, there is now strong evidence that the detection and removal of adenomatous polyps decreases the incidence of cancer [27–32].

Risk

Although colonoscopy is generally a safe procedure, risks that should be discussed with the patient as an element of informed consent include bleeding, perforation, and death. Four survey studies from the 1970s, comprising nearly 100,000 diagnostic and therapeutic colonoscopies, reported hemorrhage in 0.4% to 0.7% of patients, perforation in 0.2% to 0.4%, and procedural mortality in 0.02% to 0.05% [33–36]. Survey data relying on recall of the practitioner are likely to underestimate procedural complications; however, these surveys were also performed when the procedure was in its infancy. Subsequent studies were remarkably consistent in the complication rates reported: significant bleeding in 0.2% to 1.0%, perforation in 0.0% to 0.2%, and procedural mortality in 0.0% to 0.06% of patients [37–42].

Procedure success

Although seemingly self-evident, procedural success is an important factor. Failure to complete a colonoscopy may necessitate additional procedures, adding to the risk, cost, and discomfort of the patient. In the hands of experienced endoscopists, the frequency of total colonoscopy ranges from 91% to 99% [41,43–48]. In general, female gender appears to be predictor for incomplete or more difficult colonoscopy. Women with a low body mass index or a history of hysterectomy may be at particularly high risk for failure [43–45].

Who does colonoscopy?

It is important to note that the reported success and complication rates described above are derived from centers with experienced endoscopists. In some regions colonoscopy is usually performed by gastroenterologists, but it is also performed by general surgeons, colorectal surgeons, general internists, general practitioners, and family physicians [49]. Success rates and complication rates for colonoscopy performed by physicians who have acquired skills outside traditional training pathways (eg, gastroenterology fellowship) have not been established or validated.

It should be self-evident that competency in any aspect of medicine requires adequate training, and this is particularly true for colonoscopy. Two studies have shown that there is a learning curve to the acquisition of colonoscopic skills by endoscopic trainees [50,51]. Perhaps not surprisingly, two reports from family practice physicians describing their early experiences with colonoscopy reported cecal intubation rates of 36% and 54% in their first 300 cases [52,53]. These rates clearly fall below the current standard for colonoscopy (ie, cecal intubation rate exceeding 90%). Although endoscopic trainees are also likely to be unsuccessful in cecal intubation during the early phase of training, an important difference is that in a supervised training program, the examination will still be completed in more than 90% of patients [47]. When self-taught physicians refine their colono-scopy skills on patients during the learning curve, an incomplete examination has ramifications in terms of additional procedures, risk, patient discomfort and cost.

Summary

Colonoscopy and polypectomy, when performed by adequately trained physi-cians, is a safe and effective procedure that can decrease deaths resulting from colorectal cancer.

References

[1] Overholt BF. Clinical experience with the fibersigmoidoscope. Gastrointest Endosc 1968;15:27.

[2] Rex DK. Colonoscopy: a review of its yield for cancers and adenomas by indication. Am J Gastroenterol 1995;90:353–65.

[3] Lieberman DA, Weiss DG, Bond JH, et al. Use of colonoscopy to screen asymptomatic adults for colorectal cancer. N Engl J Med 2000;343:162–8.

[4] DiPalma JA, Brady CE III. Colon cleansing for diagnostic and surgical procedures: polyethylene glycol-electrolyte lavage solution. Am J Gastroenterol 1989;84:1008–16.

[5] Hsu C-W, Imperiale TF. Meta-analysis and cost comparison of polyethylene glycol lavage versus sodium phosphate for colonoscopy preparation. Gastrointest Endosc 1998;48:276–82.

[6] Huynh T, Vanner S, Paterson W. Safety profile of 5-h oral sodium phosphate regimen for colonoscopy cleansing: lack of clinically significant hypocalcemia or hypovolemia. Am J Gas-troenterol 1995;90:104–7.

[7] Lieberman DA, Ghormley J, Flora K. Effect of oral sodium phosphate colon preparation on serum electrolytes in patients with normal serum creatinine. Gastrointest Endosc 1996;43: 467–9.

[8] ASGE. Position statement on laboratory testing before ambulatory elective endoscopic proce-dures. Gastrointest Endosc 1999;50:906–9.

[9] ASGE. Guideline on the management of anticoagulation and antiplatelet therapy for endoscopic procedures. Gastrointest Endosc 2000;48:672–5.

[10] ASGE. Guidelines for colorectal cancer screening and surveillance. Gastrointest Endosc 2000; 51:777–82.

[11] Bond JH. Polyp guideline: diagnosis, treatment, and surveillance for patients with colorectal polyps. Am J Gastroenterol 2000;95:3053–63.

[12] Simons BD, Morrison AS, Lev R, et al. Relationship of polyps to cancer of the large intestine. J Natl Cancer Inst 1992;84:962–6.

[13] Waye JD, O'Brien MJ. Cancer in polyps. In: Cohen AM, Winawer SJ, Friedman MA, et al, editors. Cancer of the colon, rectum, and anus. New York: McGraw-Hill; 1995. p. 465–76.

[14] Chen H-S, Sheen-Chen S-M. Synchronous and "early" metachronous colorectal adenocarcinoma: analysis of prognosis and current trends. Dis Colon Rectum 2000;43:1093–9.

[15] Langevin JM, Nivatvongs S. The true incidence of synchronous cancer of the large bowel. Am J Surg 1984;147:330–3.

[16] Marshall JB, Diaz-Arias AA, Barthel JS, et al. Prospective evaluation of optimal number of

biopsy specimens and brush cytology in the diagnosis of cancer of the colorectum. Am J Gastroenterol 1993;88:1352–4.

[17] Faivre J, Tazi MA, El Mrini T, et al. Faecal occult blood screening and reduction of colorectal cancer mortality: a case-control study. Br J Cancer 1999;79:680–3.

[18] Saito H, Soma Y, Koeda J, et al. Reduction in risk of mortality from colorectal cancer by fecal occult blood screening with immunochemical hemagglutination test: a case-control study. Int J Cancer 1995;61:465–9.

[19] Selby JV, Friedman GD, Quesenberry CP Jr, et al. Effect of fecal occult blood testing on mortality from colorectal cancer: a case control study. Ann Intern Med 1993;118:1–6.

[20] Wahrendorf J, Robra BP, Wiebelt H, et al. Effectiveness of colorectal cancer screening: results from a population-based case-control evaluation in Saarland, Germany. Eur J Cancer Prev 1993; 1:221–7.

[21] Zappa M, Castiglione G, Grazzini G, et al. Effect of faecal occult blood testing on colorectal mortality: results of a population-based case-control study in the district of Florence, Italy. Int J Cancer 1997;73:208–10.

[22] Hardcastle JD, Chamberlain JO, Robinson MHE, et al. Randomised controlled trial of faecal-occult-blood screening for colorectal cancer. Lancet 1996;148:1472–7.

[23] Kronborg O, Fenger C, Olsen J, et al. Randomised study of screening for colorectal cancer with faecal-occult-blood test. Lancet 1996;348:1467–71.

[24] Mandel JS, Bond JH, Church TR, et al. Reducing mortality from colorectal cancer by screening for fecal occult blood. N Engl J Med 1993;328:1365–71.

[25] Newcomb PA, Norfleet RG, Storer BE, et al. Screening sigmoidoscopy and colorectal cancer mortality. J Natl Cancer Inst 1992;84:1572–5.

[26] Selby JV, Friedman GD, Quesenberry CP, et al. A case-control study of screening sigmoidoscopy and mortality from colorectal cancer. N Engl J Med 1992;326:653–7.

[27] Citarda F, Tomaselli G, Capocaccia R, et al. Efficacy in standard clinical practice of colonoscopic polypectomy in reducing colorectal cancer incidence. Gut 2001;48:812–5.

[28] Mandel JS, Church TR, Bond JH, et al. The effect of fecal occult-blood screening on the incidence of colorectal cancer. N Engl J Med 2000;343:1603–7.

[29] Müller AD, Sonnenberg A. Prevention of colorectal cancer by flexible endoscopy and polypectomy. Ann Intern Med 1995;123:904–10.

[30] Murakami R, Tsukuma H, Kanamori S, et al. Natural history of colorectal polyps and the effect of polypectomy on occurrence of subsequent cancer. Int J Cancer 1990;46:159–64.

[31] Thiis-Evensen E, Hoff GS, Sauar J, et al. Population-based surveillance by colonoscopy: effect on the incidence of colorectal cancer. Scand J Gastroenterol 1999;34:414–20.

[32] Winawer SJ, Zauber AG, Ho MN, et al. Prevention of colorectal cancer by colonoscopic polypectomy. N Engl J Med 1993;329:1977–81.

[33] Berci G, Panish JF, Schapiro M, et al. Complications of colonoscopy and polypectomy. Gastroenterology 1974;67:584–5.

[34] Frühmorgen P, Demling L. Complications of diagnostic and therapeutic colonoscopy in the Federal Republic of Germany: results of an inquiry. Endoscopy 1979;11:146–50.

[35] Rogers BHG, Silvis SE, Nebel OT, et al. Complications of flexible fiberoptic colonoscopy and polypectomy. Gastrointest Endosc 1975;22:73–7.

[36] Smith LE. Fiberoptic colonoscopy: complications of colonoscopy and polypectomy. Dis Colon Rectum 1976;19:407–12.

[37] Anderson ML, Pasha TM, Leighton JA. Endoscopic perforation of the colon: lessons from a 10-year study. Am J Gastroenterol 2000;95:3418–22.

[38] Basson MD, Etter L, Panzini LA. Rates of colonoscopic perforation in current practice. Gastroenterology 1998;114:1115.

[39] Eckardt VF, Kanzler G, Schmitt T, et al. Complications and adverse effects of colonoscopy with selective sedation. Gastrointest Endosc 1999;49:560–5.

[40] Macrae FA, Tan KG, Williams CB. Toward safer colonoscopy: a report on the complications of 5000 diagnostic or therapeutic colonoscopies. Gut 1983;24:376–83.

[41] Waye JD, Bashkoff E. Total colonoscopy: is it always possible? Gastrointest Endosc 1991;37: 152–4.

[42] Zubarik R, Fleischer DE, Mastropietro C, et al. Prospective analysis of complications 30 days after outpatient colonoscopy. Gastrointest Endosc 1999;50:322–8.

[43] Anderson JC, Gonzalez JD, Messina CR, et al. Factors that predict incomplete colonoscopy: thinner is not always better. Am J Gastroenterol 2000;95:2784–7.

[44] Church JM. Complete colonoscopy: how often? and if not, why not? Am J Gastroenterol 1994; 89:556–60.

[45] Cirocco WC. Factors that predict incomplete colonoscopy. Dis Colon Rectum 1995;38:964–8.

[46] Kim WH, Cho YJ, Park JY, et al. Factors affecting insertion time and patient discomfort during colonoscopy. Gastrointest Endosc 2000;52:600–5.

[47] Marshall JB, Barthel JS. The frequency of total colonoscopy and terminal ileal intubation in the 1990s. Gastrointest Endosc 1993;39:518–20.

[48] Ristikankare M, Hartikainen J, Heikkinen M, et al. The effects of gender and age on the colonoscopic examination. J Clin Gastroenterol 2001;32:69–75.

[49] Ackermann RJ. Performance of gastrointestinal tract endoscopy by primary care physicians: lessons from the US Medicare database. Arch Fam Med 1997;6:52–8.

[50] Cass OW, Freeman ML, Cohen J, et al. Acquisition of competency in endoscopic skills (ACES) during training: a multicenter study [abstract]. Gastrointest Endosc 1996;43:308.

[51] Cass OW, Freeman ML, Peine CJ, et al. Objective evaluation of endoscopy skills during training. Ann Intern Med 1993;118:40–4.

[52] Hopper W, Kyker KA, Rodney WM. Colonoscopy by a family physician: a 9-year experience of 1048 procedures. J Fam Pract 1996;43:561–6.

[53] Rodney WM, Dabov G, Cronin C. Evolving colonoscopy skills in a rural family practice. Fam Pract Res J 1993;13:43–52.

HEMATOLOGY/
ONCOLOGY
CLINICS OF
NORTH AMERICA

Hematol Oncol Clin N Am
16 (2002) 875–895

Radiologic imaging modalities in the diagnosis and management of colorectal cancer

Nora Dobos, MD, Stephen E. Rubesin, MD*

*Department of Radiology, MRI Learning Center, 1 Founders,
Hospital of the University of Pennsylvania, 3400 Spruce Street, Philadelphia, PA 19104, USA*

This article describes the roles of various radiologic modalities in the diagnosis, staging, and management of colorectal cancer. Double-contrast barium enema and CT are the primary modalities for diagnosis, staging, and follow-up of colorectal carcinoma. Ultrasound and MRI have managed to carve out specific niches in the management of rectal cancer, whereas ultrasound is the sole modality available intraoperatively. Although emerging technologies, such as positron emission tomography (PET) and CT colonography, offer hope for resolving some of the current dilemmas in diagnosis and management, it is unclear whether they will supplant or simply complement existing radiologic methods.

Screening for colon cancer and the double-contrast barium enema

In most patients, the natural history of colorectal carcinoma follows the adenoma-to-carcinoma sequence over a period of approximately 7 to 20 years, giving rise to an opportunity for early detection of cancer at a curable stage through population-wide screening. Different screening recommendations have emerged from various national organizations, each incorporating some combination of digital rectal examination, screening for fecal occult blood, and morphologic screening with flexible sigmoidoscopy, colonoscopy, or barium enema.

Routine screening is an exercise in polyp detection. Polyps smaller than 5 mm have virtually no malignant potential, whereas those measuring 5 to 10 mm harbor a 1% chance of malignancy. Polyps measuring 10 to 20 mm have a 10% chance of malignancy, and polyps larger than 2 cm have a greater than 45% chance of malignancy [1]. Therefore, the goal for screening is to consistently identify for removal all polyps larger than 10 mm. Only approximately one-third of adenomas

---

* Corresponding author.
  E-mail address: rubesin@oasis.rad.upenn.edu (S.E. Rubesin).

larger than 1 cm develop into colonic carcinoma [2]. The American College of Radiology's recommendation for screening at 5-year intervals with double-contrast barium enema (DCBE) arose out of studies showing the cost-effectiveness of screening DCBE, based on the assumption that a missed 10-mm polyp has the potential for malignant degeneration over 5 years [3,4]. A specific recommendation for a shorter interval of screening may be made if a patient has had a limited examination that precluded the detection of polyps of clinically significant size.

Polyps are detected in 10% to 12.5% of the population screened using DCBE. Overall, 50% to 60% are found in the rectum or sigmoid colon, with the remainder located more proximally [5]. The rate of polyp detection rises from 3% in the 3rd decade to 26% in the 9th decade of life [6]. At the same time, with increasing age, the distribution of polyps shifts to the proximal colon [7]. At our institution, approximately 45% of all colon cancers arise in the cecum, ascending colon, or transverse colon, well out of reach of the flexible sigmoidoscope [8]. Relatively few of these tumors have sentinel polyps in the sigmoid colon. The proximal distribution of cancer and the 5% rate of synchronous lesions argues strongly for complete colonic screening with either colonoscopy or DCBE instead of flexible sigmoidoscopy [9,10].

Debate has been ongoing regarding the efficacy of DCBE versus colonoscopy in detecting clinically significant polyps. Recognizing that both studies are operator dependent, properly performed DCBE is as accurate as colonoscopy in detecting 90% of polypoid lesions larger than 1 cm and in detecting colonic carcinomas [5]. In 1990, a quality assurance study at our hospital showed that the accuracy rate for the detection of colon cancer was 93% with DCBE, effectively identical to the 92% rate achieved with colonoscopy. Our detection rate today is even higher, after a switch to barium with superior mucosal coating. In addition, the colonoscopy detection rate was based only on those segments of the colon that were inspected and excluded the lesions that were missed because the colonoscope did not reach them. The rate of incomplete colonoscopy, prompting further investigation with barium enema, is approximately 10% at our institution, lower than other nationally quoted numbers of 25%. In a more recent series at our hospital, DCBE performed as a result of incomplete colonoscopy detected tumors larger than 1 cm in 3% of patients in areas of the colon not visualized by the endoscope [11].

The chief area of the colon with which DCBE may have difficulty is a sigmoid colon affected by diverticulosis with circular muscle thickening. Thus, in the presence of moderate to severe diverticulosis, colonoscopy is of value as a complementary study to DCBE. The supreme advantage of colonoscopy is the ability to perform a biopsy or remove a lesion. Colonoscopy is associated with a threefold higher cost and a much higher complication rate, such as colonic perforation or hemorrhage and adverse effects of anesthesia [12]. The higher cost and complications of colonoscopy make DCBE a more cost-effective study [4]. The chief drawback of DCBE is that it is not cost-effective for the radiologist. Many radiologists have little interest in performing these studies because they are time and labor intensive and are poorly reimbursed. As a result, the technical quality of DCBE varies widely.

CT colonography (virtual colonoscopy) has emerged in recent years as a potentially viable alternative for future screening for primary colorectal neoplasms. Using two- and three-dimensional surface- and volume-rendering techniques, it is designed to allow noninvasive, complete antegrade and retrograde evaluation of the entire colon. The future of CT colonography hinges on its ability to consistently detect lesions larger than 1 cm and at least approximate the track record of the DCBE [13,14]. Its efficacy is still to be determined in the general screening population. CT colonography is more costly and more time and labor intensive than DCBE. It requires meticulous colonic cleansing and insufflation, as does DCBE, but confers a higher radiation dose. Virtual colonography has significant limitations when compared to DCBE. It achieves lower spatial resolution and less colonic distention, and it precludes the manipulation of residual colonic fluid and debris in real-time, a factor essential in confidently determining the presence or absence of a lesion. There is less contrast between the tumor and

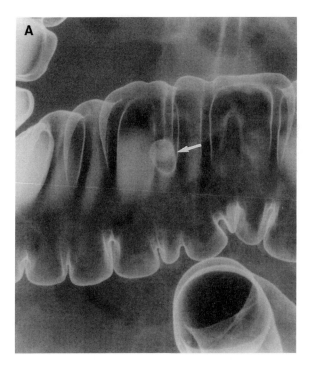

Fig. 1. Tubular adenoma detected during double-contrast barium enema performed in a 51-year-old man with a family history of colon cancer. (A) Spot radiograph obtained with the patient in the supine position shows a 1-cm diameter ring shadow (*arrow*) in the mid-transverse colon. The polyp has been "etched in white by barium." A droplet of barium lies centrally, representing a droplet of barium (stalactite) hanging off this polyp on the anterior wall. (B) Close-up spot radiograph obtained with the patient in a prone position shows a 1-cm radiolucent filling defect (*arrow*) in the barium pool, corresponding to the polyp on the anterior wall of the transverse colon.

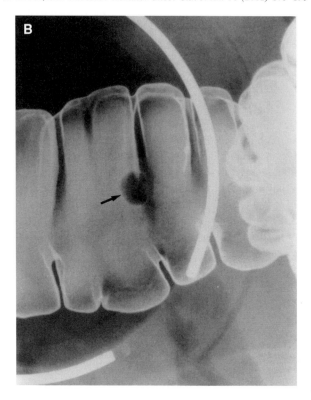

Fig. 1 (*continued*).

the adjacent wall, and the technique fails to demonstrate mucosal detail or the interstices of lesions, characteristics that are helpful in diagnosis. This author believes that CT colonography will become a secondary noninvasive screening method for debilitated patients unable to comply with the physical demands of the DCBE or colonoscopy. CT colonography may prove to be of value for examining portions of the colon proximal to an obstructing lesion that cannot be traversed by a colonoscope or by barium.

Barium enema: technique and findings

DCBE consists of 24-hour patient preparation by which the colon is cleansed of particulate debris by adhering to a 24-hour period of clear liquids followed by cathartic agents the night before and the morning of the examination. The study itself consists of insertion of an enema tip into the patient's rectum through which barium flows into the colon, followed by air insufflation to achieve double contrast. Colonic hypotonia is achieved by the injection of 1 mg glucagon intravenously, thus increasing patient comfort and ease of examination. By guiding patient positioning, the entire colon is visualized and radiographed in

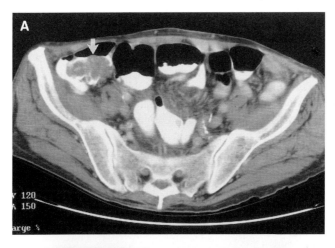

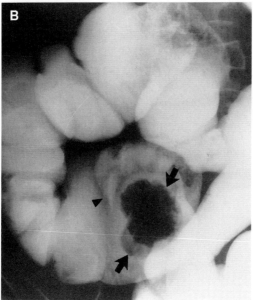

Fig. 2. Villous adenoma incidentally found on CT. CT of the chest demonstrated an adrenal lesion in a 69-year-old-man with a history of malignant thymoma for which CT of the abdomen and pelvis was obtained. (A) Axial CT through the lower abdomen shows an enhancing, polypoid, soft tissue mass (*arrow*) in the cecum. Barium fills the interstices of the tumor. (B) Single-contrast barium enema performed because of the patient's debilitated condition confirms the presence of a 4-cm multilobulated polypoid filling defect (*arrows*) in the barium-filled cecum. The tumor is separate from the ileocecal valve (*arrowhead*).

segments free of overlap, followed by several overhead radiographs. The entire examination lasts approximately 15 to 20 minutes [15].

Polyps have variable appearances on barium enema and may appear as radiolucent filling defects in the barium pool (Fig. 1), contour defects, ring shadows (see Fig. 1), carpet lesions, or bulky polypoid masses (Fig. 2) [5,16–18]. Although certain radiographic appearances suggest a particular histology, such as tubular or villous adenoma, radiographic appearance does not confidently predict histology [8]. Advanced colorectal carcinoma, more commonly detected in the

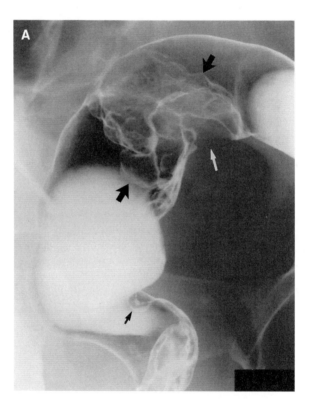

Fig. 3. Incomplete colonoscopy prompting double-contrast barium enema (DCBE) for evaluation of rectal mass before surgery. A 59-year-old woman with rectal bleeding and constipation was found to have a mass at the rectosigmoid junction. DCBE was obtained because of the failure of the colonscope to reach the cecum. (A) Oblique spot radiograph of the rectum confirms a lobulated, near-circumferential mass (*large black arrows*) at the rectosigmoid junction, demonstrating a focal contour defect (*white arrow*) and numerous barium-etched lines outlining the polypoid contours of the mass. An additional polyp (*small black arrow*) on the distal anterior rectal wall is also seen. (B) Oblique spot radiograph of the rectum obtained in a different projection shows the mass (*white arrows*) at the rectosigmoid junction en face, a 3-cm polypoid filling defect (*large black arrows*) in the mid-rectum obscured by the barium pool in panel A, and the distal rectal polyp (*small black arrow*). The patient underwent low anterior resection that showed a poorly differentiated adenocarcinoma with neuroendocrine features with lymphovascular invasion and focal invasion into pericolonic fat. The polypoid lesion in the mid-rectum and the rectal polyp represented submucosal infiltration by the primary tumor.

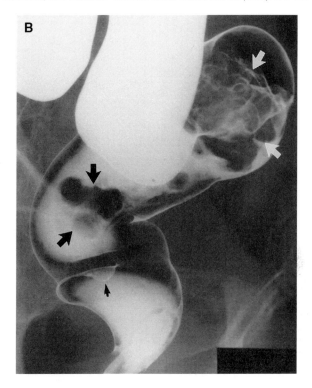

Fig. 3 (*continued*).

symptomatic population, presents on barium enema as an annular or semiannular mass (Fig. 3), polypoid mass, carpet lesion, or plaque-like lesion [5]. An atypical scirrhous pattern of carcinoma can be seen in patients with ulcerative colitis [19]. By the time an adenoma becomes a carcinoma, it is usually a large lesion. At our institution, 95% of colon cancers in symptomatic patients are larger than 2 cm [8].

CT findings

Not infrequently, CT may be the initial examination to detect colon cancer, either incidentally or in a patient evaluated for obstructive symptoms or abdominal pain. The appearance of colorectal carcinoma on CT is variable, ranging from a discrete intraluminal mass (Figs. 2, 4) to focal wall thickening (Fig. 5), whether eccentric or circumferential. Foci of calcification within a mass suggest mucinous histology, whereas areas of low attenuation indicate central necrosis or mucinous pools. Normal colonic wall thickness should not exceed 3 mm in a well-distended segment; thickness greater than 6 mm is considered clearly abnormal. CT is unreliable in determining the depth of mural invasion and, thus, in differentiating a T1 from a T2 lesion [5]. In patients with locally

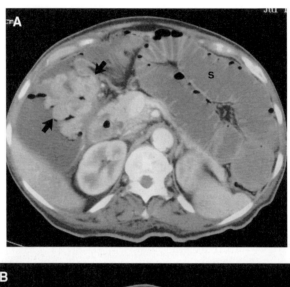

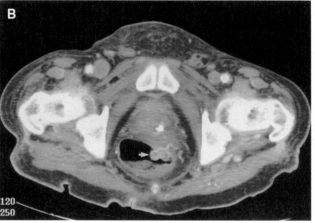

Fig. 4. Advanced colon cancer with synchronous lesion in rectum in a 78-year-old man with symptoms of bowel obstruction. (A) CT scan through the mid-abdomen at the level of the portal vein shows an enhancing polypoid mass (*arrows*) in the hepatic flexure of the colon. Dilatation of small (*s*) and large bowel indicates that this is an obstructing lesion. A moderately differentiated adenocarcinoma invading pericolonic fat, without evidence of regional lymph node metastases, was discovered at right hemicolectomy. (B) CT section through the lower pelvis demonstrates a polypoid-enhancing lesion (*arrow*) in the rectum. Biopsy revealed tubular adenoma.

advanced disease, pericolonic soft tissue stranding suggests tumor infiltration beyond the bowel wall. Visualization of local lymph nodes larger than 1 cm or a cluster of local lymph nodes suggests lymphatic spread [20]. Loss of tissue fat planes also suggests extension beyond the bowel wall, but this finding may be difficult to assess in a thin patient. The only definitive finding of invasion is direct extension into an adjacent muscle or organ. Enhancing fistulous tracts containing extraluminal gas or contrast also indicate locally advanced disease. Bony

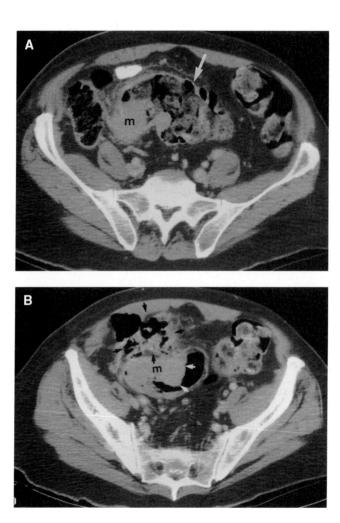

Fig. 5. Detecting and staging colon cancer with CT. A 60-year-old man had left lower quadrant abdominal pain and rectal bleeding. A CT scan was obtained for suspected diverticulitis. (A) CT image through the upper pelvis shows a partially obstructing, enhancing, near-circumferential mass (*m*) in the sigmoid colon. The colon proximal to the lesion is dilated (*arrow*), indicating obstruction. (B) An image slightly more inferior in the pelvis shows extensive pericolonic stranding and an extraluminal gas collection (*black arrows*), consistent with a contained perforation and pericolonic abscess. The edge (*white arrows*) of the colonic mass (*m*) is seen. (C) CT image through the upper abdomen shows bulky, low-attenuation, hepatic mass lesions (*m*) representing metastases. The patient underwent sigmoid colectomy that showed a moderately differentiated adenocarcinoma of the sigmoid colon with angiolymphatic invasion and infiltration of pericolonic fat. A pericolonic abscess containing feculent material was found. Intraoperative liver biopsy confirmed metastatic adenocarcinoma.

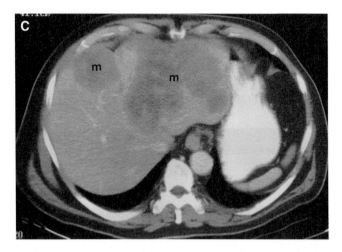

Fig. 5 (*continued*).

invasion in the pelvis ranges from subtle cortical erosion to frank destruction associated with a soft tissue mass [5].

Other colonic tumors

Other primary colonic lesions that may be specifically diagnosed by imaging include hemangiomas or lipomas. Lipomas are smooth-surfaced, variably lobulated, polypoid lesions that change size and shape and show fat attenuation on CT [21–23]. Hemangiomas appear as submucosal infiltrating lesions and are associated with phleboliths in 50% of patients [23]. Primary colonic lymphoma can be suggested by its predilection for the ileocecal region, where it may appear as a polypoid or cavitary mass [24]. Colonic lymphomas may also appear in an annular submucosal form infiltrating or, occasionally, as numerous polypoid lesions [23].

Pericolonic diseases

Many patients have extrinsic disease secondarily involving the colon, and for them CT and DCBE may offer advantages over endoscopy in the evaluation of the colon. This includes patients with diverticulitis, endometriosis, or intraperitoneal metastases. Not infrequently, secondary colonic involvement by another primary tumor can be missed entirely at endoscopy or can be misconstrued as representing a primary colorectal neoplasm (Fig. 6). In contrast, barium enema and cross-sectional imaging with CT are well suited to differentiate primary colorectal carcinoma from secondary involvement by extracolonic malignant and benign processes.

Secondary involvement of the colon by extracolonic neoplasms takes many forms, including direct invasion from contiguous or noncontiguous primary neoplasm, intraperitoneal seeding of metastases, and embolic metastases. Specific sites of involvement on barium enema are suggestive of the type of malignant dissemination.

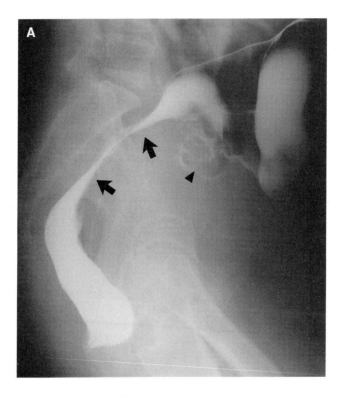

Fig. 6. Pericolonic disease secondarily involving the colon, mimicking primary colon cancer at colonoscopy. A 27-year-old woman with a history of left oophorectomy for germ-cell neoplasm sought treatment for abdominal pain and obstructive symptoms. At colonoscopy, an ulcerated obstructing lesion was encountered in the sigmoid, thought to represent a primary colon carcinoma. Biopsy revealed a poorly differentiated neoplasm. Double-contrast barium enema was then performed. (A) Lateral spot radiography of the rectum shows extrinsic mass effect (*large arrows*) compressing the anterior wall of the rectum and distal sigmoid colon. This extrinsic mass effect was not appreciated at colonoscopy. The adjacent sigmoid colon (*arrowhead*) is abnormal. (B) Coned-down oblique spot radiograph of the sigmoid colon shows destruction of the inferior wall (*arrowheads*) of the mid-sigmoid colon, thought to represent a pelvic mass secondarily invading the colon. (C) A spot radiograph of the junction of the descending and sigmoid colon shows a relatively flat, slightly lobulated, smooth-surfaced implant (*arrows*) along the inferior border of the proximal sigmoid. (D) CT section through the lower pelvis shows an enhancing, centrally necrotic, gas-containing mass (*arrows*) posterior to the urinary bladder (*b*) and to the left of the uterus (*u*), with narrowing of the rectal lumen posteriorly, corresponding to a large pelvic floor implant by recurrent germ-cell neoplasm. (E) CT section through the mid-abdomen at the level of the kidneys shows enhancing omental implants (*arrows*) in the right and left paracolic gutters and ascites in the right paracolic gutter, findings consistent with intraperitoneal seeding of metastases.

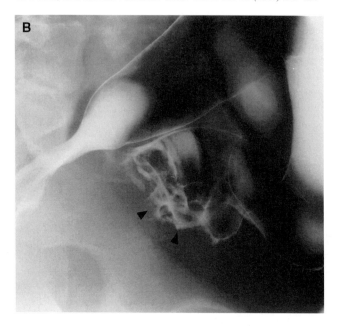

Fig. 6 (*continued*).

Invasion from contiguous primary neoplasm is common with cancers of the prostate, ovary, kidney, uterus, cervix, and gallbladder. Prostatic carcinoma spreads to the anterior border of the rectosigmoid junction and is manifested as mass effect with spiculation and mucosal pleating secondary to serosal desmoplastic reaction [25]. With advanced prostatic metastases, circumferential narrowing of the rectum and widening of the presacral space occur [26]. Left-sided ovarian carcinoma initially invades the inferior border of the sigmoid colon [27]. Carcinoma of the left kidney invades the distal transverse or proximal descending colon, whereas carcinoma of the right kidney invades the duodenum. Renal cell carcinoma usually manifests as a bulky intraluminal mass without obstruction [28].

Direct invasion from noncontiguous neoplasms occurs with gastric and pancreatic carcinomas that spread subperitoneally. Gastric carcinoma spreads through the gastrocolic ligament to the superior border of the transverse colon [27]. Pancreatic carcinoma invades the inferior border of the transverse colon through the transverse mesocolon [28]. Carcinoma of the tail of the pancreas may invade the medial border of the splenic flexure through the phrenicocolic ligament [29].

Intraperitoneal seeding of metastases is common with ovarian (see Fig. 6), gastric, pancreatic, colonic, and breast carcinomas. At sites of metastatic implants involving the colon, there is extrinsic mass effect, spiculation of the contour, and tethering and pleating of the mucosa. Characteristic sites of tumor deposition are determined by patterns of flow of ascitic fluid in the abdomen. The pouch of Douglas in women or the rectovesical space in men are the most frequent sites of

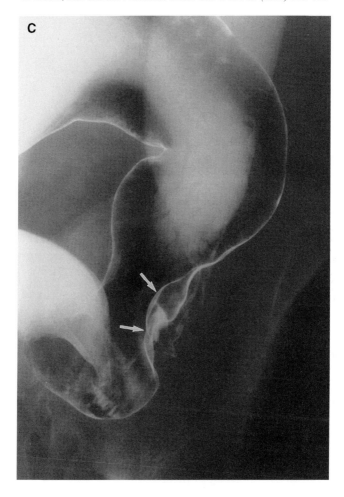

Fig. 6 (*continued*).

metastatic implants because the pelvis is the most dependent portion of the abdomen [30]. Additional sites include the superior border of the sigmoid colon, the medial border of the cecum, the mesenteric border of right lower quadrant ileal loops, and the right paracolic gutter [23]. Evidence of serosal desmoplastic reaction raises additional diagnostic considerations, including endometriosis, diverticulitis with abscess, tubo-ovarian abscess, or contiguous invasion by prostatic or gynecologic malignancy [31].

Staging of colorectal carcinoma

The goal of preoperative staging in patients with known colorectal carcinoma is to assess local disease extent, allow for surgical planning, and select patients

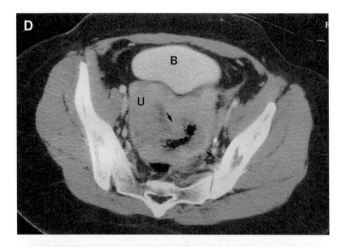

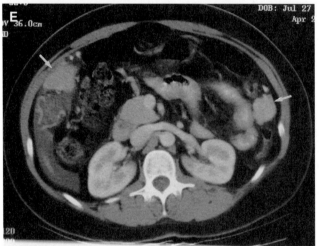

Fig. 6 (*continued*).

who may benefit from preoperative chemotherapy and radiation. Staging is of value in patients with rectal carcinoma to assess involvement of the levator ani and anal sphincter complex and to determine who is a candidate for sphincter-sparing low anterior resection versus an abdominoperineal resection and permanent colostomy.

Pelvic MRI with its exquisite soft tissue resolution is valuable in this regard, particularly in the coronal plane. Other imaging planes used on MRI allow evaluation of tumor extension into the prostate, seminal vesicles, vagina, cervix, and bladder. On T1-weighted images, carcinoma is seen as an area of wall thickening with signal intensity slightly higher than that of skeletal muscle. This presents in stark contrast to the high signal intensity of perirectal fat and the absent

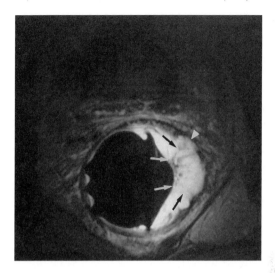

Fig. 7. MRI with endorectal coil in local staging of rectal cancer. A 75-year-old man was found to have a 5-cm ulcerated mass of the left lateral rectal wall on double-contrast barium enema. MRI with an endorectal coil was obtained to assist surgical planning. An axial T2-weighted image through the pelvis shows a shelf-like ulcerated mass (*arrows*). Mucinous histology is suggested by high signal on T2. The tumor extends deeply into the muscularis (*arrowhead*), such that microscopic perirectal fat invasion cannot be excluded. The patient underwent abdominoperineal resection that showed invasive adenocarcinoma invading through the muscularis propria, with focal extension into perirectal fat.

signal from intraluminal gas. Routine pelvic MRI cannot accurately distinguish between tumors localized to the mucosa and those that infiltrate the entire colonic wall (T1 and T2) (Fig. 7) [32]. Routine pelvic MRI cannot detect perirectal invasion or metastases to normal-sized lymph nodes [33]. Detection of nodal metastases is further hampered by the inherently lower spatial resolution of MRI compared with CT. Imaging with an endorectal coil, however, can assess the extent of tumor in the rectal wall and local adenopathy in a manner similar to endorectal ultrasound [34–37].

Patterns of lymphatic drainage for colorectal carcinoma vary by the location of the primary lesion. Rectosigmoid tumors preferentially drain to the external iliac and paraortic chains, whereas low rectal and anal carcinomas also metastasize to the inguinal lymph nodes. Left-sided colon cancer metastasizes to the left side of the superior mesenteric artery (SMA) root, and right-sided colon cancers spread to the periduodenal region to the right of the SMA root [29].

Traditionally, CT has used size criteria for determining pathologic enlargement, with 1 cm representing the cutoff between normal- and abnormal-sized lymph nodes. CT is not accurate, however, in determining whether regional lymph nodes are involved by metastatic colorectal cancer. Enlarged lymph nodes may be infiltrated by inflammatory or neoplastic cells, whereas even small lymph nodes may harbor metastatic deposits [20]. Therefore, clustered lymph nodes adjacent to known colorectal carcinoma are suspicious for metastatic involvement, despite their not meeting CT size criteria for enlargement [38]. Given that the presence of perirectal lymph nodes is highly unusual in the healthy population, any perirectal soft tissue nodules adjacent to a rectal carcinoma are highly suspicious for lymph node metastasis [5]. Furthermore, small pericolic lymph nodes adjacent to focally thickened bowel are more commonly seen in patients with colon cancer than in patients with inflammatory processes such as diverticulitis [38]. Although CT remains limited in predicting benign or malignant histology of pericolic lymph nodes, attempts to characterize lymph nodes with MRI have also proven unsuccessful [33].

Venous and lymphatic drainage of most of the colon dictates that metastatic disease is most apt to affect the liver. Hepatic metastases appear as low-attenuation masses on noncontrast-enhanced CT. In some patients, punctate calcifications indicate a mucinous histology. With dynamic contrast enhancement, colonic liver metastases demonstrate early ring enhancement but remain hypodense relative to normal liver parenchyma (see Fig. 5). With delayed imaging, colonic metastases may become isodense to liver parenchyma and, therefore, inconspicuous, particularly if the lesions are smaller than 2 cm [5]. Although the presence of hepatic metastases is unlikely to preclude surgical resection of the primary tumor, it has been shown that patients with one to four metastatic foci benefit from resection of isolated metastases and show improved survival, making preoperative detection in certain high-risk patients highly desirable [39].

Postoperative follow-up

After apparently curative resection of primary colorectal carcinoma, there is a 30% to 50% overall recurrence rate, with 50% of recurrences manifesting in the first year and 80% in the first 2 years [40]. Imaging follow-up uses a combination of CT, MRI, and barium enema or colonoscopy, with PET emerging as an increasingly valuable tool. Follow-up should not be performed for at least 3 to 4 months after surgery to allow for postoperative changes to abate. The appropriate timing of follow-up examinations is still under debate and likely varies by stage, location, and histology of the primary tumor because those factors together are most predictive of the probability of relapse [41].

Metastatic deposits have a predilection for the anastomotic site, often in a submucosal location that may be missed by endoscopic biopsy [42]; therefore, barium enema has a complementary role to colonoscopy in detecting recurrent carcinoma. CT is used in concert with the barium enema for detecting extra-colonic masses near the anastomosis and for screening for liver metastases. CT and MRI are also particularly useful for the detection of pelvic recurrences in patients after abdominoperineal resection [43]. Neither CT nor MRI, however, reliably differentiates benign from neoplastic presacral masses based on morphology, signal intensity, or enhancement pattern [44]. Their lack of specificity

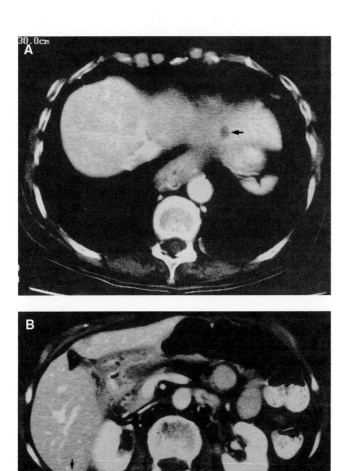

Fig. 8. Value of positron emission tomography (PET) in characterizing indeterminate lesions on follow-up imaging. After colon cancer resection, chemotherapy, and radiation treatment, a 72-year-old woman sought treatment for a rising carcinoembryonic antigen (CEA) level 1 year after surgery. (A) Axial CT image though the dome of the liver shows a 1-cm low-attenuation lesion (*arrow*) in the lateral segment of the left lobe. This lesion was inconsistently seen on serial CT because of its location, but it appeared stable. (B) Axial CT image through the inferior portion of the liver shows a low-attenuation lesion (*arrow*) in the posterior segment of the right lobe too small to characterize but thought to represent a probable cyst because of its demonstrated stability over approximately 1 year. (C) A PET scan was obtained because of a rising CEA level. Composite coronal PET images show two intense foci of fluorodeoxyglucose uptake (*large arrow and arrowhead*) in the liver, corresponding to lesions seen on CT. Biopsy confirmed metastatic adenocarcinoma. The right renal collecting system is identified with a small black arrow. (Fig. 8C courtesy of JW Sam, MD, Hospital of the University of Pennsylvania, Philadelphia, PA.)

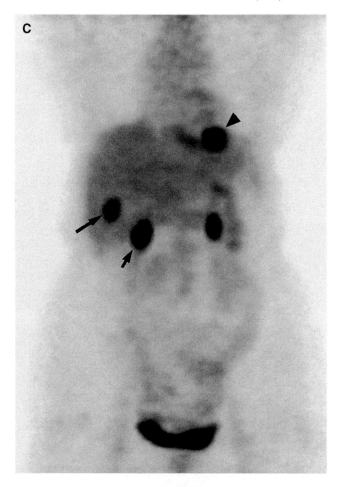

Fig. 8 (*continued*).

frequently results in either a biopsy or a follow-up study to reveal whether the perceived abnormalities remain stable or whether they regress or enlarge.

18 FDG-PET

In a patient with a rising carcinoembryonic antigen level (CEA) indicating disease progression, the challenge for imaging is to find the source, whether it is metastatic disease or local recurrence. The lack of specificity of CT and MRI when detecting soft tissue abnormalities or indeterminate liver lesions often leads to biopsy, which is sometimes limited by tissue sampling. These difficulties have provided the impetus for developing PET as a promising means for detecting distant, residual, or recurrent disease and thus resolving many clinical dilemmas.

Fluorodeoxyglucose (FDG) is a glucose analog taken up by cells and phosphorylated to FDG-6-phosphate, which, by virtue of its polarity, is trapped in malignant cells because dephosphorylation is delayed by the deficiency of glucose-6-phosphatase. The scientific basis of FDG-PET rests on the principle that malignant cells have increased glucose metabolism, increased protein synthesis, and uncontrolled cellular proliferation. Therefore, FDG uptake is proportional to true glucose metabolism. Semiquantitative analysis uses a standardized uptake value, which is the activity in a region of interest divided by patient weight and injected dose, to help discriminate benign from malignant processes [45].

In 1999 the Health Care Financing Association approved PET for the detection and localization of recurrent colorectal cancer in patients with rising CEA levels, based on the hypothesis that detecting earlier recurrence may allow for re-resection and may lead to improved patient survival. PET uses whole body imaging of the chest, abdomen, and pelvis to identify and localize local recurrences and distant metastases, altering surgical planning in up to 38% of patients [45]. It distinguishes postoperative and postradiation scarring from tumor by virtue of tumor metabolic activity [31]. It also detects unsuspected metastases not visualized on standard imaging studies (Fig. 8). In initial reports, PET achieved 95% sensitivity, 98% specificity, and 96% accuracy [45]. It remains to be seen whether PET supplants standard imaging studies for the routine follow-up of patients with colorectal carcinoma as a one stop whole body imaging study or whether, because of limitations in availability and cost, it remains a problem-solving tool in selected patients.

Summary

Colorectal carcinoma poses a serious public health threat. Detection in its early stages is the best predictor for long-term survival, which is the impetus for population-based screening programs. We believe that full-colon imaging by either DCBE or colonoscopy is necessary for colon cancer screening because flexible sigmoidoscopy, even if perfect, only detects 50% to 60% of colon cancers, a rate far worse than even the worst rate reported for single-contrast barium enema. Screening for colon cancer with flexible sigmoidoscopy is equivalent to performing a "left" mammogram for the detection of breast cancer. The role of CT colonography is still to be determined.

When confronted with a symptomatic patient, barium enema is applied in conjunction with CT to detect primary colorectal carcinoma, to differentiate it from other benign and malignant processes involving the colon, and to assess for disease extent before surgery in selected high-risk patient populations. Pelvic MRI may be useful in the preoperative assessment of patients with rectal carcinoma as a means for assisting surgical planning. CT, MRI, and barium enema are used in postoperative follow-up for detecting local recurrence and distant spread. In response to known difficulty in discriminating between normal postoperative changes and tumor recurrence and in determining the nature of certain liver lesions, FDG-PET has been approved for the detection and localization of recurrent colorectal cancer in patients with rising CEA levels and indeterminate findings on standard imaging studies. Given its current promise of offering high sensitivity, specificity, and accuracy, the indications for PET may well expand in the future, but its final role is still to be determined.

References

[1] Muto T, Bussey HJR, Morson BC. The evolution of cancer of the colon and rectum. Cancer 1975;36:2251–70.
[2] Winawer SJ, Zauber AG, O'Brien MJ, et al. The national polyp study: design, methods, and characteristics of patients with newly diagnosed polyps. Cancer 1992;70:1236–45.
[3] Eddy DM, Nugent FW, Eddy JF, et al. Screening for colorectal cancer in a high-risk population. Gastroenterology 1987;92:682–92.
[4] Glick S, Wagner JL, Johnson CD. Cost-effectiveness of double-contrast barium enema in screening for colorectal cancer. AJR Am J Roentgenol 1998;170:629–36.
[5] Thoeni RF, Laufer I. Polyps and carcinoma of the colon. In: Gore RM, Levine MS, editors. Textbook of gastrointestinal radiology. 2nd edition. Vol 1. Philadelphia: WB Saunders; 2001. p. 1009–48.
[6] Laufer I. The double contrast enema: myths and misconceptions. Gastrointest Radiol 1976;1: 19–31.
[7] Bernstein MA, Feczko PJ, Halpert RD, et al. Distribution of colonic polyps: increased incidence of proximal lesions in older patients. Radiology 1985;155:35–8.
[8] McCarthy PA, Rubesin SE, Levine MS, et al. Colon cancer: morphology detected by barium enema examination versus histopathologic stage. Radiology 1995;197:683–7.
[9] Fischel RE, Dermer R. Multifocal carcinoma of the large intestine. Clin Radiol 1975;26:495–8.
[10] Lieberman D. How to screen for colon cancer. Ann Rev Med 1998;49:163–72.
[11] Chong A, Shan JN, Levine MS, Rubesin SE, Laufer I, Ginsberg GG, et al. Diagnostic yield of barium enemas after incomplete colonoscopy. Radiology 2002;223:620–4.
[12] Habr-Gama A, Waye JD. Complications and hazards of gastrointestinal endoscopy. World J Surg 1989;13:193–201.
[13] Hara AK, Johnson CD, Reed JE, et al. Detection of colorectal polyps by computed tomographic colography: feasibility of a novel technique. Gastroenterology 1996;110:284–90.
[14] Hara AK, Johnson CD, Reed JE. Colorectal lesions: evaluation with CT colography. Radiographics 1997;17:1157–68.
[15] Laufer I. Barium studies of the colon. In: Gore RM, Levine MS, editors. Textbook of gastrointestinal radiology. 2nd edition, Vol 1. Philadelphia: WB Saunders; 2001. p. 892–904.
[16] Iida M, Iwashita A, Yao T, et al. Villous tumor of the colon: correlation of histologic, macroscopic, and radiographic features. Radiology 1988;167:673–7.
[17] Miller W Jr, Levine MS, Rubesin SE, et al. Bowler hat sign: a simple principle for differentiating polyps from diverticula. Radiology 1989;173:615–7.
[18] Rubesin SE, Sul SH, Laufer I, et al. Carpet lesions of the colon. Radiographics 1985;5:537–52.
[19] Raskin MM, Viamonte M, Viamonte M Jr. Primary linitis plastica carcinoma of the colon. Radiology 1974;113:17–22.
[20] Farouk R, Nelson H, Radice E, et al. Accuracy of computed tomography in determining resectability for locally and advanced primary or recurrent colorectal cancers. Am J Surg 1998;175: 283–7.
[21] Hurwitz MH, Redleaf PD, Williams HJ, et al. Lipomas of the gastrointestinal tract. AJR Am J Roentgenol 1967;99:84–9.
[22] Megibow AJ, Redmond PE, Bosniak MA, et al. Diagnosis of gastrointestinal lipomas by CT. AJR Am J Roentgenol 1979;133:743–5.

[23] Rubesin SE, Furth EE. Other tumors of the colon. In: Gore RM, Levine MS, editors. Textbook of gastrointestinal radiology, 2nd edition. Vol 1. Philadelphia: WB Saunders; 2001. p. 1049–74.

[24] O'Connell DJ, Thompson AJ. Lymphoma of the colon: the spectrum of radiologic changes. Gastrointest Radiol 1978;2:377–85.

[25] Becker JA. Prostatic carcinoma involving the rectum and sigmoid colon. AJR Am J Roentgenol 1965;94:421–8.

[26] Rubesin SE, Levine MS, Bezzi M, et al. Rectal involvement by prostatic carcinoma: radiographic findings. AJR Am J Roentgenol 1989;152:53–57.

[27] Meyers MA. Intraperitoneal spread of malignancies and its effect on the bowel. Clin Radiol 1981;32:129–46.

[28] Meyers MA, McSweeney J. Secondary neoplasms of the bowel. Radiology 1972;105:1–11.

[29] Meyers MA. Dynamic radiology of the abdomen: normal and pathologic anatomy. 3rd edition. New York: Springer-Verlag; 1988.

[30] Meyers MA. Distribution of intra-abdominal malignant seeding: dependency on dynamics of flow of ascitic fluid. AJR Am J Roentgenol 1973;119:198–206.

[31] Kim EE, Chung SK, Haynie TP, et al. Differentiation of residual recurrent tumors for post-treatment changes with F-18 FDG PET. Radiographics 1992;12:269–79.

[32] Butch RJ, Stark DD, Wittenberg J, et al. Staging rectal cancer by MR and CT. AJR Am J Roentgenol 1986;146:1155–60.

[33] Dooms GC, Hricak H, Crooks LE, et al. Magnetic resonance imaging of the lymph nodes: comparison with CT. Radiology 1984;153:710–38.

[34] Kim NK, Kim NJ, Yun SH, et al. Comparative study of transrectal ultrasonography, pelvic computerized tomography, and magnetic resonance imaging in preoperative staging of rectal cancer. Dis Colon Rectum 1999;42:770–5.

[35] Schnall MD, Furth EE, Rosato EF, et al. Rectal tumor stage: correlation of endorectal MR imaging and pathologic findings. Radiology 1994;190:709–14.

[36] Zagoria RJ, Schlarb CA, Ott DJ, et al. Assessment of rectal tumor infiltration utilizing endorectal MR imaging and comparison with endoscopic rectal sonography. J Surg Oncol 1997;64:312–7.

[37] Zerhouni EA, Rutter C, Hamilton SR, et al. CT and MR imaging in the staging of colorectal carcinoma: report on the Radiology Diagnostic Oncology Group II. Radiology 1996;200:443–51.

[38] Chintapalli KN, Esola CC, Chopra S, et al. Pericolic mesenteric lymph nodes: an aid in distinguishing diverticulitis from cancer of the colon. AJR Am J Roentgenol 1997;169:1253–5.

[39] Fong Y, Kemeny N, Paty P, et al. Treatment of colorectal cancer: hepatic metastases. Semin Surg Oncol 1996;12:219–52.

[40] Cass AW, Million RR, Pfaff W. Patterns of recurrence following surgery alone for adenocarcinoma of the colon and rectum. Cancer 1976;37:1861–5.

[41] Olson RM, Perencevich P, Malcolm AW, et al. Patterns of recurrence following curative resection of adenocarcinoma of the colon and rectum. Cancer 1980;45:2969–74.

[42] Thoeni RF, Moss AA. The gastrointestinal tract. In: Moss AA, Gamsu G, Genant H, editors. Computed tomography of the body. Philadelphia: WB Saunders; 1992. p. 643–734.

[43] Lee JKT, Stanley RJ, Sagel SS, et al. CT appearance of the pelvis after abdomino-perineal resection for rectal carcinoma. Radiology 1981;141:737–41.

[44] Ebner F, Amendola MA, Gefter WB. MR imaging of recurrent colorectal carcinoma versus fibrosis. J Comput Assist Tomogr 1988;12:521–3.

[45] Tan TXL, Klein MY, Tabib VT, Turner C, Forde JM. Oncologic applications of PET: an updated review. Appl Radiol 2000;29:18–25.

Hematol Oncol Clin N Am
16 (2002) 897–906

HEMATOLOGY/
ONCOLOGY
CLINICS OF
NORTH AMERICA

Endoscopic ultrasound and endoscopic mucosal resection for rectal cancers and villous adenomas

Nuzhat A. Ahmad, MD, Michael L. Kochman, MD, FACP,
Gregory G. Ginsberg, MD*

*Division of Gastroenterology, Department of Medicine, University of Pennsylvania Cancer Center,
University of Pennsylvania Medical School, 3 Ravdin, 3400 Spruce Street,
Philadelphia, PA 19104, USA*

The prognosis for patients with cancer of the colon or rectum is strongly correlated with the pathologic stage at the time of diagnosis. For these tumors, optimal management of the carcinoma is predicated on curative resection of the primary tumor. It is here, however, that treatment of these two lesions differ. Unlike more proximal colonic tumors, rectal neoplasms may be resected by a wide variety of surgical techniques associated with disparate rates of post-operative morbidity. Superficial lesions may be resected transanally or by endoscopic mucosal resection. Alternatively, more advanced lesions generally require extensive resection. Transmural tumors superior to the peritoneal reflection may potentially be treated with sphincter-sparing, low-anterior resec-tion, whereas more distal tumors may require abdominoperineal resection. In addition, advanced lesions may also be considered for neoadjuvant chemo-radiation. Thus, unlike more proximal colon cancer, the optimal method of resection for rectal carcinoma is critically dependent on accurate preoperative staging of the disease. It is precisely for this reason that endoscopic ultrasound has become an important addition to the preoperative evaluation of rectal lesions.

Equipment for rectal endosonography

Ultrasound evaluation of rectal lesions can be performed with rigid, non-optically guided probes or with flexible fiberoptic echoendoscopes that have integrated ultrasound transducers. The most commonly used echoendoscope is an

---

* Corresponding author.
E-mail address: gregory.ginsberg@uphs.upenn.edu (G.G. Ginsberg).

oblique-viewing instrument, the tip of which contains the ultrasound transducer that provides a 360° image perpendicular to the long axis of the scope at an ultrasound frequency of 7.5 MHz, 12 MHz, or 20 MHz. Fine-needle aspiration can be performed using curvilinear array echoendoscopes that provide a scan parallel to the axis of the scope. Rigid rectal imaging probes that produce an image perpendicular or parallel to the long axis of the probe are also available with biopsy capability. High-frequency catheter ultrasound probes, which have a frequency of 20 MHz or 30 MHz and produce a 360° image, perpendicular to the axis of the probe, are available. These catheter ultrasound probes can be passed through the accessory channel of a conventional videoendoscope, also allowing the probe to be positioned within the rectum under direct endoscopic vision.

Endosonographic staging of rectal cancer

A number of staging systems have been proposed for rectal cancers. Several organizations, including the National Institutes of Health and the American Joint Committee of Cancer, have identified the tumor, node, metastasis, or TNM, classification as the preferred staging system [1]. This system is based on the determination of depth of tumor invasion (T-classification), presence of regional lymph node metastases (N-classification), and presence of distant metastases (M-classification). Individual classifications are combined to provide an overall stage. The resultant overall stage and the individual components have been demonstrated to be predictive of 5-year survival. Endosonographic staging can define which lesions may be resected through endoscopic mucosal resection, transanal excision (T1), or surgical resection with or without neoadjuvant therapy.

Endosonographic tumor staging

Endosonographically, the rectal wall appears as five alternating hyperechoic and hypoechoic layers. The histologic correlation of the echolayers is as follows:

First layer (hyperechoic)—interface between water or balloon and superficial mucosa
Second layer (hypoechoic)—deep mucosa and muscularis mucosa
Third layer (hyperechoic)—submucosa and its interfaces
Fourth layer (hypoechoic)—muscularis propria
Fifth layer (hyperechoic)—interface between serosa and perirectal fat

Tumors generally appear as homogeneous hypoechoic masses with disruption of the normal wall echolayer pattern on endosonographic examination. The longitudinal and circumferential extent of tumor, along with depth of invasion into the surrounding structures, can be assessed by endoscopic ultrasound (EUS). A tumor that by EUS appears to be limited to the mucosa or the submucosa (first three echo layers) is classified as a T1 lesion. A tumor that invades the muscularis propria (hypoechoic fourth EUS layer) is a T2 lesion. A T3 lesion penetrates the rectal wall, extending beyond the five echo layers and into the surrounding perirectal tissue. A T4 lesion is a colorectal cancer that locally invades an adjacent organ, such as the prostate gland, sacrum, or vagina. EUS can also determine involvement of the internal and external anal sphincters.

Endosonographic nodal staging

Endosonographically, lymph nodes appear as round or oval structures that are hypoechoic compared with the surrounding perirectal fat. The nodal area that may be evaluated is limited to the perirectal space; nodes in the iliac and mesenteric chains may not be detected. Endosonographic criteria for the determination of malignant nodal involvement in rectal cancer are not as well reported as they are for other gastrointestinal malignancies, though there are no data to suggest that there should be a distinction. Data obtained primarily in patients with esophageal carcinoma have identified four sonographic criteria predictive of malignancy: large size (>1 cm), hypoechoic echodensity, sharply demarcated borders, and round (rather than ovoid or flat) shape [2]. The likelihood of malignancy is highly correlated with the number of these criteria that are present [2]. These criteria may not apply to rectal carcinoma because in these patients many metastatic lymph nodes are smaller than 5 mm [3–5]. The specificity of endosonographic staging of nodal involvement may be improved by the use of EUS-guided fine-needle aspiration (FNA) of the individual lymph node.

Accuracy of EUS in staging rectal cancer

Accuracy of tumor and nodal staging is dependent on the expertise of the endosonographer [6]. The overall accuracy of T-staging for rectal cancer ranges between 78% and 92% [7–15] (Table 1), though it is reported to be as low as 60% to 69% in some studies [16,17]. When EUS is incorrect for T-staging, it is typically because of overstaging rather than understaging [9–15]. EUS tends to overstage cancers because high-resolution ultrasound can detect, but not separate,

Table 1
Accuracy of rectal ultrasound in staging rectal cancer compared with surgical abnormality

Authors (y)	*n*	T stage (%)	N stage (%)	Type of ultrasound probe
Marone (2000) [7]	63	81	70	CF-UM20 (7.5 MHz)
Gualdi (2000) [8]	26	77	–	
Glaser (1993) [9]	154	86	81	Rigid, radial (7 MHz)
Herzog (1993) [10]	118	89	80	Rigid, radial (7 MHz)
Cho (1993) [11]	76	82	70	Flexible, radial (7.5 MHz)
Boyce (1992) [12]	45	89	79	Flexible, radial (7.5, 12 MHz)
Yamashita (1988) [13]	122	78	–	Rigid, radial (7.5 MHz)
Beynon (1988) [14]	100	93	83	Rigid, sector/linear (5.5–7 MHz)
Feifel (1987) [15]	79	89	–	Rigid, radial (3–7 MHz)

inflammation adjacent to the malignancy from the tumor itself. Accuracy is generally lowest for lesions classified as T2 by EUS, which may be overstaged as T3 lesions. Overstaging is apt to occur during imaging of tumors located on a haustral fold because of artifact induced by tangential imaging. When understaging occurs, it is usually because of undetected microscopic invasion of cancer cells beyond that observed by EUS [13].

The overall accuracy of N-staging by EUS is 73% to 83% (see Table 1) [7–15]. This low accuracy results because EUS cannot reliably distinguish between inflammatory and malignant lymph nodes. Data with other malignancies have suggested that the performance of needle aspiration cytology can markedly increase the accuracy and specificity of EUS for nodal classification [18]; however, there is little published experience for EUS-FNA for rectal cancer. The paucity of data likely reflects the fact that nodal classification rarely alters treatment plans. Plans are altered only if nodal spread is identified in patients in whom T-classification would otherwise suggest the possibility of local endoscopic or transanal resection as a curative option. In this instance, needle aspiration of a sonographically visible node may be clinically appropriate. In one preliminary report, nodal disease was suspected by EUS in only 33% of patients with pathologically node-positive tumors at resection. In contrast, EUS-FNA correctly predicted nodal status in 87% of patients [19].

Nontraversable stenoses will be encountered in 14% of rectal cancers [3]. Although few series have addressed this issue, extrapolation from data with esophageal malignancies suggest that imaging from below the obstruction may be prone to understaging [20]; however, one group has reported an accuracy rate of 82% using this technique with a rigid probe [21]. As with esophageal cancer, however, if a tumor is near obstructing, it is most likely at an advanced stage and would not be amenable to local resection, though no data exist to support this possibility in colorectal cancer.

Interobserver agreement for EUS rectal cancer staging

There is interobserver variability in both T- and N-stage interpretation. In a group of patients with rectal cancer, there was 88% agreement for T-stage but only 78% agreement for N-stage [22]; however, nearly all tumors in this study were stage T3. Palazzo and Burtin [23] found that agreement was fair for T1 tumors and poor for T2 tumors but good for T3 and T4 tumors. They also found that intraobserver agreement was good with respect to the subjective appearance of a malignant perirectal lymph node.

Accuracy of rectal EUS compared with CT and MRI

Endoscopic ultrasound has been reported to be equal or superior to CT. Among several comparative studies, EUS has a greater accuracy than CT for staging of rectal cancer—67% to 93% versus 53% to 86% for T-stage [10,16,24–27] and 80% to 87% versus 57% to 72% for N-stage [10,14,16,27]. CT cannot discriminate between wall layers of the rectum; therefore, it is not helpful in discriminating between T1 and T2 tumors for local resection.

MRI has been compared with EUS in a few small studies and appears to be similar in accuracy [28–30]. Although the accuracy rates for both imaging techniques are similar, however, MRI is more expensive than transanal ultrasound. Endorectal MRI has been introduced but is not widely available. Theoretically, endorectal MRI offers some advantages compared to EUS. It permits a larger field of view, may be less operator and technique dependent, and allows study of stenotic tumors. Comparison studies have shown EUS and endorectal MRI to be similar in accuracy for T-staging of rectal cancers [8,31] though in one report of 21 patients, EUS appeared to be superior to endorectal MRI for determination of T-stage [32]. In summary, EUS and endorectal MRI may be complementary for primary tumor staging and more accurate than CT for tumor and nodal staging.

Restaging after neoadjuvant therapy

Neoadjuvant chemoradiation is often used for downstaging of rectal cancer before surgical resection and for facilitating resection. Neoadjuvant therapy of rectal cancer may result in significant inflammatory and fibrotic changes in the rectal wall, which may be sonographically indistinguishable from the original tumor. As such, T-staging after radiation therapy is significantly less accurate as a result of overstaging. One recent study suggested an accuracy rate of only 52%, with overstaging occurring in 44% of patients [33]. Similar results were noted with regard to N-classification [33]. Thus, there is no standard for EUS imaging after neoadjuvant therapy. EUS can direct therapy in patients who have undergone neoadjuvant therapy as a prelude to possible sphincter-sparing surgery.

EUS for local recurrence of colorectal carcinoma

Local recurrence of rectal cancer after attempted curative resection occurs in 10% to 15% of patients, usually within the first 2 years of surgery. It is conceivable that early detection of recurrent local tumor, prompting early retreatment, would improve survival. Although this concept may be reasonable, it remains unproven. EUS may be useful in the detection of suspected local recurrence when no intramucosal lesions are seen during surveillance sigmoidoscopy. Initial data obtained using rigid ultrasound probes suggested that rectal ultrasound was highly sensitive for the detection of anastomotic recurrence [34,35]. Unfortunately, sonographic changes that may represent recurrence are not highly specific and may simply represent postoperative or postradiation inflammatory or fibrotic changes [36]. A recent study by investigators in Germany described EUS as highly sensitive (>90%) in the detection of local rectal tumor recurrence [37]. At the time of this writing, however, the use of EUS alone to justify surgical reexploration cannot be recommended. Local recurrence suspected by EUS can be confirmed by EUS-guided fine-needle aspiration.

Endoscopic mucosal resection of rectal lesions

Endoscopic mucosal resection (EMR), a technique devised by Japanese endoscopists, refers to the removal of sessile or flat neoplasms confined to the mucosa (Fig. 1). EMR provides an alternative to surgical resection for the management of sessile colorectal villous adenomas, adenomas with carcinoma in situ, and some T1 lesions. It represents an important advance for endoscopists in technical and oncologic terms. Compared with endoscopic methods of tumor destruction, EMR has the advantage of providing a complete or piecemeal specimen for analysis that allows histopathologic assessment. Histopathology combined with endoscopic assessment of completeness of resection allows treatment to be adjusted accordingly. Sessile rectal lesions and rectal cancers

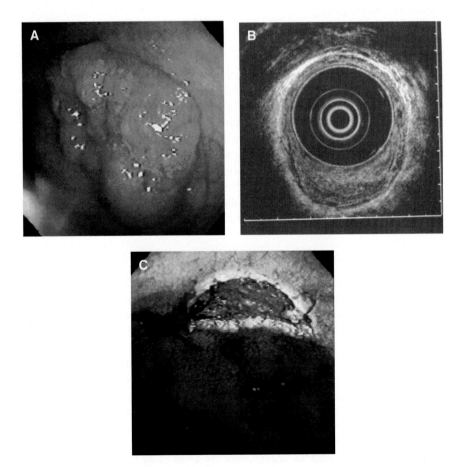

Fig. 1. (A) A sessile lesion in the rectum. (B) Endoscopic ultrasound of the lesion shows the lesion to be limited to the mucosa with an intact muscular muscosa. (C) The resection site post-endoscopic mucosal resection.

that are limited to the mucosa or have discrete submucosal invasion as determined by pre-EMR EUS are suitable for EMR.

Technique

EMR was developed to address flat, depressed, or sessile mucosal lesions not amenable to standard electrocautery snare polypectomy techniques. EMR uses adjunctive techniques to facilitate this, the most common of which is submucosal injection. Injection of solution into the submucosa lifts the lesion onto a cushion of injectate, thus creating a pseudostalk. The distance between the mucosa and the muscularis propria is increased, which decreases the risk for perforation or transmural burn. A snare is placed over the base of the raised area, and the lesion is resected with electrocautery. Lesions are resected as a single specimen or in a piecemeal fashion, depending on the size. En bloc retrieval of the resected specimen permits detailed histopathologic analysis and provides the basis for stratification of patient outcomes.

Endoscopic findings of superficial early cancers of the gastrointestinal tract are often subtle. When the lesions are visible, the borders between lesions and the normal tissue can often be hard to distinguish. Chromoendoscopy, which refers to the topical application of chemical stains or pigment, is the most reliable and widely used method for improving visualization, localization, and characterization of these subtle lesions. In the colon and rectum, indigo-carmine or methylene-blue solution enhances the contours and topography of the lesion. This "highlighter function" often reveals lesion edges that are not visible without staining.

Patient Selection for EMR

Determination of the depth of invasion of the lesion and the presence or absence of lymph node metastasis is critical for initial patient selection for EMR treatment. EUS, either with an echoendoscope or a through-the-scope ultrasound probe, is key in facilitating this selection. Conventional EUS using an echoendoscope is accurate in determining tumor depth and lymph node metastasis of large or bulky lesions. It may be less precise, however, to diagnose the depth of invasion of small, flat, or depressed tumors. In these instances, the high-frequency ultrasound probe may be particularly useful. In a study of 49 patients with colorectal cancer, using a 20-MHz ultrasound probe, the invasion depth was accurately diagnosed in 88% of patients [38].

Outcomes of EMR

Results of EMR in large colorectal polyps and early cancers have been favorable [39–42]. Kudo [43] reported his experience of 674 patients with early colorectal cancer on colonoscopy. EMR was performed in 633 patients, and surgery was performed exclusively in 44 patients because of massive submucosal invasion. In the EMR group, 10 patients subsequently underwent surgery because of submucosal invasion of the tumor on histopathologic assessment;

residual tumor tissue in the surgical resection specimens was noted in 20% and lymph node metastases in 30%. In the group treated successfully with EMR, none had local or distant recurrence [43]. Binmoeller et al [39] reported that only 19 (16%) of 117 patients who had sessile adenomatous polyps larger than 3 cm required further endoscopic treatment for recurrent adenoma during a follow-up of at least 6 months. Furthermore, among seven patients who had malignant polyps with favorable characteristics (well-differentiated carcinoma with no lymphatic or vascular invasion), five had no recurrence during a mean follow-up of 24 months [39]. Similarly, Kanamori et al [40], in their study of 33 patients with large sessile colorectal polyps who underwent EMR, found no tumor recurrence after a minimum follow-up of 1 year. Seventeen of these 33 patients had mucosal cancer, and 5 had cancer invading the submucosa [40]. Outcomes in patients with laterally spreading tumors of the large intestine ranging from 1 to 5 cm have been reported recently [42]. EMR was completed in 22 of 23 of these patients. En bloc resection was completed in 15 patients; the rest had piecemeal resection, which is less desirable for histologic interpretation. During a mean follow-up of 14 months with colonoscopy and biopsy, they found recurrence in one patient who had a large (45-mm) lesion; this patient required a repeat EMR.

Complications

The main complications of EMR are bleeding, perforation, and transmural burn syndrome. Bleeding during endoscopic resection of colorectal polyp is common; it occurs in 24% of patients with polypectomy of large (more than 3 cm) colorectal polyps [39]. Bleeding during EMR is almost always easily controlled by endoscopic techniques [44]. The reported rate of colon perforation is less than 1% [45]. Although perforation attributed to EMR is uncommon, the reported perforation rates in some series are many times greater than those reported for standard polypectomy. Transmural burn syndrome, also known as post-poly-pectomy syndrome, occurs when thermal energy during electrocoagulation extends to the muscularis propria and serosa, producing thermal injury and inflammation without perforation. It occurs in 0.5% to 1% of patients who undergo colonoscopic polypectomy [46,47].

Summary

EUS is the most accurate tool for local staging of rectal carcinoma. In addition to providing accurate T- and N-stages, EUS allows assessment of the internal and external anal sphincters. Accurate endosonographic staging directs the optimal method of management of rectal carcinoma, type of resection, and candidacy for neoadjuvant therapy. EMR may be applied to large rectal adenomas as an alternative to surgical resection in selected patients. EUS is important in discriminating lesions suitable for EMR.

References

[1] Behrs DH, Hansen DE, Hutter RVP et al, editors. American Joint Committee on Cancer. Colon and rectum: manual for staging of cancer. 4th edition. Philadelphia: JB Lippincott; 1992. p. 75–9.

[2] Catalano MF, Sivak Jr MV, Rice T, et al. Endosonographic features predictive of lymph node metastasis. Gastrointest Endosc 1994;40:442–6.

[3] Savides TJ, Hawes RH. Endoscopic ultrasound staging of rectal cancer. Van Dam J, Sivak Jr MV, editors. Gastrointestinal Endosonography. Philadelphia: WB Saunders; 1999. p. 279–89.

[4] Spinelli P, Schiavo M, Meroni E, et al. Results of EUS in detecting perirectal lymph node metastases of rectal cancer: the pathologist makes the difference. Gastrointest Endosc 1999; 49:754–8.

[5] Herrera-Ornelas L, Justiniano J, Castillo N, et al. Metastases in small lymph nodes from colon cancer. Arch Surg 1987;122:1253–6.

[6] Orrom WJ, Wong WD, Rothenberger DA, et al. Endorectal ultrasound in the preoperative staging of rectal tumors: a learning experience. Dis Colon Rectum 1990;33:654–9.

[7] Marone P, Petrulio F, de Bellis M, et al. Role of endoscopic ultrasonography in the staging of rectal cancer: a retrospective study of 63 patients. J Clin Gastroenterol 2000;30:420–4.

[8] Gualdi GF, Casciani E, Guadalaxara A, et al. Local staging of rectal cancer with transrectal ultrasound and endorectal magnetic resonance imaging: comparison with histologic findings. Dis Colon Rectum 2000;43:338–45.

[9] Glaser F, Kuntz C, Schlag P, et al. Endorectal ultrasound for control of preoperative radiotherapy of rectal cancer. Ann Surg 1993;217:64–71.

[10] Herzog U, von Flue M, Tondelli P, et al. How accurate is endorectal ultrasound in the preoperative staging of rectal cancer? Dis Colon Rectum 1993;36:127–34.

[11] Cho E, Nakajima M, Yasuda K, et al. Endoscopic ultrasonography in the diagnosis of colorectal cancer invasion. Gastrointest Endosc 1993;39:521–7.

[12] Boyce GA, Sivak MV, Lavery IC, et al. Endoscopic ultrasound in the preoperative staging of rectal cancer. Gastrointest Endosc 1992;38:468–71.

[13] Yamashita Y, Machi J, Shirouzu K, et al. Evaluation of endorectal ultrasound for the assessment of wall invasion of rectal cancer: report of a case. Dis Colon Rectum 1988;31:617–23.

[14] Beynon J. An evaluation of the role of rectal endosonography in rectal cancer. Ann R Coll Surg Eng 1989;71:131–9.

[15] Feifel G, Hildebrandt U, Dhom G. Assessment of depth of invasion of rectal cancer by endosonography. Endoscopy 1987;19:64–7.

[16] Rifkin MD, Ehrlich SM, Marks G. Staging of rectal carcinomas: prospective comparison of endorectal ultrasound and CT. Radiology 1989;170:319–22.

[17] Hulsmans FJ, Tio TL, Fockens P, et al. Assessment of tumor infiltration depth in rectal cancer with transrectal sonography: caution is necessary. Radiology 1994;190:715–20.

[18] Wiersema MJ, Vilman GM, Giovannini M, et al. Endosonography-guided fine-needle aspiration biopsy: diagnostic accuracy and complication assessment. Gastroenterology 1997;112:1087–95.

[19] Park HH, Nguyen PT, Tran Q, et al. Endoscopic ultrasound-guided fine needle aspiration in the staging of rectal cancer [abstract]. Gastrointest Endosc 2000;51:AB171.

[20] Van Dam J, Rice TW, Catalano MF, et al. High-grade malignant stricture is predictive of esophageal tumor stage: risks of endosonographic evaluation. Cancer 1993;71:2910–7.

[21] Nielson MB, Pederson JF, Christiansen J. Rectal endosonography in the evaluation of stenotic rectal tumors. Dis Colon Rectum 1993;36:275–9.

[22] Roubein LD, Lynch P, Glober G, et al. Interobserver variability in endoscopic ultrasonography: a prospective evaluation. Gastrointest Endosc 1996;44:573–7.

[23] Palazzo L, Burtin P. Interobserver variation in tumor staging. Gastrointest Endosc Clin North Am 1995;5:559–67.

[24] Beynon J, Mortensen NJMC, Foy DMA, et al. Pre-operative assessment of local invasion in rectal cancer: digital examination, endoluminal sonography or computed tomography? Br J Surg 1986;73:1015–7.

[25] Kramann B, Hildebrandt U. Computed tomography versus endosonography in the staging of rectal carcinoma: a comparative study. Int J Colorect Dis 1986;1:216–8.

[26] Romano G, deRosa P, Vallone G, et al. Intrarectal ultrasound computed tomography in the pre- and postoperative assessment of patients with rectal cancer. Br J Surg 1985;72:S117–9.

[27] Pappalardo G, Reggio D, Frattaroli FM, et al. The value of endoluminal ultrasonography and computed tomography in the staging of rectal cancer: a preliminary study. J Surg Oncol 1990;43:219–22.

[28] Waizer A, Powsner E, Russo I, et al. Prospective comparative study of MRI versus transrectal ultrasound for pre-operative staging and follow-up of rectal cancer. Dis Colon Rectum 1991;34:1068–72.

[29] Thaler W, Watzka S, Martin F, et al. Preoperative staging of rectal cancer by endoluminal ultrasound vs. magnetic resonance imaging: preliminary results of a prospective, comparative study. Dis Colon Rectum 1994;37:1189–93.

[30] Schaefer H, Gossmann A, Heindel W, et al. Comparison of endorectal MR imaging and trans-rectal ultrasound with pathology in rectal tumors. Endoscopy 1996;28:S9–13.

[31] Hunerbein M, Pegios W, Rau B, et al. Prospective comparison of endorectal ultrasound, three-dimensional endorectal ultrasound, and endorectal MRI in the preoperative evaluation of rectal tumors: preliminary results. Surg Endosc 2000;14:1005–9.

[32] Meyenberger C, Huch Boni RA, Bertschinger P, et al. Endoscopic ultrasound and endorectal magnetic resonance imaging: a prospective, comparative study for preoperative staging and follow-up of rectal cancer. Endoscopy 1995;27:469–79.

[33] Napoleon B, Pujol B, Berger F, et al. Accuracy of endosonography in staging of rectal cancer treated by radiotherapy. Br J Surg 1991;78:785–8.

[34] Beynon J, Mortensen NJMC, Foy DMA, et al. The detection and evaluation of locally recurrent rectal cancer with rectal endosonography. Dis Colon Rectum 1989;32:509–17.

[35] Feifel G, Hildebrandt U. Diagnostic imaging in rectal cancer: endosonography and immunoscintigraphy. World J Surg 1992;16:841–7.

[36] Hunerbein M, Dohmoto M. Haensch: evaluation and biopsy of recurrent rectal cancer using three-dimensional endosonography. Dis Colon Rectum 1996;39:1373–8.

[37] Muller C, Kahler G, Scheele J. Endosonographic examination of gastrointestinal anastamoses with suspected locoregional tumor recurrence. Surg Endosc 2000;14:45–50.

[38] Saitoh Y, Obara T, Einami K, et al. Efficacy of high-frequency ultrasound probes for the pre-operative staging of invasion depth in flat and depressed colorectal tumors. Gastrointest Endosc 1996;44:34–9.

[39] Binmoeller KF, Bohnacker S, Seifert H, et al. Endoscopic snare excision of "giant" colorectal polyp. Gastrointest Endosc 1996;43:183–8.

[40] Kanamori T, Itoh M, Yokoyama Y, et al. Injection-incision-assisted snare resection of large sessile colorectal polyp. Gastrointest Endosc 1996;43:189–95.

[41] Yokota T, Sugihara K, Yoshida S. Endoscopic mucosal resection for colorectal neoplastic lesions. Dis Colon Rectum 1994;37:1108–11.

[42] Yoshikane H, Hidano H, Sakakibara A, et al. Endoscopic resection of laterally spreading tumors of the large intestine using a distal attachment. Endoscopy 1999;31:426–30.

[43] Kudo S. Endoscopic mucosal resection of flat and depressed types of early colorectal cancer. Endoscopy 1993;25:455–61.

[44] Ahmad NA, Kochman ML, Long WB. et al. Endoscopic mucosal resection: efficacy, safety and clinical outcomes: a study of 101 cases. Gastrointest Endosc 2002;55:390–6.

[45] Inoue H, Kawano T, Tani M, et al. Endoscopic mucosal resection using a cap: techniques for use and preventing perforation. Can J Gastroenterol 1999;13:477–80.

[46] Christie JP, Marrazzo J. Mini-perforation of the colon: not all postpolypectomy perforations require laparotomy. Dis Colon Rectum 1991;34:132–5.

[47] Waye JD, Lewis BS, Yessayan S. Colonoscopy: a prospective report of complications. J Clin Gastroenterol 1992;15:347–51.

provides the best long-term results for primary tumors and for isolated recurrences in the colon, liver, or lung. The occasional patient requires resection of contiguous organs involved by tumor extension. Furthermore, surgical intervention has a significant role in the palliation of advanced or recurrent colorectal cancer. Resection or diversion for bleeding or obstruction is almost always indicated and provides significant symptomatic relief.

Hepatic metastases from colorectal cancer are a common clinical problem. As with primary tumors, surgical resection offers the best long-term outcome; however, only a minority of patients has resectable disease. When resection is not possible, growing evidence suggests that regionally-directed therapy to the liver in the form of ablative procedures, such as cryotherapy and radiofrequency ablation, and hepatic artery infusion pumps offer increased disease-free and potentially overall survival.

This article reviews the various roles of surgical intervention in the curative and palliative treatment of patients with colorectal cancer. Preoperative evaluation, primary resection techniques, and postoperative care of the patient who has undergone colorectal surgery are discussed, as are the controversial and evolving topics of laparoscopic resection, sentinel lymph node mapping, and liver-directed therapy.

Preoperative evaluation

All patients with biopsy-proven colorectal cancer should be evaluated for surgical intervention, unless their overall surgical risk from preexisting comorbid disease would make the risk for death from surgery prohibitively high. When evaluating a patient before surgery, key points should be addressed in the history and physical examination. Careful review of exercise tolerance and presence of cardiac risk factors should be noted because cardiac complications remain the principal cause of patient morbidity and mortality after abdominal surgery [3]. In addition, risk factors for poor pulmonary performance, such as cigarette smoking, should be addressed before surgery because pulmonary complications contribute to perioperative morbidity. However, routine preoperative pulmonary function testing is not indicated because it has not been found to be a reliable predictor of postoperative complications [4]. A history of bleeding or easy bruising or, conversely, of prior thromboembolic events should be elicited before surgery because possible bleeding diatheses or prothrombotic conditions may not be evident on routine coagulation studies. If present, these conditions require careful attention and management in the perioperative period. It should be recognized, however, that surgery for colorectal cancer is not purely elective, and undue delay in performing preoperative studies is not warranted.

Physical examination should stress important factors, such as body habitus (eg, obesity, narrow pelvis), that would have an impact on surgical technique (eg, construction of a low rectal anastomosis after surgery for rectal cancer). It is also important to note previous abdominal incisions in planning the operation. In

HEMATOLOGY/
ONCOLOGY
CLINICS OF
NORTH AMERICA

Hematol Oncol Clin N Am
16 (2002) 907–926

Surgical treatment of colon and rectal cancer

Robert J. Canter, MD, Noel N. Williams, MD*

*Department of Surgery, Hospital of the University of Pennsylvania, 4 Silverstein, 3400 Spruce Street,
Philadelphia, PA 19104, USA*

Cancer of the colon and rectum is a significant health problem in the United States and other Western nations. Nearly 50% of the 186,000 patients diagnosed annually with colorectal cancer in the United States eventually die of their disease. The colon is the site of the third highest incidence of new malignancies and is second only to lung cancer in mortality. Because colorectal cancer is frequently preceded by development of a premalignant lesion, an adenomatous polyp, screening modalities have been shown to have significant impact on the incidence of and mortality from this disease. Population screening through digital rectal examination, fecal occult blood testing, and, more recently, endoscopic examination of the large intestine have been shown to significantly reduce the risk for death from colorectal cancer [1,2]. The frequency and selection of screening modalities is an evolving process. Recent trials suggest that all patients older than 50 should undergo screening colonoscopy [1,2]. Clearly, patients who are at higher risk, such as those with a positive family history, should undergo colonoscopic surveillance at regular intervals. Similarly, patients who have been treated for colorectal cancer or a polyp should have regular and frequent surveillance.

The polyp–cancer relationship has been well demonstrated for the past 25 years. Although not all polyps become cancers, prophylactic removal of all polyps is felt to be indicated. Moreover, familial adenomatous polyposis, an autosomal dominant condition characterized by diffuse intestinal polyposis, predisposes to colorectal cancer. Left untreated, this condition develops into colorectal cancer in all patients during early adulthood.

Early detection and surgical intervention for primary tumors are of the utmost importance. Although endoscopic removal of small polypoid cancers has been advocated, most colorectal carcinomas require surgical resection. The ability to perform en bloc resection with removal of the tumor and adjacent lymph node-bearing areas provides the optimal chance for cure. Resection for cure clearly

---

* Corresponding author.

E-mail address: williamn@uphs.upenn.edu (N.N. Williams).

women, careful bimanual gynecologic examination is of particular relevance because the ovaries are a frequent site of metastasis in colon cancer.

Laboratory evaluation should be dictated by the patient's comorbid condition(s). The value of the measurement of carcinoembryonic antigen (CEA) remains controversial [5–7], but most centers use this as a guide to the success of total resection of cancer. Credible evidence suggests that following the CEA level post-resection does not impact on ultimate survival [7,8], but many surgeons believe that it offers a guide to the presence of an occult recurrence and may improve survival for a subset of patients.

Endoscopy and biopsy are mandatory before surgery. Not only do they establish a definitive diagnosis, but they enable the entire colon to be inspected for possible synchronous lesions that occur in approximately 5% of patients. Polyps may also be noted; they are present in up to 20% of patients. During colonoscopy, if mucosal or submucosal lesions are present, India ink tattooing can be performed to aid in intraoperative localization of the tumor, which can be a difficult maneuver even in conventional, open procedures.

Cross-sectional imaging with CT or MRI may show evidence of metastasis to regional nodes or the liver. Questionable lesions noted in the liver are an indication for intraoperative sonography of the liver. Endoscopic ultrasound (EUS) is important for the preoperative staging of rectal cancer for assessment of local invasion and for potential regional lymph node involvement. EUS is reported to be 95% accurate in distinguishing T1 and T2 lesions from T3 and T4 tumors and 80% accurate in detecting lymph node positivity [9,10]. This information is helpful in determining the need for neoadjuvant chemoradiation, which has been shown to increase the rate of success in the ability to perform sphincter-preserving surgery.

Nichols [11] originally described and emphasized the importance of preoperative mechanical and antibiotic preparation of the bowel before colon resection. Cleansing enemas and laxatives and oral antibiotics are administered to provide significant reduction in the bacterial population of the colon before resection. Some surgeons also advocate on-table colon irrigation, particularly for low rectal lesions. These preoperative maneuvers are widely believed to decrease the incidence of wound infection, intraabdominal abscesses, and anastomotic leaks. For the last 30 years, they have been regarded as standards of care for colorectal operations. Studies have demonstrated that there is actually little statistical evidence to support their practice [12], but they are so commonly performed that failure to follow them is considered iconoclastic. Moreover, though some patients may acquire hypovolemia after preoperative bowel preparation, there is little evidence to suggest that these practices have an overall negative effect on the patient's course.

Techniques of primary resection

The fundamental principle in surgery for cancer of the colon and rectum is an anatomic, en bloc resection of the primary tumor, with adequate margins and removal of the regional lymph nodes. Because the pericolonic mesenteric lymph nodes are, with rare exception, the initial site of metastatic spread of colon cancer, regional lymphadenectomy carries diagnostic and therapeutic value. In addition, the blood vessels and regional lymph node basins follow a parallel course so that the goals of en bloc resection and lymph node retrieval are typically interrelated (Fig. 1). For intraperitoneal tumors, the extent of the resection is dictated by the vascular supply, and the question of adequate margins of bowel is rarely an issue.

Colonic tumors

Tumors of the cecum and right colon require resection of the terminal ileum and ascending colon, including the hepatic flexure (Fig. 2). This involves freeing the colon from its lateral retroperitoneal attachments and then retracting it medially. In so doing, care must be taken to identify the right ureter and duodenum and to avoid injury to these structures. The bowel is then divided several centimeters proximal to the ileocecal valve and approximately one third

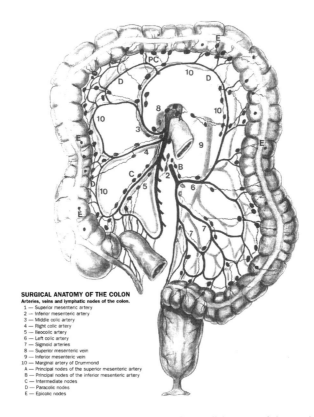

SURGICAL ANATOMY OF THE COLON
Arteries, veins and lymphatic nodes of the colon.
1 — Superior mesenteric artery
2 — Inferior mesenteric artery
3 — Middle colic artery
4 — Right colic artery
5 — Ileocolic artery
6 — Left colic artery
7 — Sigmoid arteries
8 — Superior mesenteric vein
9 — Inferior mesenteric vein
10 — Marginal artery of Drummond
A — Principal nodes of the superior mesenteric artery
B — Principal nodes of the inferior mesenteric artery
C — Intermediate nodes
D — Paracolic nodes
E — Epicolic nodes

Fig. 1. Surgical anatomy of the colon and rectum. The parallel course of the arteries, veins, and lymphatics is demonstrated. (*From* Etala E. Atlas of gastrointestinal surgery. Baltimore: Williams & Wilkins; 1997. p. 1729; with permission.)

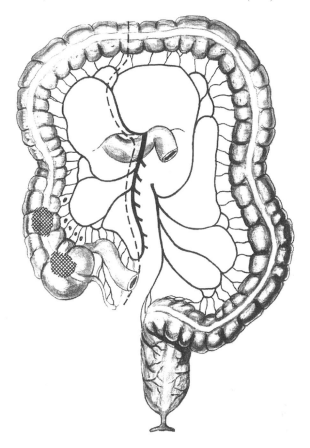

Fig. 2. Technique of right hemicolectomy. Ligation of the ileocolic, right colic, and right branch of the middle colic arteries is performed, thereby determining the extent of bowel resection. (*From* Etala E. Atlas of gastrointestinal surgery. Baltimore: Williams & Wilkins; 1997. p. 1757; with permission.)

of the distance along the transverse colon, depending on the course of the middle colic artery. The ileocolic artery and right branch of the middle colic artery are then ligated, and an anastomosis is performed. For resection of the right colon, most surgeons use stapling instruments, resulting in a side-to-side anastomosis that is functionally end-to-end.

Tumors of the transverse colon are generally treated by resection from the hepatic flexure to the splenic flexure, ligating the middle colic artery close to its origin from the superior mesenteric artery. Proximal ligation of the vessels supplying these portions of the colon results in wide removal of the lymph node-bearing areas. When reestablishing intestinal continuity, it important to construct a tension-free anastomosis to reduce the risk for anastomotic leak or dehiscence. For this reason, mid and distal transverse colon tumors can be technically challenging given the fixed retroperitoneal attachments of the right and left colon. In these patients, extended right hemicolectomy (Fig. 3) may be needed to anastomose the ileum to the descending colon.

Left colon and sigmoid colon cancers above the peritoneal reflection require mobilization of the splenic flexure and removal of the entire left colon (Fig. 4). Care must be taken to avoid injury to the spleen in such procedures because this may cause significant bleeding. Debate as to the efficacy of radical left colectomy versus segmental resection for left colon cancers has never been satisfactorily resolved. Most surgeons make the decision intraoperatively based on the extent of the tumor and the possibility of lymph node metastasis.

It is important to reiterate that tumors attached to other organs require en bloc resection, including of the adjacent organ, to achieve curative resection. In the presence of obstruction, cancers of the right colon may be safely removed with a one-stage operation, with reestablishment of intestinal continuity at the time of

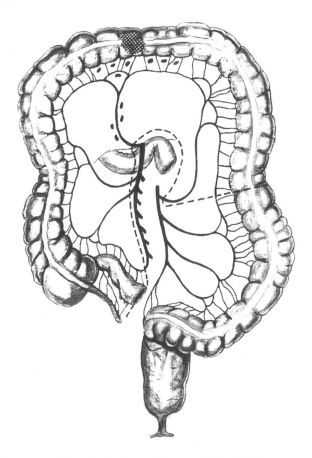

Fig. 3. Technique of extended right hemicolectomy. In cases of mid and distal transverse colon tumors, to construct a tension-free anastomosis, an extended right hemicolectomy may be needed, anastomosing the ileum to the descending colon. (*From* Etala E. Atlas of gastrointestinal surgery. Baltimore: Williams & Wilkins; 1997. p. 1761; with permission.)

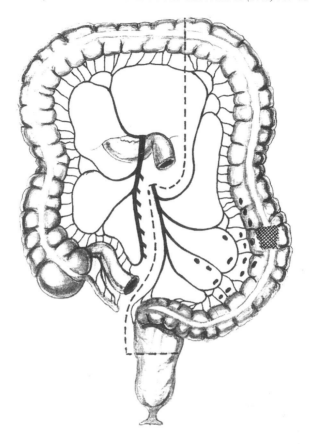

Fig. 4. Technique of left hemicolectomy. Tumors of the descending colon require resection from the distal transverse colon to the rectum. Tumors of the sigmoid colon may be treated by sigmoidectomy alone. (*From* Etala E. Atlas of gastrointestinal surgery. Baltimore: Williams & Wilkins; 1997. p. 1765; with permission.)

surgery without the need for temporary colostomy. Even if perforation occurs, it is feasible to perform a primary anastomosis for right-sided lesions because of the reduced bacterial contamination. On the other hand, left-sided obstructing lesions may require a staged operation depending on the degree of obstruction and the degree of proximal bowel dilatation [13]. If perforation and peritonitis result from left-sided lesions, most surgeons perform resection with creation of a temporary end-colostomy and a Hartmann pouch because of the risk for ongoing sepsis and poor anastomotic healing.

Rectal tumors

Below the peritoneal reflection, the extent of resection is a greater issue that varies from center to center. Early lesions of the rectal mucosa and submucosa may be adequately treated by transanal excision with a surrounding margin of normal tissue [14]. This technique provides adequate resection of T1 and T2 lesions and spares patients the morbidity of an extensive rectal resection. Although there is a risk for local recurrence with this treatment, repeat resection can often be performed with the possibility of a successful long-term outlook.

The surgical approach to invasive tumors of the rectum is contingent on the location of the tumor in relation to the anal verge and on whether there is an adequate distal margin to safely restore intestinal continuity. Digital rectal examination is an important maneuver before surgery because palpable lesions generally require abdominoperineal resection (APR), a procedure that encompasses resection of the rectum, sigmoid colon, and both anal sphincters, with creation of a permanent colostomy. Preoperative endoscopy, in conjunction with endoscopic ultrasound, also localizes the tumor in relation to the anal verge and guides operative management. It is important to remember that, given the curvilinear course of the rectum, endoscopy can be unreliable in predicting tumor distance from the anal verge.

For purposes of the surgical approach, the rectum can be divided into three sections. The upper third begins at the sacral promontory and is completely intraperitoneal. Tumors in this location are amenable to low anterior resection (LAR) in which the anal sphincters are preserved and intestinal continuity is reestablished in an end-to-end fashion. The transition from intraperitoneal to extraperitoneal occurs in the middle third of the rectum. Tumors in this location are also generally resectable by LAR, but these tumors can be technically challenging, especially in the presence of unfavorable patient characteristics such as obesity or a narrow male pelvis. Tumors of the lower third, located 5 cm or less from the anal verge, have historically been treated by APR. Recognition that smaller margins of uninvolved bowel are adequate from an oncologic perspective has helped spur a trend toward more frequent performance of low anterior resection for rectal cancer.

For adequate removal of the cancer, it appears that negative margins of 2 cm do not adversely affect long-term survival. Pathology studies have shown that fewer than 6% of tumors demonstrate intramural spread beyond 2 cm, and those that do are aggressive Dukes C and D tumors in which death typically occurs as a consequence of distant disease rather than local recurrence [15]. The movement from APR to LAR has also been fueled by the advent and widespread use of circular staplers, which enable performance of a low or an ultra-low anastomosis with less technical difficulty than a sutured anastomosis. Since the introduction of the so-called end-to-end anastomosis (EEA) stapler, which simplifies the construction of a low rectal anastomosis, the rate of APR for tumors of the mid-rectum has dropped from 60% to 7% [15]. At the time of LAR, it is often necessary to perform a temporary ileostomy or colostomy to divert the fecal stream proximally to allow for good healing of a low anastomosis.

Considerable debate has centered on the importance of widely resecting the entire mesorectum when performing LAR or APR. Several studies, including a recent randomized, prospective trial, have emphasized the importance of total mesorectal excision (TME) in the surgical treatment of low rectal cancers [16,17].

Data from these studies suggest that TME, predicated on the sharp dissection under direct vision of the mesorectum posteriorly and laterally down to the pelvic floor and the midline anococcygeal raphe, decreases local recurrence and improves overall survival. Although these authors report no difference in morbidity with TME versus less radical resections of the mesorectum [16–18], it should be remembered that extensive mobilization of the rectum, especially posteriorly along the presacral fascia, carries a risk for injury to the autonomic nerves responsible for bowel, bladder, and sexual function. Rates of significant sexual and voiding dysfunction after LAR and APR range from 5% to 15%.

Although LAR may sometimes be technically possible for tumors in the distal third of the rectum, most tumors in this location are treated with APR; however, for tumors just proximal to the anal verge, intestinal continuity may be restored and a permanent colostomy avoided through the creation of a coloanal anastomosis [19]. This technique involves suturing the proximal colon directly, or after folding it into a pouch, to the anal mucosa. Most authors acknowledge that coloanal anastomoses are technically difficult, and sphincter control after this procedure is variable. Nevertheless, some surgeons advocate this technique for patients who do not want a permanent colostomy.

Postoperative patient care

Postoperative care of the colorectal surgery patient has undergone significant modifications in recent years. Nasogastric tubes, for example, are no longer considered routine by some surgeons. Many surgeons still advocate the use of these tubes after colon resection, but the length of time that they are left in place is extremely variable. Although data exist to support early and late removal of nasogastric tubes [20,21] in practice, early removal has become more common. At our institution, nasogastric tubes are placed during surgery. If drainage remains minimal (less than 250 mL for 24 hours), they are typically removed on the first or second postoperative day to improve patient comfort, facilitate mobilization, and improve pulmonary function.

Consistent with the growing trend toward earlier mobilization after surgery, which is of particular importance, early removal of bladder catheters has been advocated. This is also important for reducing the risk for nosocomial urinary tract infection. At our institution, urinary catheters are left in place for no more than 24 hours after surgery unless considerable manipulation of the bladder has occurred, as in a LAR or APR. However, even prolonged urinary catheterization after LAR or APR has been subjected to debate. A recent randomized, prospective trial of 126 patients comparing 1-day and 5-day bladder catheterization after rectal resection demonstrated a 2.5-fold increase (25% versus 10%) in urinary retention for patients undergoing 24 hours of catheterization. This was offset by a 2-fold increase (42% versus 20%) in urinary tract infections for patients undergoing 5 days of catheterization [22]. Studies such as this have supported the current trend of early removal of bladder catheters even after LAR or APR, with the recognition that reinsertion may be required for a subset of patients who experience urinary retention. Similarly, the presence of an epidural catheter for postoperative pain control should not be considered an absolute indication for ongoing bladder catheterization because only a minority of patients using that treatment experience urinary retention.

There is a recent trend toward more rapid resumption of oral intake among patients in the postoperative period [23]. The passage of flatus is usually accepted as indicative of the return of sufficient bowel function to institute liquid oral intake. This more aggressive approach is based on the theory that gastrointestinal motility, and perhaps even immune function, is increased by small amounts of enteral intake. Obviously, this must be closely monitored so that the occasional patient who is unable to tolerate oral intake is not pushed to the point of nausea or vomiting. In addition, resumption of a full solid diet is not thought to be a prerequisite for hospital discharge because many patients can regulate the advancement of their diet at home. Conversely, early institution of total parenteral nutrition (TPN) should be provided for patients who are unable to resume enteral nutrition 7 days after surgery. Moreover, despite the restrictive regulations of managed care organizations, patients with severe malnutrition should receive 1 week of preoperative TPN for improved outcome [24].

As do all patients undergoing major abdominal surgery, patients with colorectal cancer should receive postoperative low-dose heparin therapy during hospitalization as prophylaxis against thromboembolic events [25]. Support hose with intermittent compression have been found to be equally important, particularly for patients who are kept in the lithotomy position for several hours while undergoing rectal resection.

Laparoscopy for colorectal cancer

Surgery of the biliary tract and gastroesophageal junction has been revolutionized by laparoscopic techniques that have now become firmly established. Similarly, there are growing proponents for laparoscopic and laparoscopic-assisted (requiring mini-laparotomy for extracorporeal anastomosis) colorectal surgery for benign diseases of the colon. Since 1991, when laparoscopic colorectal surgery was first performed, multiple series on the use of laparoscopic techniques for colorectal resection have been reported [26–29]. Concern, however, about the ability to adequately resect regional lymph nodes with the laparoscopic approach in patients with colon cancer and early reports of recurrent cancer at sites of port placement [30] has made laparoscopic resection for colorectal cancer a highly controversial topic.

The growth of minimally invasive techniques in all fields of surgery has been fueled by the intuitive concept that smaller incisions are less traumatic to patients and provide for a faster postoperative recovery. In the realm of colorectal surgery, multiple studies have shown that after laparoscopic resection, postoperative pain is reduced, hospital stay is shortened, and return to work appears to be faster [26–28]. Overall 30-day morbidity and mortality rates are generally equivalent between laparoscopic and conventional procedures, and conversion from laparoscopy to open surgery is required in approximately 10% to 20% of patients. Moreover, for technical reasons, laparoscopic procedures are limited to resection of the upper rectum and of the right, left, and sigmoid colon.

To a greater degree than other intraabdominal procedures, laparoscopic colorectal resection is technically difficult because blood vessels within the mesentery must be ligated and the bowel must be transected and reanastomosed. Consequently, many surgeons believe that laparoscopic resection is less optimal than conventional open surgery because the ability to retrieve lymph nodes and obtain wide margins of uninvolved bowel may be limited by technical constraints. In addition, because the surgeon loses the ability to palpate the bowel with laparoscopy, it is possible to remove an incorrect segment of bowel if adequate preoperative localization has not been performed. This is important to remember, especially with smaller lesions. Consequently, laparoscopic colorectal resection for a neoplastic lesion mandates the availability of intraoperative colonoscopy.

Initial series of laparoscopic resection of colorectal cancer reported rates of port-site implantation as high as 20% [30], prompting some authors to hypothesize that the process of pneumoperitoneum required for intraabdominal visualization somehow led to tumor dissemination. Much subsequent attention was therefore paid to careful handling of the specimens and to protection of port sites from contact with tips of instruments. Hence, recent series have reported an approximate 2% rate of port-site recurrence, comparable to rates of incisional recurrence for open procedures [29,31].

Data from several studies suggest that laparoscopic colorectal resection is as effective as conventional open surgery for malignant diseases of the large bowel, including the ability to resect mesenteric lymph nodes [26–29]. These studies are limited, however, by various methodological flaws such as small sample sizes, data from single institutions, and retrospective reviews. Preliminary analysis from a National Institutes of Health-sponsored multiinstitutional, randomized trial comparing laparoscopy with open resection for colorectal cancer has shown no significant difference between the two techniques for adequacy of surgical margins or number of lymph nodes removed [31]; however, follow-up data regarding overall and disease-free survival are not yet available. Consequently, the current recommendation of the American College of Surgeons is that curative resection for colorectal cancer should be performed laparoscopically only as part of a prospective clinical trial [32]. Nevertheless, there remains a definite and growing role for laparoscopy in the diagnosis, staging, and palliation of patients with carcinoma of the colon and rectum.

Sentinel lymph node evaluation

Extensive clinical studies have validated the concept that the sentinel node or nodes are the first to receive the lymphatic drainage from a tumor and, therefore, that they can be used to predict with high sensitivity and specificity whether a regional nodal basin will be positive or negative for metastatic disease. This technique has become standard practice in the surgical treatment of melanoma and breast cancer because it allows for equivalent cancer staging while sparing patients the morbidity resulting from extended regional lymphadenectomy, which can be significant for the axilla and the groin. In addition, because there are fewer of them, the sentinel lymph node or nodes can be examined pathologically with greater detail than the nodes in a formal regional lymphadenectomy. This allows for identification and "upstaging" of patients with micrometastatic disease, who may then benefit from formal lymph node dissection and become candidates for adjuvant chemotherapy.

In colon cancer, the potential benefits of sentinel lymph node biopsy are less apparent. In contrast to the inguinal and axillary regions, regional lymphade-nectomy is performed as part of the primary bowel resection because of the parallel course of the bowel's vascular supply and the nodal drainage. Lmphadenectomy adds little to the complexity or duration of the surgical procedure. Moreover, because final pathologic analysis of the sentinel lymph node(s) is not available at the time of surgery, few practitioners would support harvesting only the sentinel lymph nodes during primary resection and submitting patients to reoperation because of a positive sentinel node in order to resect more lymph nodes. Consequently, unlike biopsy for breast cancer and melanoma, sentinel lymph node biopsy for carcinoma of the colon and rectum does not offer the potential to limit surgical morbidity. Any benefit of the procedure, therefore, would depend on whether the upstaging of patients through detailed immunohistochemical analysis of the sentinel node(s) provides therapeutic advantage in the adjuvant treatment of patients with colorectal cancer. Although small, single-institution series have reported an approximate 30% rate of detecting the presence of micrometastatic disease when immuno-histochemical or reverse transcription–polymerase chain reaction techniques are applied to conventionally node-negative specimens, the biologic and clini-cal significance of these findings remain to be determined [33–36]. To this end, the American College of Surgeons Oncology Group is initiating a trial to determine the potential role of sentinel lymph node mapping in the treatment of colorectal cancer.

Palliative surgery

Patients with advanced colorectal cancer are at risk for local and intraperitoneal recurrence despite maximal surgical and adjuvant therapy. Intraperitoneal recur-rence is often complicated by intestinal obstruction, which can entail significant morbidity and mortality, including possible perforation if high-grade obstruction goes untreated. Although recurrence is frequently the harbinger of progressive disease for which a poor prognosis exists, surgical intervention should not be denied to patients if it offers the potential for significant palliation.

Patients with a confined local recurrence, such as at the site of a prior anastomosis, should be viewed as having potentially surgically curable disease. Alternatively, patients with unresectable recurrence causing bowel obstruction may be treated with intestinal bypass to restore intestinal continuity and the ability to eat. For patients with multiple foci of recurrence, who are therefore not amenable to bypass, colonic or distal small bowel diversion through creation of an ostomy allows for decompression of the bowel. This enables the patient to resume oral alimentation, with an improved quality of life. Patients with proximal small bowel obstruction or multiple points of obstruction will not benefit from bypass or diversion to restore oral alimentation. In these patients, if intractable nausea and vomiting are present, a gastrostomy tube, inserted either open or by percutaneous endoscopy, can provide significant relief, though it does not allow the resumption of oral intake.

Patients with disseminated intraperitoneal carcinomatosis are a subset for whom limited treatment options exist. Patients without extraabdominal disease have been treated with various experimental therapies, including intraperitoneal chemotherapy, hyperthermic continuous peritoneal perfusion, and intraperitoneal photodynamic therapy (PDT). At our institution, a phase 2 trial combining surgical debulking to less than 5 mm with the delivery of intraoperative PDT is under way [37]. This therapy is based on the ability of photosensitizing agents to concentrate in tumor cells. Laser light then transforms the photosensitizing agent to reactive-oxygen species, which are cytotoxic to the tumor cells. Interim analysis has shown a median survival of 12 months for patients with carcinomatosis secondary to colorectal cancer treated with PDT. These results represent a modest improvement compared to the historical survival of 6 to 8 months for this group of patients.

Postoperative surveillance

The nature and extent of postoperative follow-up is controversial. CT and colonoscopy 1 year after surgery have been shown to help detect early recurrence [5,6]. Beyond that interval, in the absence of symptoms, no improvement in survival has been demonstrated between yearly history and physical examination and yearly CT and colonoscopy [38]. As mentioned above, follow-up CEA monitoring is controversial, but it often helps to detect recurrent disease before it is clinically evident [7]. Further randomized studies are necessary to establish a standard of care for postoperative surveillance after surgery for colorectal cancer. At this time, most would agree that surveillance endoscopy, especially proctoscopy for rectal cancer, is important in the first year after surgery. After that, at a minimum, careful history taking and physical examination, combined with selected laboratory studies, should be performed on an annual basis. A low threshold should be maintained for investigating symptoms or laboratory abnormalities with more invasive tests. More specific guidelines for postoperative surveillance after resection for colorectal cancer are inherently empirical and vary among practitioners. At our institution, careful history taking and physical examination, along with liver function tests and CEA levels, are performed annually. In addition, lower endoscopy and CT are performed routinely within the first year of resection and every 2 to 3 years thereafter.

Liver metastases

Every year, approximately 50,000 patients in the United States are diagnosed with colorectal cancer metastatic to the liver [39]. For many of these patients, the liver is the only site of spread. Without treatment, survival is typically measured in months, and liver failure contributes substantially to their demise. Surgical resection offers the only chance for cure, and in some patients (approximately 25%) for whom liver metastases are resectable with curative intent, the 5-year survival is approximately 30% [39,40]. In contrast, for most patients, colorectal metastases to the liver are unresectable because of the number of lesions, their proximity to major vascular structures, or advanced preexisting liver disease. Recent liver-directed surgical therapies including cryoablation, radiofrequency ablation (RFA), and hepatic artery infusion (HAI) of chemotherapy have shown promise for limiting progression of regional disease and arguably for extending survival.

Liver resection

There is no question that surgical resection of colorectal liver metastases offers the best outcome if disease is confined to a resectable portion of the liver. No other therapy can approach the 25% to 35% 5-year survival rate that has been demonstrated in multiple studies [39]. In addition, for this group of patients, 10-year survival remains at approximately 20%, and overall median survival is between 28 and 40 months. Even patients who have previously undergone hepatic resection for colorectal liver metastasis benefit from repeat resection if it is technically possible. A recent series of 64 patients reported a 41% 5-year survival rate for this subset of patients [40]. For these reasons, unless there is an absolute prohibitive medical risk, all patients with potentially resectable liver metastases should be considered for surgery. However, though it is generally well tolerated, there exists significant morbidity (8–12%) and mortality (1–4%) with liver resection, and patients should undergo careful evaluation to determine whether they have potentially resectable disease [5].

Preoperative evaluation of patients with liver disease is similar to that for patients with primary colorectal tumors, with the exception of specific hepatic cross-sectional and nuclear imaging. Although CT is sensitive for identifying liver lesions, its specificity for distinguishing benign from malignant lesions is less accurate. In contrast, MRI is sensitive and specific for malignant hepatic lesions and, as such, is the study of choice in evaluating potentially metastatic colorectal cancer. In addition, MRI provides valuable information on the relationship between liver lesions and the hepatic vasculature, which becomes important in the technical aspects of liver resection. Before surgery, it is necessary to evaluate for extrahepatic disease because its presence significantly changes the management strategy. Consequently, positron emission tomography (PET) is a valuable adjunct in the radiologic evaluation of potential candidates for liver resection. PET technology is based on the observation that malignant cells have a higher affinity for glucose, so the active compound used is a radioactive glucose analogue. Several studies have shown PET scanning to be the most sensitive modality for detecting extrahepatic metastases [41,42].

Despite these techniques for preoperative evaluation, some patients who undergo laparotomy for planned resection are found to be unresectable because of unrecognized carcinomatosis or because of technical factors related to the location or number of hepatic metastases. Intraoperative ultrasound (IOUS) is a necessary component in the evaluation of any patient with liver metastases undergoing planned liver resection with curative intent. IOUS provides superior imaging detail for deep lesions, nonpalpable lesions, and lesions within the dome of the liver that are often obscured in other imaging studies. In addition, IOUS delineates the precise relation to major vessels to guide operative strategy.

For patients in whom resection is not possible, other regionally directed modalities have been used, including cryoablation, RFA, HAI pump (HAIP) placement, and isolated hepatic perfusion. These therapies have been studied in multiple scenarios, singly and in combination, after liver resection and in unresectable patients. As a result, definitive conclusions regarding their efficacy are difficult to make [39,44–46].

Ablative therapies

In cryotherapy, the ablation of liver tumors is based on the cytotoxic effects of multiple freeze–thaw cycles. A probe is inserted into the lesions with ultrasound guidance, and the tumors are treated until they obtain a characteristic homogenous appearance on ultrasound. If lesions are in proximity to vascular structures, there is the potential for the cold therapy to be drawn away by convective currents, thereby limiting efficacy. Alternatively, vascular structures can be damaged by the cold therapy, possibly leading to massive hemorrhage. Cryotherapy has been studied as an isolated therapy and in combination with resection and HAIP placement. Retrospective analysis of cryotherapy with or without resection of all liver lesions reported a median survival of 26 to 30 months [46]. Despite these results, a key factor limiting the availability of cryotherapy is its expense—machines cost in excess of $300,000.

RFA uses heat-generated energy to cause tumor necrosis. Similar to cryotherapy, it is performed under ultrasound guidance, and tumors are ablated until a characteristic necrotic appearance is obtained. Because the probes used for RFA are smaller and easier to manipulate than those for cryotherapy, the technology can also be performed by a percutaneous approach. In RFA, the zone of necrosis is limited to a 3-cm diameter because the burned tissue does not conduct the energy required to produce heat necrosis outside this zone. To treat lesions larger than 3 cm, multiple passages of the probe are necessary, with the potential for nonuniform delivery of therapy.

RFA is more readily available than cryoablation, primarily because, at approximately $20,000 for the machine, it represents a significantly smaller capital expense. To improve effectiveness, smaller probes delivering energy at higher frequency are being designed to create larger and more uniform zones of necrosis. In studies to date, RFA has been well tolerated, even in patients with severe preexisting parenchymal liver disease. Its most frequent morbidity is abscess formation in the necrotic lesions, which occurred in 8% of patients in a recent series [45]. In current clinical practice, RFA is frequently combined with intraarterial chemotherapy, and studies have reported median survival in the range of 18 to 22 months [46].

Regional chemotherapy

Liver-directed chemotherapy through a hepatic artery infusion pump was initially used in the 1970s and 1980s. The theoretical benefits supporting the development of this technique included the potential to deliver higher doses of agents directly to the target tissue while minimizing systemic toxicity. In addition, experimental studies demonstrated that metastatic tumor deposits within the liver derive their blood supply from branches of the hepatic artery. It was therefore felt that intraarterial chemotherapy would more selectively target tumors while sparing normal liver tissue. Technically, implantation of a HAIP is relatively straightforward; however, it is important to obtain a preoperative visceral angio- gram because only two thirds of patients have conventional vascular anatomy. In most patients, cannulation of the gastroduodenal artery (GDA) is sufficient to obtain bilobar delivery of agents. It is necessary to divide the small arterial branches of the GDA to the stomach and proximal duodenum to prevent perfusion of these organs with chemotherapy that can lead to ulceration, bleeding, and perforation. Anomalous vessels should be ligated and cholecystectomy should be performed to further prevent extrahepatic delivery of the drug(s). After the catheter has been secured within the GDA, fluorescein is injected and visualized with a Wood lamp to verify bilobar liver perfusion without perfusion of the adjacent organs, such as the stomach or duodenum. After surgery, this perfusion pattern is again confirmed with a nuclear medicine study. The pump itself is tunneled into a subcutaneous pocket in the abdominal wall and secured in place with sutures. Ideally, the pump should be placed away from the incision at a location that is as comfortable and unobtrusive for the patient as possible.

Early studies of the HAIP, in the absence of liver resection or ablation, revealed an increased response rate within the liver when compared to systemic chemotherapy. However, these studies failed to demonstrate a survival benefit. Advocates of HAIP argue that these studies were limited by methodological problems, such as a high rate of crossover from the systemic arm to the HAIP arm

[43,44]. Moreover, there might have been inadequate statistical power within the sample sizes to detect a small but clinically significant difference between the treatments. In addition, in these trials many HAIP patients did not receive adequate intraarterial therapy because of technical complications with the device or liver toxicity from the chemotherapeutic agents. Nevertheless, the data from these studies suggested that the presumed regional benefit of HAIP was offset by systemic progression of the disease and surgical and medical complications from the therapy.

Recent studies have focused on HAIP as an adjuvant therapy to liver resection or ablation. For example, in 1999, a randomized, prospective trial was reported comparing liver resection, systemic chemotherapy, and HAIP therapy to resection and systemic chemotherapy alone [43]. This study found an increased median survival time of 13 months in the HAIP group. In addition, the 2-year survival rate was 86% in the group receiving HAIP versus 72% for the group receiving conventional therapy. These results suggest that HAIP has a benefit in the adjuvant treatment of metastatic colorectal cancer to the liver when combined with resection and systemic chemotherapy. No prospective data exist comparing the outcome of radiofrequency ablation or cryoablation with HAIP to ablation alone, but retrospective series using these techniques have reported a median survival time in the range of 18 to 22 months [45,46]. Compared with the historical survival time of 14 months for HAIP alone, these results suggest a potential survival benefit when the regional treatment modalities are combined.

Another technique of regional surgical therapy that has been applied to the liver is isolated hepatic perfusion (IHP). It is a technically complicated procedure that requires complete vascular control of the liver through cannulation of the hepatic artery and inferior vena cava with concurrent venovenous bypass. Like HAIP, it delivers regional high-dose chemotherapy while minimizing systemic toxicity. With IHP, however, chemotherapy is delivered through a recirculating bypass pump and is limited to the duration of the surgery. Phase 1 and 2 clinical trials of IHP have been performed using melphalan and tumor necrosis factor (TNF) as a corollary to studies of isolated limb perfusion with this combination of agents for the treatment of advanced melanoma of the extremities. Preliminary studies of IHP with melphalan and TNF have achieved response rates of 75% to 85%, with occasional complete responses [47]. Although technically challenging, this therapy has the potential to significantly improve the treatment of a large number of patients with unresectable colorectal liver metastases and therefore warrants further study in phase 3 trials.

Summary

There are many indications for surgical intervention in the current treatment of cancer of the colon and rectum. The hallmark of surgical therapy remains en bloc resection of the primary tumor, accompanied by removal of the mesenteric lymph nodes. Surgical resection is also the principal and most successful treatment for local recurrences and isolated metastases. Although the application of minimally invasive techniques is growing in all aspects of surgery and is accepted in the treatment of benign lesions of the colon, laparoscopic resection for colorectal cancer cannot be recommended apart from randomized, controlled trials. Similarly, the role of sentinel lymph node biopsy in the surgical treatment of colorectal cancer remains to be defined. Various surgical modalities have been developed for the treatment of unresectable colorectal cancer metastatic to the liver. Further studies should help to elucidate the exact role of these therapies in the treatment of this common clinical problem. In summary, surgical treatment plays an important role in multiple aspects of the care of the patient with colorectal cancer.

References

[1] Imperiale TF, Wagner DR, Lin CY, et al. Risk of advanced proximal neoplasms in asymptomatic adults according to the distal colorectal findings. N Engl J Med 2001;343:169–74.
[2] Lieberman DA, Weiss DG. One-time screening for colorectal cancer with combined fecal occult-blood testing and examination of the distal colon. N Engl J Med 2001;345:555–60.
[3] ACC/AHA Task Force. Special report: guidelines for perioperative cardiovascular evaluation for noncardiac surgery. Report of the American College of Cardiology/American Heart Association Task Force on practice guidelines (Committee on perioperative cardiovascular evaluation for noncardiac surgery). J Cardiothor Vasc Anesth 1996;10:540–52.
[4] Smetana GW. Preoperative pulmonary evaluation. N Engl J Med 1999;340:937–44.
[5] Goldberg RM, Fleming TR, Tangen CM, et al. Surgery for recurrent colon cancer: Strategies for identifying resectable recurrence and success rates after resection. Ann Int Med 1998;129: 27–35.
[6] Graham RA, Wang S, Catalano PJ, et al. Postsurgical surveillance of colon cancer: preliminary cost analysis of physician examination, carcinoembryonic antigen testing, chest x-ray, and colonoscopy. Ann Surg 1998;228:59–63.
[7] MacDonald JS. Carcinoembryonic antigen screening: pros and cons. Semin Oncol 1999;26: 556–60.
[8] Moertel CG, Fleming TR, MacDonald JS, et al. An evaluation of the carcinoembryonic antigen (CEA) test for monitoring patients with resected colon cancer. JAMA 1993;270:943–7.
[9] Hildebrandt U, Schuder G, Feifel G. Preoperative staging of rectal and colonic cancer. Endoscopy 1994;26:810–2.
[10] Lindmark G, Elvin A, Pahlman L, et al. The value of endosonography in preoperative staging of rectal cancer. Int J Colorectal Dis 1992;7:162–6.
[11] Nichols RL, Broido P, Condon RE, et al. Effect of preoperative neomycin-erythromycin intestinal preparation on the incidence of infectious complications following colon surgery. Ann Surg 1973;178:453–62.
[12] Platell C, Hall J. What is the role of mechanical bowel preparation in patients undergoing colorectal surgery? Dis Colon Rectum 1998;41:875–82.
[13] Lau PW, Lo CY, Law WL. The role of one-stage surgery in acute left-sided colonic obstruction. Am J Surg 1995;169:406–9.
[14] Bleday R, Breen E, Jessup JM, et al. Prospective evaluation of local excision for small rectal cancers. Dis Colon Rectum 1997;40:388–92.
[15] McArdle CS, Hole D. Impact of variability among surgeons on post-operative mortality and ultimate survival. BMJ 1991;302:1501–5.
[16] Heald RJ, Moran BJ, Ryall RD, et al. Rectal cancer: the Basingstoke experience of total mesorectal excision, 1978–1997. Arch Surg 1998;133:894–8.

[17] Kapiteijn E, Marijnen CA, Nagtegaal ID, et al. Preoperative radiotherapy combined with total mesorectal excision for resectable rectal cancer. N Engl J Med 2001;345:638–46.

[18] Havenga K, Deruiter MC, Enker WE, et al. Anatomical basis of autonomic nerve-preserving total mesorectal excision for rectal cancer. Br J Surg 1996;83:384–8.

[19] Cavaliere F, Pemberton JH, Cosimelli M, et al. Coloanal anastomosis for rectal cancer: long-term results at the Mayo and Cleveland Clinics. Dis Colon Rectum 1995;38:807–12.

[20] Meltvedt R Jr, Knecht B, Gibbons G, et al. Is nasogastric suction necessary after elective colon resection? Am J Surg 1985;149:620–2.

[21] Wolff BG, Pembeton JH, van Heerden JA, et al. Elective colon and rectal surgery without nasogastric decompression: a prospective, randomized trial. Ann Surg 1989;209:670–3.

[22] Benoist S, Panis Y, Denet C, et al. Optimal duration of urinary drainage after rectal resection: a randomized controlled trial. Surgery 1999;125:135–41.

[23] Detry R, Ciccarelli O, Komlan A, et al. Early feeding after colorectal surgery: preliminary results. Acta Chir Belg 1999;99:292–4.

[24] Anonymous. Perioperative total parenteral nutrition in surgical patients: the Veterans Affairs total parenteral nutrition cooperative study group. N Engl J Med 1991;325:525–32.

[25] Collins R, Scrimgeour A, Yusuf S, et al. Reduction in fatal pulmonary embolism and venous thrombosis by perioperative administration of subcutaneous heparin: overview of results of randomized trials in general, orthopedic, and urologic surgery. N Engl J Med 1988;318:1162–73.

[26] Falk PM, Beart Jr. RW, Wexner SD, et al. Laparoscopic colectomy: a critical appraisal. Dis Colon Rectum 1993;36(1):28–34.

[27] Fielding GA, Lumley J, Nathanson L, et al. Laparoscopic colectomy. Surg Endosc 1991;11: 745–9.

[28] Milsom JW, Kim SH. Laparoscopic vs. open surgery for colorectal cancer. W J Surg 1997;21: 702–5.

[29] Milsom JW, Bohm B, Hammerhofer KA, et al. A prospective, randomized trial comparing laparoscopic versus conventional techniques in colorectal cancer surgery: a preliminary report. J Am Coll Surg 1998;187:46–54.

[30] Kazemier G, Bonjer HJ, Berends FJ, et al. Port site metastases after laparoscopic colorectal surgery for cure of malignancy. Br J Surg 1995;82:1141–2.

[31] Stocchi L, Nelson H. Laparoscopic colectomy for colon cancer: trial update. J Surg Oncol 1998; 68:255–67.

[32] Greene F. Laparoscopic management of colorectal cancer. CA Cancer J Clin 1999;49:221–8.

[33] Merrie AE, van Rij AM, Phillips LV, et al. Diagnostic use of the sentinel node in colon cancer. Dis Colon Rectum 2001;44:410–17.

[34] Waters GS, Geisinger KR, Garske DD, et al. Sentinel lymph node mapping for carcinoma of the colon: a pilot study. Am Surg 2000;66:943–5.

[35] Wong JH, Steineman S, Calderia C, et al. Ex vivo sentinel node mapping in carcinoma of the colon and rectum. Ann Surg 2001;233:515–21.

[36] Wood TF, Saha S, Morton DL, et al. Validation of lymphatic mapping in colorectal cancer: In vivo, ex vivo, and laparoscopic techniques. Ann Surg Oncol 2001;8:150–7.

[37] Hendren SK, Hahn SM, Spitz FR, et al. Phase II trial of debulking surgery and photodynamic therapy for disseminated intraperitoneal tumors. Ann Surg Oncol 2001;8:65–71.

[38] Schoemaker D, Black R, Giles L, et al. Yearly colonoscopy, liver CT, and chest radiography do not influence 5-year survival of colorectal cancer patients. Gastroenterology 1998;114:7–14.

[39] Fong Y. Surgical therapy of hepatic colorectal metastasis. CA Cancer J Clin 1999;49:231–55.

[40] Adam R, Bismuth H, Castaing D, et al. Repeat hepatectomy for colorectal liver metastases. Ann Surg 1997;225:51–62.

[41] Akhurst T, Larson SM. Positron emission tomography imaging of colorectal cancer. Semin Oncol 1999;26:577–83.

[42] Fong Y, Saldinger PF, Akhurst T, et al. Utility of 18F-FDG positron emission tomography scanning on selection of patients for resection of hepatic colorectal metastases. Am J Surg 1999; 178:282–7.

[43] Kemeny N, Huang Y, Cohen A, et al. Hepatic arterial infusion of chemotherapy after resection of hepatic metastases from colorectal cancer. N Engl J Med 1999;341:2039–48.

[44] Koea J, Kemeny N. Hepatic artery infusion chemotherapy for metastatic colorectal carcinoma. Semin Surg Oncol 2000;19:125–34.

[45] Wood TF, Rose DM, Chung M, et al. Radiofrequency ablation of 231 unresectable hepatic tumors: indications, limitations, and complications. Ann Surg Oncol 2000;7:593–600.

[46] Yoon SS, Tanabe KK. Multidisciplinary management of metastatic colorectal cancer. Surg Oncol 1998;7:197–207.

[47] Alexander HR, Bartlett DL, Libutti SK, et al. Isolated hepatic perfusion with tumor necrosis factor and melphalan for unresectable cancers confined to the liver. J Clin Oncol 1998;16: 1479–90.

Hematol Oncol Clin N Am
16 (2002) 927–946

HEMATOLOGY/
ONCOLOGY
CLINICS OF
NORTH AMERICA

Surgical treatment of rectal cancer

Sonia L. Ramamoorthy, MD,
James W. Fleshman, MD, FACRS, FACS*

*Section of Colorectal Surgery, Washington University and Barnes Jewish Hospital,
St. Louis, MO 63108, USA*

The surgical treatment of rectal cancer has evolved dramatically over the past century. Indeed, initially thought to be only a surgical disease, it is now best approached from a multi-disciplinary standpoint. The correct staging of the tumor, selection of appropriate adjuvant therapy and timing of surgery in relation to adjuvant therapy ultimately determines outcome. Surgical approaches toward preoperative evaluation of rectal cancer, operative decision-making, and post-operative outcomes such as tumor recurrence, bowel function, and complications will be addressed.

Anatomy

Understanding the surgical approach to the treatment of rectal cancer requires knowledge of the anatomy of the rectum. The rectum is defined as the distal aspect of the large intestine where the teniae of the colon converge and is generally accepted to begin at the sacral promonotory. The National Cancer Institute (NCI)-sponsored consensus conference on rectal cancer for all patients participating in National Institutes of Health (NIH) and NIH-sponsored inter-group trials describe the rectum as the last 12 cm of bowel proximal to the anal verge. The upper third is covered by peritoneum anteriorly and the lower third is an extraperitoneal structure. The rectum is bounded by the sacrum and coccyx posteriorly, anteriorly by the bladder and prostate in men, and the uterus and vagina in women. It is surrounded laterally by the pelvic sidewall within the abdomen and distally by the levator ani muscles. The surrounding structures are often involved with advanced rectal cancer and can have a profound effect on the surgical management. The rectum receives its blood supply from both the inferior mesenteric artery and branches of the internal iliac artery. The venous

---

* Corresponding author.
E-mail address: fleshmanj@msnotes.wustl.edu (J.W. Fleshman).

blood drains into both the systemic system via the middle and inferior hemorrhoidal veins and the portal venous system via the superior rectal vein. Lymphatic drainage of the proximal two thirds of the rectum drains toward nodes that lie along the path of the inferior mesenteric artery (Fig. 1). Lymphatics from the distal third of the rectum flow along any of the feeding arterial paths. This can lead to lymphatic spread both locally and laterally along the middle and inferior hemorroidal arterial path, posteriorly along the middle sacral artery, or anteriorly through the channels in the rectovaginal or rectovesicular septums [1], and eventually into para iliac and para aortic nodes. Because

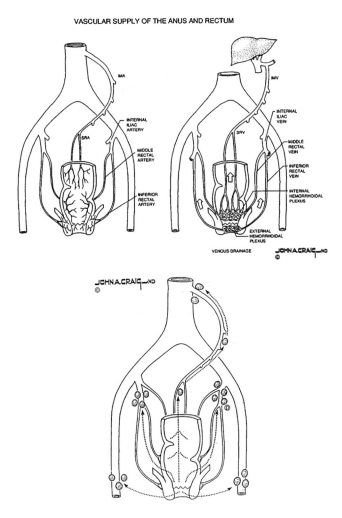

Fig. 1. Vascular supply of the rectum and anus. (A) Arterial. (B) Venous. (C) Lymphatic drainage. (Courtesy of the Section of Colorectal Surgery, Washington University School of Medicine/Barnes Jewish Hospital.)

of this joint drainage system, rectal cancer metastases can occur along both the systemic and portal-venous pathways. The fat and lymphatics of the mesorectum are enveloped in the visceral fascia (fascia propria) and separated from the parietal fascia (presacral fascia) by an avascular arelolar tissue plane. Splanchnic and presacral nerves, the basivertebral venous plexus, and the sacral arteries are posterior to the presacral fascial layer all the way to the pelvic floor. The reflection of the presacral fascia onto the fascia propria below the coccyx is called Waldeyer's fascia. Division of this layer admits entry to the true pelvic floor and anal canal.

Preoperative staging

Accurate preoperative staging is essential to plan treatment and provide prognostic information. Rectal cancer is staged using the tumor node metastasis (TNM) classification (uTNM for ultrasound or pTNM for pathology) (Fig. 2). Preoperative staging begins with the determination of the depth of invasion through the rectal wall. The "T and N" stage can be defined by transrectal endoluminal ultrasound (TRUS). TRUS, in experienced hands, is a simple, quick outpatient office procedure with high sensitivity and specificity [2]. It can be performed on most rectal lesions but is most accurate for mid to low rectal cancers. Fleshman et al showed that an accurate depth of invasion could be determined in 90% of cases, with a negative predictive value of 90% for lymph node involvement and an accuracy of 70% for the detection of local lymph node involvement (Fig. 3) [3]. In conjunction with proctoscopy and digital rectal exam, TRUS provides information that influences the decision to give preoperative neoadjuvent therapy. Findings of extensive adenopathy or advanced local disease invading adjacent organs in the pelvis are examples of situations benefiting from neoadjuvent chemoradiation. MR imaging may also be used to stage rectal cancer. Usually, an endoluminal coil is required. Images are very clear, and accuracy is high. CT scan to evaluate for intrabdominal and distant disease, a full colonoscopic evaluation to rule out

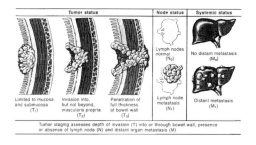

Fig. 2. Rectal cancer tumor node metastasis staging. (The Clinical Symposia, 41:1989.)

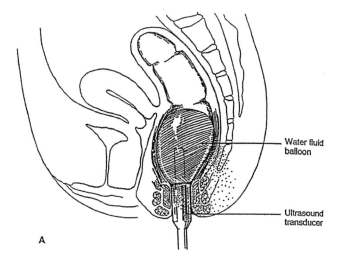

A

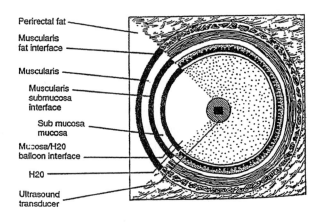

B

Fig. 3. (A) Transrectal ultrasound technique of insertion. (B) Ultrasound images showing layers of the rectal wall. (The Clinical Symposia, 41:1989.)

synchronous disease, and laboratory studies are needed to complete the preoperative staging workup.

Rectal cancer staged using the TNM classification

Depth of tumor (T) stage of rectal cancer is reported as follows:

T1 Tumor confined to the mucosa and submucosa
T2 Tumor invading through the submucosa into the muscularis propria

T3 Tumor invading the perirectal fat, or through the serosa for upper rectal cancer

T4 Tumor invading adjacent structures

Histology

Histologic factors including differentiation, mucinous/signet cell component, and vascular or lymphatic invasion can alter treatment plans in patients with seemingly early rectal cancers. Willett et al demonstrated that poor histologic characteristics lead to more aggressive rectal cancers and are therefore best treated aggressively at any stage [4]. Morson [5] found that poorly differentiated rectal cancers are associated with lymphatic involvement in up to 80% of cases.

At the time of surgery, the appropriate procurement and histologic evaluation of the cancer specimen is critical to stage the cancer accurately. Lymph node retrieval and evaluation by the pathologist is critical to staging patients with rectal carcinoma. A complete resection of all lymph node-bearing material in the mesorectum up to 5 cm below the level of the tumor with an intact fascia propria envelope is considered an appropriate resection. The mesorectum should be resected at right angles to the bowel and a "shaving" of the mesorectum should be avoided. Several studies have shown an inverse relationship between the number of positive lymph nodes and long-term survival. The number of lymph nodes obtained at the time of resection affect the accuracy of the staging (N0 versus N1 or N2), and thus the local recurrence and long-term survival for a group of patients with a similar stage of rectal cancer. Pathologists should be asked to perform lateral margin evaluation for all rectal cancers. This either requires inking of the enveloping mesorectum at the time of specimen retrieval or "bread loafing" of the specimens as described by Quirke [6]. Positive lateral or radial margins influence local recurrence and survival.

Clincial decision-making

The initial surgical consultation for a patient with rectal cancer is extremely important. A history of the patient's disease process is obtained, and certain pertinent findings will affect operative decision-making. For example, a patient with sporadic rectal cancer is approached much differently from the patient with a cancer in the setting of a polyposis syndrome or inflammatory bowel disease. Furthermore, an assessment of the patient's bowel function and continence is critical to determine the affect of the tumor on the sphincter mechanism, and whether the patient may suffer from sphincter compromise from previous surgical or obstetrical trauma. Sphincter preservation should not be attempted in those patients with anal incontinence unless the sphincter can be repaired and yield a reasonable possibility for return of normal function.

The physical exam should be tailored toward identifying evidence of distant disease, as well as locally advanced disease. The key aspect of the anorectal examination is the digital rectal exam (DRE) and proctoscopy. Experienced surgeons can often determine the degree of invasion of low rectal cancers with DRE [7]. A lesion that is freely mobile over the underlying muscle may be treated with local excision or endocavitary radiation. The tumor that is tethered to the rectal wall most likely has invaded the muscle, or even through the wall into the surrounding fat, and will require a more radical surgical approach. Lesions that are fixed to the surrounding tissues indicate a more advanced tumor and may require neoadjuvent therapy to free the tumor and allow resection with clear margins. The rectal exam can also provide information about sphincter function and involvement of surrounding structures such as prostate or vagina. Even so, TRUS has become the standard of care for determining depth of invasion or extent of advanced disease. Patients with symptoms of fecal incontinence and tumor in the area of the sphincter complex may have invasion into the muscle, thus making sphincter preservation unlikely. Rigid proctoscopy is routinely performed by many surgeons because it allows visualization of the lesion and confirmation of the distance from the anal verge or dentate line. Colonoscopic estimation of tumor distance from the anal verge is notoriously inaccurate because of the flexible nature of the colonoscope; even so, a complete evaluation of the remaining colon is essential to rule out synchronous lesions. After neoadjuvant treatment, a follow-up exam is sometimes recommended to re-evaluate the size, extent of fixation, and sphincter function of the preoperative patient. It is at this time that the patient and surgeon can have a candid discussion about the operation, potential outcomes, and the possibility of additional treatment postoperatively.

A patient with a completely or nearly obstructing colon or rectal cancer poses several problems in management. The evaluation of these patients is slightly different. Complete colonoscopic evaluation of the colon may not be possible. In these cases, water-soluble contrast studies are required to localize the tumor and evaluate the proximal colon. In recent years, endoscopic stenting of obstructing rectal lesions has served as a bridge to the operating room [8]. Only 10–30% of colorectal cancers present as obstructing lesions [9]. Stenting of obstructing lesions not only allows for better physiologic and mechanical bowel prepping of patients but relieves symptoms long enough for patients to undergo neoadjuvant treatment when indicated. Recent literature has shown a growing number of indications for colorectal stenting, with fewer complications and improved patient outcomes [10]. Emergency subtotal colectomy and ileorectal anastomosis or resection of the rectosigmoid and a colostomy are the two usual surgical alternatives. On-table colonic washout, resection, and primary anastomosis can be performed safely but are rarely indicated in rectal cancer, being more often used in colon cancer patients.

Preoperative preparation

If any form of ostomy is being considered, an evaluation by an enterostomal nurse is warranted. Preparing the patient for all the possible surgical outcomes, including change in bowel habits, temporary or permanent stoma, involvement of surrounding structures that may require resection, loss of sexual function, unresectability, or advanced local disease, is as important as any other aspect of preoperative care. The decision to perform sphincter-preserving radical resection of the rectum is influenced by position of the tumor relative to the anal sphincter and the function of the sphincter. Adequate distal margins and radial margins are necessary to reduce local recurrence. A distal margin of 2 cm is recommended [11]. After neoadjuvant therapy, however, a negative distal margin of any length and a negative radial margin by microscopic examination are acceptable.

Involvement of the anal sphincter by tumor dictates a complete removal of the rectum and anus (abdominoperineal resection, [APR]). The policy at our institution is to base this decision on the staging performed before neoadjuvant therapy (ie, a uT3 lesion invading into the sphincter will undergo APR even if it shrinks to a T2 or T1 lesion after treatment with preoperative radiation and chemotherapy). There is evidence to suggest that certain individuals may be candidates for expectant observation if the tumor responds completely to the neoadjuvent therapy [12]. This needs prospective evaluation in a randomized trial to identify selection criteria for this management.

Anal sphincter dysfunction that results in anal incontinence and that is not influenced by the presence of the rectal tumor should be considered a relative contraindication for sphincter-sparing surgery after removal of almost the entire rectum (low or extended low anterior resection of the rectum). The incapacitating loss of fecal control and change in the quality of life of the patients is devastating, even though bowel continuity has been restored. Pelvic floor or anal sphincter reconstruction is attempted in some instances, but results are variable [13]. The elderly patient with an already incompetent sphincter who may require post-operative chemotherapy should strongly consider an APR.

Adjuvant therapy

The use of adjuvant therapy in rectal cancer has been shown to improve local control of rectal cancer. At the same time, it may allow for preservation of the rectum and bowel function. In 1990, the NIH consensus on rectal cancer recommended postoperative radiation and chemotherapy for the treatment of stage 2 and 3 rectal cancer [14–17]. At the time, local recurrence was high after surgical treatment, and survival was influenced by the reduction of local recurrence. Since that time, however, the use of preoperative radiation with or without chemotherapy has been advocated by many for its ability to "down-stage" large locally invasive rectal cancers, potentially allowing surgical resection for cure and, in one study, improved local recurrence rates [18].

In recent years, the benefit of adjuvant therapy has also been called into question with the refinement of surgical technique. Total mesorectal excision (the removal of all of the rectal mesentery) has been advocated by some to have similar results as adjuvant therapy [19,20]. More recently, the Dutch Colorectal Cancer Group has shown an additional reduction in local recurrence when both adjuvant therapy and total mesorectal excision are combined [21]. These studies show that improving surgical technique and appropriate use of adjuvant therapy can lead to better outcomes.

The type of adjuvant therapy remains a debated issue as well. Current acceptable preoperative treatment for stage 3 and 4 rectal cancer is 4–5 weeks of preoperative chemoradiation, followed by surgical resection 6–8 weeks later. This delay in surgery allows resolution of the acute radiation-induced inflammation within the pelvis and shrinkage of the tumor. In some cases, this allows a change in the planned surgery, ie, a sphincter sparing procedure is performed. There is no evidence that the delay results in metastasis of the tumor. There are no intraoperative complications that can be attributed to this dose of preoperative radiation [22].

Though there has been no consensus on adjuvant therapy for stage 1 and 2 rectal cancers, studies that attempt to identify patients in this category who would benefit from chemoradiation are ongoing. A randomized controlled study in the Netherlands has shown a lower local recurrence rate for stage 2 rectal cancers when treated with 2500cGY of preoperative radiation, followed by surgery within 10 days [21]. At Washington University, patients with lymph node involvement on TRUS (N1 or N2) or large T3 tumors invading through the rectal wall in whom tumor shrinkage is desired receive 4500cGY in 5 weeks of preoperative radiation with surgery 6–8 weeks later and may receive 5-FU chemotherapy with the radiation to achieve greater shrinkage. Patients with tumors confined to the rectal wall (uT2 or small uT3), and not considered amenable to local treatment, but in whom we want the benefit of reduction of local recurrence receive 2000cGY in 5 days of radiation preoperatively, followed immediately by surgical resection [23]. A clinical scoring system is utilized that includes high-risk factors of localization < 5 cm from the anal verge, circumferential lesion, near obstruction, and tethered or fixed tumor. A score of 0–1 indicates a candidate for short course radiation, whereas a score of 2 or more indicates the need for a more aggressive regimen [24]. Kim et al reported a series of patients with T2 and T3 tumors treated with chemoradiation followed by local excision [25]. Patients were offered only local excision if they had a complete clinical response to adjuvant therapy regardless of the pretreatment stage. In this small group of patients, no local recurrences were identified at 19 months. Though there is early data suggestive of better local control rates, long-term survival rates from these new protocols have yet to be determined.

Early favorable rectal cancer

Early favorable rectal cancer is confined to the rectal wall (T1 or T2), has no evidence of distant disease (lung, liver, or lymph nodes), and shows well-differentiated pathology without lymphovascular or neural invasion. On digital rectal examination, these lesions are freely mobile and have no fixation to the muscular wall. Ultrasound staging reveals a T1 or T2 invasion. Current thinking suggests that these tumors may be treated with a less radical approach such as local excision, endocavitary radiation, or transanal endoscopic microsurgery (TEM). Tumors that are best suited for standard transanal local excision are within 8 cm of the anal verge. The need for palliation, or associated severe comorbid conditions, may make some patients who are not ideal, from a rectal cancer point of view, candidates for local therapy. In these rare cases, local excision may be supplemented with additional modalities of treatment.

Transanal endoscopic microsurgery

TEM is a technique designed to allow for local excision of rectal tumors that were once thought inaccessible transanally. It is performed by a small number of surgeons and, to date there are no randomized studies that document similar recurrence and survival. The surgical principle is similar to that of colposcopy for cervical cancer. An endoscope is passed transanally, the rectum is insufflated with CO_2 and a seal created. Then, microsurgical techniques are utilized to perform partial or full thickness resections [26–28]. Early results have shown that approximately 97% of early cancers can be resected this way. In a study by Heinz et al, "favorable" T1 rectal cancers had similar local recurrence rates as those treated with radical surgery. With T1 lesions, the local recurrence rates in the TEM treatment group were 36%, as compared with no recurrence in the radical surgery group [28]. Though this may represent a viable option for local excision of early rectal cancers that were once thought too proximal to treat locally, the long-term survival and recurrence rates have yet to be determined. Once again, this may be a minimally invasive method of treating ideal or nonideal tumors in the rectum depending on the patient comorbidities and tumor characteristics.

Endocavitary radiation

The need for curative local therapy for early rectal cancers without the morbidity of radical surgery has prompted the use of such modalities as endocavitary radiation (ECRT). The technique involves the local delivery of a low-energy electron beam source to the tumor bed transanally (Fig. 4). The treatments are administered as 1500cGY over 2 minutes, with a reconfirmation of placement and followed by a second 1500cGY over 2 minutes for a total of 3000cGY per session. A full treatment course at our institution is 6000cGY in conjunction with 4500cGY of external beam radiation. Treatments are performed as outpatient surgeries under local anesthesia [3]. Patients received 25 fractions of 45cGY 5–7 weeks before ECRT. A recent review of 199 patients with rectal cancer who received endocavitary radiation at Washington University over a 14-year follow-up period showed an overall local control rate of 71% after treatment with ECRT and external beam radiation to the pelvis [29]. The local control rate for a favorable T1 lesion was 100%, 85% for T2 lesions, and 56% for T3 lesions in this series. The true benefit of endocavitary radiation coupled with

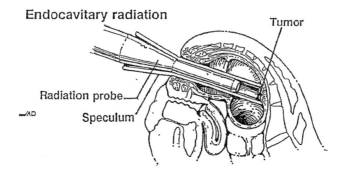

Fig. 4. Endocavitary radiation. (The Clinical Symposia, 41:1989.)

external beam radiation is the preservation of the end organ and bowel function without compromising local control or long-term survival. This modality has not been used with combined external beam radiation and chemotherapy to determine whether higher stage lesions (T2 and T3) would respond better.

Transanal excision

Tumors appropriate for transanal excision are stage I tumors (T1 or T2, N0) that are freely mobile on examination. Small tumors that are well- to moderately differentiated and show no evidence of lymphovascular invasion are most appropriate for this surgical approach. Though no specific standard exists, rigorous attempts to stage such tumors accurately are of paramount importance to avoid an inadequate resection. Transrectal ultrasound provides the best method of staging at present. MR imaging with rectal coil may become more feasible in the future and provide a nonoperator-dependent staging technique available to everyone. A biopsy proven adenocarcinoma (uT1 or uT2) within 8 cm of the anal verge, and no larger than one-third the circumference of the rectum is appropriate for local excision. Minsky et al showed local excision to be adequate treatment for T1 rectal cancers with a zero incidence of lymph node involvement when examined pathologically [30]. Increased incidence of lymph node involvement was found with higher stages of disease. A prospective study by Bleday and Steele confirmed that local excision should not be considered for T3 lesions, and T2 lesions probably need adjuvant therapy [31]. Mellgren et al have shown a high incidence of local recurrences in T2 lesions [32]. The 10% local recurrence rate after transanal resection of T1 lesions may indicate that a better selection criterion is needed, or adjuvant therapy is justified if high-risk indicators can be identified.

Local excision is a relatively simple operation, using only a spinal anesthetic. The excision is performed with the patient in either the prone or lithotomy position depending on the location of the tumor. A full-thickness incision through the rectal wall is necessary to ensure an adequate deep margin. Once the tumor is excised with a 1-cm lateral margin, the rectal wall is reapproximated and the lumen checked for stenosis. It is not unusual for this opening in the rectal wall to open after several days. This scar will close over time with conservative treatment (elemental diet and oral antibiotics).

Operative techniques

Sphincter perservation in rectal cancer

The ability to treat rectal cancer and preserve bowel continuity with sufficient continence is the goal of every colorectal surgeon. Surgical technique and instrumentation continue to evolve, making restoration of bowel continuity less complicated than in years past. Preservation of sexual and bladder function must all be taken into consideration when performing extensive surgery in the pelvis. The size of the tumor, its extension into the surrounding organs, and involvement of the sphincter complex are important preoperative considerations. The patient's preoperative bowel habits must be considered when discussing the expected postoperative function. Preoperative radiation in high doses given in a short course (2500cGY in 5 days) has been shown to affect fecal control adversely after sphincter sparing proctectomy [33]. But 4500cGY over 5 weeks has very little affect on the sphincter after a low anterior resection of the rectum [34]. This may be because of a higher "biological" dose of radiation delivered in the 2500cGY regimen.

Low anterior resection

Low anterior resection (LAR) is a segmental resection of the sigmoid and rectum with re-establishment of bowel continuity (Fig. 5). This operation is suited for high to mid rectal cancers but can also be used for low rectal cancers when the sphincter is not involved with tumor. The operation requires mobilization of the left colon and splenic flexure in addition to the sigmoid and rectum. The rectum is mobilized below the anterior peritoneal reflection as low as the levator ani muscles to provide a distal margin of 2 cm. The inferior mesenteric artery (IMA) is ligated just distal to the takeoff of the left colic artery or at the origin depending on the need for left colon mobility. The inferior mesenteric vein (IMV) is taken as proximally as possible also to facilitate mobility of the left colon. Care is taken to protect the ureters during this dissection. Anastomosis is most often accomplished with a stapling device, especially in a lower anastomosis. Several studies have shown that local recurrence and long-term survival rates are similar for mid rectal cancers when comparing LAR with APR [35,36]. In fact, our most recent experience suggests a higher local recurrence after an APR [22]. This is most likely caused by the fact that APR is reserved for the largest and most-advanced tumors. Reanastomosis following resection includes colorectal anastomosis, coloanal anastomosis with or without pouch reconstruction. Unlike preoperative radiation alone, preoperative chemoradiation may produce more inflammatory changes and result in a higher complication rate after a low anterior resection. Complications associated with this technique were evaluated by Enker et al [37]. The overall perioperative mortality rate was 0.6% in 681 patients. The length of

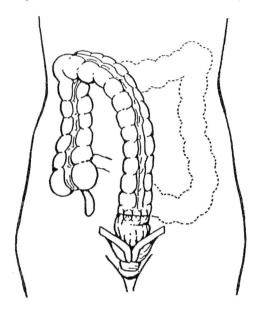

Fig. 5. Low anterior resection. (*From* Archives of Surgery 1999;134:670–7; with permission.)

stay was similar in both groups; however, a slightly longer operative time, higher estimated blood loss, and more frequent pelvic abscess formation were seen in patients who received preoperative chemoradiation. For this reason, it is our policy to utilize a protecting loop ileostomy when low anastomosis or colonic J pouch is constructed after chemoradiation [22].

Coloanal anastomosis

A coloanal J pouch is technically performed by suturing the colon to the anal canal at or just above the level of the dentate line. An ultra-low anterior resection of the rectum with a double-stapled anastomosis within the surgical anal canal is technically a coloanal anastomosis. Some surgeons consider only those anastomoses performed by hand sewing the colon to the dentate line as a true coloanal anastomosis. Controversy exists with regard to oncologic adequacy of resection and functional outcomes when the technique of coloanal anastomosis is utilized. In a study by Gamagami et al, 174 patients who had undergone either abdominoperineal resection or coloanal anastomosis for distal-third rectal cancers were followed for local and distant recurrence rates [38]. With a mean follow-up of 66 months, their study showed no difference (74% versus 78%) in 5-year survival or local/distal recurrence (12.9% versus 7.9%), respectively.

The low mobile cancer invading only the internal sphincter can be mobilized first from a transanal approach, beginning at the dentate line and progressing to the pelvis. An abdominal procedure to remove the entire rectum is then performed before constructing a hand-sewn coloanal anastomosis [39]. These patients benefit from neoadjuvant therapy and achieve excellent local control with preservation of sphincter function.

Studies evaluating functional results have shown increased stool frequency, fragmentation, and incontinence to gas and liquids in the early postoperative period, but improved bowel function in the late postoperative period. Most patients improve significantly, however, by 1 year after surgery [40]. Seow-Choen and Goh showed that all patients reconstructed with a colonic pouch reported near-normal continence and bowel function at 1 year compared with less than 70% in the coloanal group [41]. Overall, coloanal patients complained of more frequent bowel movements (6 versus 3) per day and higher rates of incomplete evacuation symptoms. The early bowel function problems experienced by patients with straight coloanal anastomosis are believed to be caused by the lack of a "reservoir." But many surgeons use the distal left and sigmoid as the proximal component of the anastomosis which may increase the frequency, etc, as compared with a mid left colon to anal anastomosis. This is only possible if the splenic flexure is mobilized and the inferior mesenteric artery and vein are divided at the origin.

Originally described by Lazorthes et al in 1986, the creation of a neorectum using the colon is widely used after LAR of rectal cancers [42]. Recreating the rectum after resection of low rectal cancers primarily serves to reduce the symptoms of urgency and incontinence and improve quality of life in the first year after the operation. The J pouch is created by folding the end of the colon and dividing the intervening septum using a linear stapling instrument to create a 7–8 cm reservoir (Fig. 6). A larger reservoir results in emptying dysfunction. The technique involves mobilization of the splenic flexure. Potential problems exist when the patients have foreshortened mesenteries that prevent the apex of the pouch from reaching the pelvis without tension. Many surgeons automatically divert patients with low pouches with a temporary ileostomy to avoid perioperative leak and pelvic sepsis. This is controversial because there is some evidence to suggest blood supply is better and leak rate is lower for the J pouch than for the straight coloanal [43].

An alternative to the J pouch is the coloplasty technique. This avoids the problem of tension with J pouches, or of fitting a bulky mesentery in a narrow male pelvis. The coloplasty is performed similarly to a stricturoplasty for Crohn's disease in that an 8–10 cm colotomy is made in the colon 4–6 cm from the transected end and is closed transversely [44]. Coloplasty has been shown to yield similar functional results in the early postoperative period [45].

Abdominoperineal resection

The abdominoperineal resection has been the definitive operation of choice for low rectal cancers. The operation involves complete removal of the rectum, mesorectum, and anus with surgical closure of the perineal defect. Ligation of the IMA is performed at the takeoff of the left colic artery, with care being taken to preserve blood supply to the proximal colostomy. A permanent end colostomy is

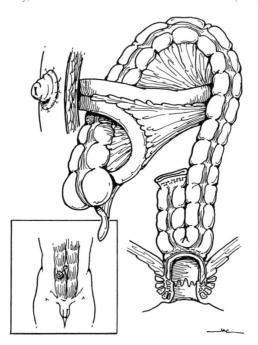

Fig. 6. Coloanal anastomosis with colonic J-Pouch and temporary diverting loop ileostomy. (Archives of Surgery 1999;134:670–7; with permission.)

performed. The APR, having once been the gold standard for mid to low rectal cancers, is now performed in less than 5% of all patients with rectal cancer, and only in patients with advanced low rectal cancers invading the sphincter or in patients with compromised sphincter function. A laparoscopic approach to the APR may allow a procedure to be performed with no abdominal incision other than the colostomy as the specimen is removed through the perineal wound. Early experience suggests this to be a potential alternative to open APR [46]. Several trials, both retrospective and prospective, have shown encouraging results for laparoscopically assisted resection of colorectal cancer [7]. The laparoscopic approach to rectal cancer presents a unique set of technical challenges. Rectal cancers located high in the rectum are technically easier than those that are deep in the pelvis located within the mid to low rectum. Access to this area is often limited by both the size of the pelvis and instrumentation. Large or invasive rectal cancers that involve the pelvic side-wall or surrounding structures may pose a difficult problem when attempting to obtain negative radial margins.

Total mesorectal excision

In the early 1980s, interest in the anatomic approach to rectal cancer was reintroduced in Europe under the name total mesorectal excision (TME). The removal of all of the mesorectal lymph node-bearing tissue should be standard for all types of radical resections for rectal cancer, LAR, or APR (Fig. 7). The current version of the technique removes the entire circumferentially intact rectal mesentery and rectum to 5 cm below the tumor. This technique was developed in response to the significant rate of local recurrence with traditional nonanastomotic surgical approaches to rectal cancer. Local recurrence rates as high as 15–45% have been reported with nonanatomic dissection techniques [47,48]. This was previously believed to be partly caused by discontinuous lymphovascular spread of rectal cancer. Kockerling et al, however, showed a reduced local recurrence rate from 39% to 10% with the introduction of TME for the treatment of rectal cancer [49]. This has been confirmed by other investigators [50]. Some authors suggest that TME would obviate the need for adjuvant therapy [51]. Several studies since that time have shown how the benefit from TME can be further augmented by adjuvant therapy [52]. The superiority of anatomic tumor-specific dissection over conventional surgery without adjuvant therapy has been shown in retrospective studies by the Mayo Clinic [53] and reinforces the fact that both colorectal surgeons and surgeons with an interest and extensive experience in dealing with rectal cancer have better outcomes. The controversy now surrounds which form of treatment, neoadjuvant therapy versus postoperative adjuvant therapy in addition to tumor-specific dissection, will be more effective in preventing local recurrence and prolonging long-term survival.

Unresectable rectal cancer

Unresectability can often be predicted by radiographic, endoscopic, and physical exam findings. Most surgeons agree that every attempt should be made, when possible, to downstage or shrink the tumor in an attempt to offer these patients a chance for resection. In studies by Mendenhall and Minsky, patients initially thought to be unresectable were sufficiently downstaged by adjuvant therapy that resection was possible in up to 89% of cases [52,54]. In the Sloan Kettering series, 20% of unresectable cases were resected for cure after neo-adjuvant therapy. In cases where the tumor is found to be unresectable at operative exploration despite neoadjuvant therapy, intraoperative radiation therapy or brachytherapy have been used to achieve short-term local control after a debulking procedure [55]. Results for both these techniques are better if margins are clear but close rather than grossly positive.

Obstructed patients can often be palliated with endoscopic stents when prognosis is poor, more than 50% of the liver replaced by tumor, or comorbid conditions preclude operative intervention. In cases where endoscopic stenting is not feasible, endoscopic laser therapy and or radiation treatment should be considered to maintain lumen patency before proceeding to colostomy. Medically unfit patients can consider local therapy to a rectal cancer that would otherwise require more radical approaches (ie, local excision or endocavitary radiation with

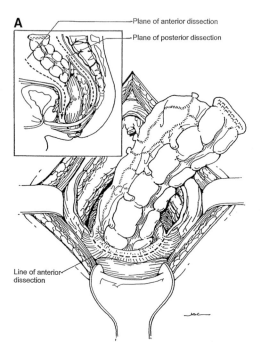

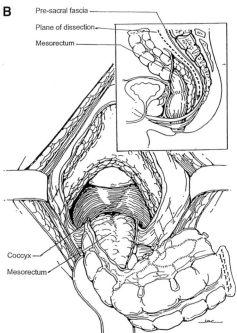

chemoradiation). These patients are best served by a multidisciplinary discussion regarding treatment options and long-term prognosis.

Pelvic exenteration

Pelvic exenteration is defined as the resection of the pelvic visceral organs, including the distal colon and rectum, lower ureters and bladder, reproductive organs, and all associated lymph nodes and peritoneum. Indications for pelvic exenteration include rectal cancer that is locally invasive and limited to the pelvis and recurrent rectal cancer. Pelvic exenteration results in a lower recurrence rate when done for primary disease as compared with recurrent disease (36% versus 66%) [56]. Pelvic exenteration is associated with a median survival of 20–30 months and a 5-year survival of up to 50%; however, perioperative morbidity is significant and hospital morbidity and mortality may approach 40–50% [56]. Perioperative complications include intra-abdominal hemorrhage, renal insufficiency, urethral injury, anastomotic leak or intestinal fistula formation, and overwhelming infection. Careful selection of patients who would benefit from pelvic exenteration is enhanced by the use of radiographic imaging techniques such as positron emission tomography (FDG-PET) scans.

Recurrent rectal cancer

The best chance to cure rectal cancer is at the time of initial presentation. Surgery alone for the treatment of locally advanced rectal cancer carries recurrence rates greater than 25%, even in the face of pathologically negative margins. Scheduled endoscopies, carcinoembryonic antigen (CEA) levels, and office visits may help identify patients with recurrent cancer. There is no consensus for the best method of following patients after resection of rectal cancer. Recently, FDG-PET has been shown to be an effective test for identifying additional local and distal recurrence in patients in whom a resection of recurrent disease is being considered. Libutti et al showed that PET scan was a more reliable method when compared with CEA scan and exploration for predicting resectable disease [57]. In a recent retrospective article by Strasberg and Linehan, FDG-PET correctly identified surgically resectable liver metastasis in patients with colorectal cancer more often than the standard imaging techniques [58]. The use of PET imaging has also helped avoid unnecessary surgery and predicts good outcomes after resection of recurrent disease in those patients with no other disease in PET preoperatively [59].

Fig. 7. Total mesorectal excision involves complete resection of the soft tissue mesentery surrounding the rectum. (A) Anterior dissection of the rectum starts behind the bladder and prostate. (B) The posterior dissection begins at the sacral promintory behind the mesorectum. (Courtesy of the Archives of Surgery/American Medical Association.)

Summary

Rectal cancer should no longer be thought of as only a surgically treated disease. Centers that treat large numbers of rectal cancer patients should provide state of the art radiotherapy and chemotherapy as well as offer anatomic tumor-specific operations for advanced-stage cancers and local treatment options for favorable, early lesions.

References

[1] Fry R, Fleshman J, Kodner I. Cancer of colon and rectum. Ciba Clinical Symposia. 1989; 41:5.
[2] Fleshman J, Myerson R, Fry R, Kodner I. Accuracy of transrectal ultrasound in predicting pathologic stage if rectal cancer before and after preoperative radiation therapy. Dis Colon Rectum 1992;35:823–9.
[3] Fleshman J, Kodner I. Rectal cancer: transrectal ultrasound staging and endocavitary irradiation. Problems in General Surgery. 1996;12:18–26.
[4] Willett CG, Compton C, Shellito P, Efird J. Selection factors for local excision vs. abdomino-perineal resection of early stage rectal cancer. Cancer 1994;73:2716–20.
[5] Morson BC. Factors influencing the prognosis of early cancer of the rectum. Proc R Soc Med 1966;59:607–8.
[6] Quirke P, Dixon MF, Durdey P, Williams NS. Local recurrence of rectal adenocarcinoma due to inadequate surgical resection. Histopathological study of lateral tumor spread and surgical excision. Lancet 1986;2(8514):996–9.
[7] Mason A. Rectal cancer: the spectrum of selective surgery. Aust Nz J Surg 1976;46(4):322–9.
[8] Stamos M, Tolmos J, Fleshman J, Sweeney W, Bailey H. Large-bowel obstruction: a multicenter experience of colonic stenting: (27). Dis Colon Rectum 2001;44(4):A13.
[9] Harris GJ, Senagore AJ, Lavery IC, Fazio VW. The management of neoplastic colorectal obstruction with colonic endoluminal stenting devices. Am J Surg 2001;181:499–506.
[10] Tamim W, Ghellai A, Counihan T, Swanson R. Experience with endoluminal colonic wall stents for the management of large bowel obstruction for benign and obstructing lesions. Arch Surg 2000;135:434–8.
[11] Vernava AM III, Moran M, Rothenberger DA, Wong WD. A prospective evaluation of distal margins in carcinoma of the rectum. Surg Gynecol Obstet 1992;175(4):333–6.
[12] Haber-Gama A, de Souza PM, Ribeiro Jr. U, et al. Low rectal cancer: impact of radiation and chemotherapy on surgical treatment. Dis Colon Rectum 1998;41(9):1087–96.
[13] Williams NS, Ogunbiyi OA, Scott SM, Fajobi O, Lunniss PJ. Rectal augmentation and stimulated gracilis anal neosphincter: a new approach in the management of fecal urgency and incontinence. Dis Colon Rectum 2001;44(2):192–8.
[14] Fisher B, Wolmark N, Rockette H, et al. Postoperative adjuvent chemotherapy or radiation for rectal cancer: results from NSABP protocol R-01. Journal of the National Cancer Institiute 1988;80:21–9.
[15] Gastrointestinal Tumor Study Group. Prolongation of the disease-free interval in surgically treated rectal carcinoma. N Engl J Med 1985;312:1465–72.
[16] Krook JE, Moertel CG, Genderson LL, et al. Effective surgical adjuvent therapy for high risk rectal carcinoma. N Engl J Med 1991;324:709–15.
[17] NIH consensus conference. Adjuvant therapy for patients with colon and rectal cancer. JAMA 1990;264:1444–50.
[18] Frykholm GJ, Glimelius B, Pahlman L. Preoperative or postoperative irradiation in adenocarcinoma of the rectum: final treatment results of a randomized trial and an evaluation of late secondary effects. Dis Colon Rectum 1993;36:564–72.

[19] Enker WE, Thaler HT, Craner ML, et al. Total mesorectal excision in the operative treatment of carcinoma of the rectum. J Am Coll Surg 1995;181:335–46.

[20] Heald RJ. Rectal cancer: the surgical options. Eur J Cancer 1995;31A:1189–92.

[21] Kapiteijn E, Marijen CA, Nagtegaal ID, et al. Preoperative radiotherapy combined with total mesorectal excision for resectable rectal cancer. N Engl J Med 2001;345:638–46.

[22] Read TE, Ogunbiyi OA, Fleshman JW, et al. Neoadjuvant external beam radiation and proctectomy for adenocarcinoma of the rectum. Dis Colon Rectum 2001;44(12):1778–90.

[23] Myerson RJ, Genovesi D, Lockett MA, et al. Five fractions of preoperative radiotherapy for selected cases of rectal carcinoma: long-term tumor control and tolerance to treatment. Int J Radiat Oncol Biol Phys 1999;43(3):537–43.

[24] Myerson RJ, Singh A, Birnbaum EH, et al. Pretreatment clinical findings predict outcome for patient preoperative radiation for rectal cancer. International Journal of Radiation Oncology. Biology and Physics. 2001;50:665–74.

[25] Kim CJ, Yeatman TJ, Coppola D, et al. Local excision of T2 and T3 rectal cancers after downstaging chemoradiation. Annals of Surgery 2001;234(3):352–8.

[26] Kreis ME, Jehle EC, Haug V, et al. Functional results after transanal endoscopic microsurgery. Dis Colon Rectum 1996;39:1116–21.

[27] Buess G, Mentges B, Manncke K, Starlinger M, Becker HD. Technique and results of transanal endoscopic microsurgery in early rectal cancer. Am J Surg 1992;163:63–70.

[28] Heintz A, Morschel M, Junginger T. Comparison of results after transanal endoscopic microsurgery and radical resection for T1 carcinoma of the rectum. Surg Endosc 1998;12:1145–8.

[29] Aumock A, Birnbaum E, Fleshman J, et al. Treatment of rectal adenocarcinoma with endocavitary and external beam radiation therapy: results for 199 patients with localized tumors. Int J Radiat Oncol Biol Phys 2001;51:363–70.

[30] Minsky BD, Rich T, Recht A, et al. Selection critieria for local excision with or without adjuvant radiation therapy for rectal cancer. Cancer 1989;63:1421.

[31] Bleday R, Steele G Jr. Current protocols and outcomes of local therapy for rectal cancer. Surg Oncol Clin N Am 2000;9(4):751–8.

[32] Mellgren A, Sirivongs P, Rothenberger DA, Madoff RD, Garcia-Aguilar J. Is local excision adequate therapy for early rectal cancer? Dis Colon Rectum 2000;43(8):1064–71.

[33] Swedish Rectal Cancer Trial. Improved survival with preoperative radiotherapy in resectable rectal cancer. N Engl J Med 1997;336(14):980–7.

[34] Birnbaum EH, Myerson RJ, Fry RD, Kodner IJ, Fleshman JW. Chronic effects of pelvic radiation therapy on anorectal function. Dis Colon Rectum 1994;37:909–15.

[35] Manson PN, Corman ML, Coller JA, Veidenheimer MC. Anterior resection for adenocarcinoma: Lahey Clinic experience from 1963 through 1969. Am J Surg 1976;131:434.

[36] Slanetz CA, Herter FP, Grinnell RS. Anterior resection versus abdominoperineal resection for cancer of the rectum and rectosigmoid. Am J Surg 1972;123:110–7.

[37] Enker WE, Merchant N, Cohen AM, et al. Safety and efficacy of low anterior resection for rectal cancer: 681 consecutive cases from a speciality service. Ann Surg 1999;230:1–18.

[38] Gamagami RA, Liagre A, Chiotasso P. Coloanal anastomosis for distal third rectal cancer: prospective study of oncologic results. Dis Colon Rectum 1999;42:1272–5.

[39] Bannon JP, Marks GJ, Mohiuddin M, Rakinic J, Jian NZ, Nagle D. Radical and local excisional methods of sphincter-sparing surgery after high-dose radiation for cancer of the distal 3 cm of the rectum. Ann Surg Oncol 1995;2(3):221–7.

[40] Barrier A, Martel P, Gallot D, et al. Long term functional results of colonic J pouch versus straight coloanal anastomosis. Br J Surg 1999;86:1176–9.

[41] Seoh- Choen F, Goh HS. Prospective randomized trial comparing J colonic pouch-anal anastomosis and straight coloanal reconstruction. Br J Surg 1995;82:608–10.

[42] Lazorthes F, Fages P, Chiotasso P, et al. Resection of the rectum with construction of a colonic reservoir and colo-anal anastomosis for carcinoma of the rectum. Br J Surg 1986;73:136–8.

[43] Joo JS, Latulippe JF, Alabaz O, Weiss EG, Nogueras JJ, Wexner SD. Long-term functional

evaluation of straight coloanal anastomosis and colonic J-pouch: is the functional superiority of colonic J-pouch sustained? Dis Colon Rectum 1998;41(6):740–6.

[44] Fazio VW, Mantyh CR, Hull TL. A novel technique to enhance low colorectal or coloanal anastomosis. Dis Colon Rectum 2000;43:1448–50.

[45] Mantyh CR, Hull TL, Fazio VW. Coloplasty in low colorectal anastomosis: manometric and functional comparison with straight and colonic J-Pouch anastomosis. Dis Colon Rectum 2001;44:37–42.

[46] Fleshman J, Wexner S, Anvari M, et al. Laparoscopic vs. open abdominoperineal resection for cancer. Dis Colon Rectum 1999;42:930–9.

[47] Phillips RK, Hittinger R, Blesovsky L, Fry US, Fielding LP. Local recurrence following "curative" surgery for large bowel cancer. I. The overall picture. Br J Surg 1984;71:12–6.

[48] Kapiteijn E, Marijnen C, Colenbrander AC, et al. Local recurrence in patients with rectal cancer, diagnosed between 1988 and 1992: a population based study in the west Netherlands. Eur J Surg Oncol 1998;24:528–35.

[49] Kockerling F, Reymond MA, Altendorf-Hofman A, Dworak O, Hohenberger W. Influence of metachronous distant metastases and survival in rectal cancer. J of Clin Oncol. 1998; 16: 324–9.

[50] Kapiteijn E, Kranenberg EK, Steup WH, et al. Total mesorectal excision (TME) with or without preoperative radiotherapy in the treatment of primary rectal cancer: prospective randomized trial with standard operative and histopathological technique. Eur J Surg 1999;165:410–20.

[51] Heald RJ, Moran BJ, Ryall, RD, Sexton R, MacFarlane JD. Rectal cancer: the Basingstoke experience of total mesorectal excision, 1978–1997. Archives of Surgery 1998;133(8):894–8.

[52] Mendenhall WM, Souba WW, Bland KI, et al. Preoperative irrdiation and surgery for initially unresectable adenocarcinoma of the rectum. Am Surg 1992;58:423–9.

[53] Zaheer S, Pemberton JH, Farouk R, Dozois R, Wolff, BG, Ilstrup D. Surgical treatment of adenocarcinoma of the rectum. Annals of Surgery 1998;227(6):800–1.

[54] Minsky BD, Cohen AM, Kemeny N, et al. The efficacy of preoperative 5-FU, high dose leucovorin, and sequential radiation therapy for unresectable rectal cancer. Cancer 1993;71: 3486–92.

[55] Beart RW Jr, Streeter OE Jr. IOHDR brachytherapy in recurrent or metastatic colorectal carcinoma. Ann Surg Oncol 1998;5(1):2–3.

[56] Hafner GH, Herrera L, Petrelli NJ. Morbidity and mortality after pelvic exenteration for colorectal adenocarcinoma. Ann Surg 1992;215:63–7.

[57] Libutti SK, Alexander HR Jr, Choyke P, et al. A prospective study of 2-[18F] fluoro-2-deoxy-D-glucose/positron emission tomography scan, 99mTc-labeled arcitumomab (CEA-scan), and blind second-look laparotomy for detecting colon cancer recurrence in patients with increasing carcinoembryonic antigen levels. Ann Surg Oncol 2001;8(10):779–86.

[58] Strasberg SM, Dehdashti F, Siegel BA, Drebin JA, Linehan D. Survival of patients evaluated by FDG-PET before hepatic resection for metastatic colorectal carcinoma: a prospective database study. Ann Surg 2001;233(3):293–9.

[59] Whiteford MH, Whiteford HM, Yee LF, et al. Usefulness of FDG-PET scan in the assessment of suspected metastatic or recurrent adenocarcinoma of the colon and rectum. Dis Colon Rectum 2000;43(6):759–67.

Hematol Oncol Clin N Am
16 (2002) 947–967

HEMATOLOGY/
ONCOLOGY
CLINICS OF
NORTH AMERICA

Regional therapy of hepatic metastases

Douglas L. Fraker, MD[a,b,*], Michael Soulen, MD[b]

[a]*Department of Surgery, University of Pennsylvania Medical School, 1 Silverstein,
3400 Spruce Street, Philadelphia, PA 19104, USA*
[b]*Department of Radiology, University of Pennsylvania Medical School, 3400 Spruce Street,
Philadelphia, PA 19104, USA*

Regional cancer therapies target a specific organ or area of the body in contrast to systemic therapies, which treat the entire patient [1]. For various reasons, the treatment of primary and metastatic disease to the liver is a paradigm for regional cancer therapy. First, the liver is a common site for metastatic disease—in fact, often the liver is the sole site of cancer in this patient population. Colorectal metastases account for most tumors of metastatic disease limited to the liver. Several reasons account for the predominance of colorectal cancer metastasis. First, colorectal cancer is the third most common cancer in the United States; the incidence was 142,000 cases in 2001 [2]. Second, the natural history of this malignancy produces hepatic metastases in limited numbers. Third, the overall growth kinetics of colorectal cancer is slower than that for other gastrointestinal malignancies. For these reasons, the treatment of colorectal metastases accounts for most information in the literature regarding various regional hepatic therapies. Other malignancies with similar natural histories and metastases limited to the liver include gastrointestinal and pancreatic neuro-endocrine tumors, ocular melanoma, and some gastrointestinal stromal tumors. The list below categorizes the appropriateness of regional hepatic therapy, depending on metastasis:

Often appropriate for regional hepatic therapy
    Colorectal cancer
    Pancreatic neuroendocrine tumor
    Carcinoid
    Ocular melanoma
    Gastrointestinal stromal tumor

* Corresponding author. Department of Radiology, University of Pennsylvania Medical School, 3400 Spruce Street, Philadelphia, PA 19104.
   E-mail address: frakerd@uphs.upenn.edu (D.L. Fraker).

Occasionally appropriate for regional hepatic therapy
  Renal cell carcinoma
  Breast cancer
  Cutaneous melanoma
  Thyroid cancer
Rarely appropriate for regional hepatic therapy
  Lung cancer
  Pancreatic cancer
  Gastric cancer
  Esophageal cancer
  Prostate cancer
  Ovarian cancer

Other common tumor types—lung cancer, prostate cancer, gastric cancer, breast cancer, and pancreatic cancer—have different natural histories that rarely make them appropriate targets for regionally directed therapy to the liver.

A second reason the liver is an outstanding target for regional therapy is its vascular anatomy and accessibility. The vascular anatomy of the liver encompasses a dual blood supply from the hepatic artery and portal vein, and the accessibility of this organ to percutaneous techniques and to vascular access by interventional radiology allows for a variety of approaches to tumors within the liver. Other organs or regions of the body in which locally recurrent or metastatic disease occurs, such as the brain, pelvis, and extremities, are less easily approached than the liver. The lung may be the sole site of metastatic disease in many types of malignancies; however, regional treatment of pulmonary metastases is rarely undertaken because of the difficulty in accessing the bronchial arteries and the problem of multiple treatment with bilateral organs as opposed to a single organ such as the liver.

A final reason why the liver is an excellent target for regional cancer therapy relates to its physiology. One of the primary functions of the liver is drug metabolism and excretion [3,4]. The ability of the liver to metabolize infused agents greatly increases the opportunity to escalate drug doses because often the liver is able to metabolize the infused agent to a great extent, limiting systemic exposure. This function of the liver allows regional infusion of chemotherapeutics with a significant therapeutic index because of high local concentration and minimal systems exposure.

The types of liver-directed regional therapies may be categorized as vascular-based treatments or direct ablative techniques [1]. Vascular-based treatments deliver agents through inflow vessels, typically to treat the entire liver or at least large regional areas such as the right or left lobe of the liver. Ablative techniques use heat, cold, or local injection of toxic agents in individual tumor nodules to destroy the tumor. The box below lists the various approaches that have been used to deliver regional therapy to the liver. A second way to classify regional cancer treatments is by type of agent used to cause tumor destruction. The most important category treatment is standard chemotherapeutic drugs. An advantage of regional therapy, however, is that certain agents may be difficult to deliver effectively by systemic administration because the pharmacokinetics or trafficking patterns do not permit adequate concentration at the site of tumor. These agents may be delivered regionally with more success. One example of this type of drug would be gene therapy vectors, which could be given either by vascular infusion or intratumoral-directed injection into the liver [5]. Other treatment modalities used in ablative techniques include cold temperatures from cryosurgery, heat from radiofrequency ablation, and ethyl alcohol and other chemicals used as direct toxic agents.

Categorization of types of hepatic regional therapies and agents used for tumor destruction

Type of treatment

Vascular treatment
  Hepatic artery infusion
  Chemoembolization
  Isolated hepatic perfusion
  Percutaneous hepatic perfusion with hemofiltration

Direct treatment

  Resection
  Radiofrequency thermal ablation
  Cryosurgery
  Direct injection

Agent

  Standard chemotherapeutics
  Gene therapy vectors
  Radiolabeled compounds
  Slow-release compounds
  Heat by radiofrequency electrodes
  Cold by liquid nitrogen
  Chemical ablation with ethyl alcohol

Hepatic intraarterial chemotherapy

The benchmark for comparing outcomes of any regional therapeutic techniques is the best-achievable results with available systemic chemotherapeutic agents. For several decades, the standard systemic chemotherapy treatment for metastatic colorectal cancer was 5-fluorouracil (5-FU)–based regimens; however, 5-FU–based chemotherapy treatments produced objective tumor regression in only 11% to 20% of patients, with a median duration of response of 6 to 8 months [6]. There was no approved second-line chemotherapeutic agent until irinotecan was shown to produce objective responses in 15% and 22% of patients with metastatic colon cancer and in whom 5-FU failed [6,7]. Recent phase 3 trials have shown that the combination of 5-FU, irinotecan, and leucovorin results in a 37% overall response rate and a median duration of response of 9 to 10 months [8,9]. This combination of drugs, administered as either the Saltz regimen [8] or the De Gramont regimen [9], is considered standard therapy for metastatic colorectal cancer. Various other systemic agents, including standard investigational chemotherapy drugs such as oxaliplatin, and agents that target tyrosine kinase growth factor receptors, such as C225 and iressa, are actively under investigation as additional agents that may be beneficial in systemic colorectal cancer therapy [10]. Results of regional cancer therapy for metastatic disease in the liver has to be significantly better in terms of response rates or the toxicity has to be significantly less than the outcome from systemic regimens for regional treatment to be a useful strategy.

Two discoveries in the 1970s regarding drug delivery to the liver initiated the use of intraarterial chemotherapy as a regional treatment for colorectal metastases in the liver. First, though the liver receives most of its blood flow from the portal vein, it has been demonstrated that from 90% to 100% of the blood supply to metastatic cancer growing in the liver is from the hepatic arterial system [11,12]. Second, pharmacologic studies demonstrate that between 97% and 99% of the 5-FU analog, 5-fluoro-2′-deoxy-β-uridine (FUDR), was cleared or metabolized during the first pass of perfusion through the liver [4]. These two findings led to clinical trials of continuous infusion of FUDR into the hepatic artery, potentially achieving extremely high concentrations of the drug in the tumor microenvironment with minimal systemic exposure.

Initial trials of infusion FUDR in the liver were performed by using indwelling percutaneous catheters with continuous infusion between 1 and 5 days. This percutaneous approach was cumbersome and costly and made it difficult to administer repetitive courses of drug. More than 20 years ago, an implantable pump system was developed for continuous hepatic arterial infusion [13]. The indwelling pump, which continues to be used today, has a reservoir and is placed entirely below the skin with no external attachments. The current models of implantable pumps reliably deliver between 1.0 and 1.5 mL perfusate per day. The device also has a bolus infusion port for delivering a rapid infusion of drug and for imaging purposes.

Surgical techniques

The hepatic arterial infusion pump is placed during open surgery through a midline or a right subcostal incision. The hepatic arterial vasculature to the liver is completely dissected, skeletonizing the common hepatic artery, the proper common hepatic artery, and the gastroduodenal artery. Side branches from these vessels, including the right gastric artery, are ligated. For patients with standard hepatic arterial anatomy, the distal gastroduodenal artery is ligated and the tip of the catheter is placed by a cut-down in this vessel such that the catheter delivers agents at the origin of the proper common hepatic artery. If accessory or replaced right or left hepatic arteries exist, these vessels are ligated and that lobe of the liver is eventually fed that crossover collateral perfusion from the other arterial system, which is cannulated through the gastroduodenal artery. Correct placement of this device is verified during surgery with a fluorescein injection and after surgery by a nuclear medicine technique using macroaggregated albumin. Postoperative imaging is used to evaluate any collateral arterial branches not lighted during surgery that could deliver chemotherapy to the stomach or duodenum. It also can identify the degree of shunt of drug through the liver to the lung, resulting in systemic exposure. Systemic exposure occurs most frequently when there is bulky disease in the liver.

Initial phase 3 trials

Initial trials using the intraarterial infusion pump defined a dose regimen of 0.30 mg/kg/day of FUDR, delivered in a regimen of 2 weeks of chemotherapy followed by 2 weeks of heparinized saline [13]. Objective response rates with this regimen were three to four times greater than those achieved with systemic 5-FU. With this clear difference in response rates, appropriate prospective, randomized, phase 3 trials were initiated in a variety of institutions comparing the standard agent 5-FU to intraarterial FUDR (Table 1). Results of these studies confirm the significant differences in response rates between systemic therapy with 5-FU (9–21%) and intraarterial FUDR (42–68%) [14–19]. Significant improvement in response translated to improvement in survival in only 2 of 6 trials [18,19], however, and in a small subset of patients with negative portal hepatic lymph nodes in another trial [15].

Table 1
Randomized trials of intraarterial chemotherapy for colorectal metastases to the liver

Institution	n	Objective response rate (%)			Survival (median, mo)		
		Systemic	intraarterial	P	Systemic	intraarterial	P
UCSF [14]	110	10	42	<0.0001	NA - crossover	—	—
NCI [15]	64	17	68	<0.003	15 mo	22 mo	2 yr survival
MSKCC [16]	99	20	50	<0.001	NA - crossover	—	—
Mayo Clinic [17]	69	21	48	<0.05	11 mo	13 mo	NS
Paris [18]	163	9	43	NA	11 mo	15 mo	—
England [19]	100	—	NA	—	7.5 mo	13.5 mo (P<.05)	—

NA, not available; NS, not significant.

These trials have been thoroughly reviewed, analyzed, and criticized by advocates and opponents to hepatic intraarterial therapy [20]. A large number of design flaws in these trials make interpretation of the true value of the intraarterial infusion difficult. First, most of these trials allowed for crossover from the intravenous treatment arm to insertion of a pump for intraarterial therapy when patients progressed on systemic therapy. Allowing this crossover to occur makes it difficult to demonstrate a survival advantage for the intraarterial infusion group. Second, the initial regimens of FUDR using 0.3 mg/kg/day led to severe chemical hepatitis and biliary sclerosis (discussed below). In some trials, patients in the intraarterial infusion arm discontinued therapy because of hepatic toxicity, not because of tumor progression, and experienced considerable morbidity and some mortality from the treatment [14]. Third, opponents of the concept of intraarterial therapy point out that patients were not appropriately balanced between the two arms of treatment. Specifically, patients who underwent hepatic intraarterial infusion pump insertion underwent surgical staging to evaluate for extrahepatic disease, such as nodal disease, local recurrence, and carcinomatosis during laparotomy for pump input. Patients who were randomized to systemic therapy did not undergo laparotomy and, therefore, might have extrahepatic disease that went unrecognized by imaging studies. Opponents of hepatic intraarterial therapy point out that most trials produced negative findings, leading to no survival benefits and considerable hepatic toxicity. Advocates of this approach point out that design flaws and small sample size prevented demonstration of a survival advantage that might have been present because of the significantly better response rates.

Second-generation intraarterial drug regimens

While the data from the initial randomized trials of intraarterial chemotherapy for hepatic metastases matured, the next phase was the development of different regimens to try to limit hepatotoxicity (Table 2). Two institutions developed alternative regimens that maintained a high level of response rates while limiting chemical hepatitis [21,22]. The group at Memorial Sloan-Kettering Cancer Center decreased the FUDR dose significantly, added leucovorin and dexametha-

Table 2
Disease hepatotoxicity approaches with intraarterial therapy

Regimen	Response rate (%)	Biliary sclerosis (%)
FUDR 0.3 mg/kg/d for 14 d Every 4 wk [13–19]	42–68	8–50
FUDR 0.3 mg/kg/d + dexamethasone 20 mg × 14 d every 4 wk [21]	71	8
FUDR 0.18 mg/kg/d + leucovorin 200 mg + dexamethasone 20 mg for 14 days every 4 wk [21]	75	3
FUDR 0.1 mg/kg/d for 7 days with bolus IA 5 FU 15 mg/kg q y d × 4 [22]	50	0

sone, and reported a 78% overall response rate with a 3% rate of biliary sclerosis [21]. This new regimen used the same plan—2 weeks of chemotherapy and 2 weeks of saline infusion—with the FUDR dose of 0.18 mg/kg/day combined with 200 mg leucovorin and 20 mg dexamethasone. Investigators at the University of California at San Francisco significantly decreased the dose of FUDR to 0.1 mg/kg/day for only 1 week and, in the intervening weeks, gave a bolus 5-FU through the pump side-port [22]. This alternative phase 2 regimen produced a 50% objective response rate with a 0% reported incidence of biliary sclerosis. Based on these phase 2 data, a new phase 3 trial comparing intraarterial chemotherapy with systemic chemotherapy was initiated that attempted to address all the flaws in the previous studies. First, the new Memorial Sloan-Kettering regimen of decreased doses of FUDR was used to decrease hepatotoxicity. Second, the trial was written requiring that patients who entered the study sign a consent form stating that no crossover treatment was allowed. In other words, a patient for whom systemic therapy failed was not to receive placement of an intraarterial infusion pump. Third, the study was powered to detect a smaller difference than could be achieved in the earlier phase 3 trials by randomizing more than 300 patients. This intergroup study has achieved its accrual goals; data are maturing but have yet to be reported.

Continuous intraarterial therapy with systemic treatment

The third phase of hepatic intraarterial therapy while data from this current randomized trial are maturing has been to develop new combinations of intraarterial therapy with systemic therapy. A recent study [23] combined intraarterial FUDR and systemic irinotecan, attempting to reproduce the benefits of combining 5-FU and irinotecan in systemic regimens [8,9]. The phase 1 study defined the maximum tolerated dose of irinotecan as 100 mg/m^2 weekly for 3 weeks at 4-week intervals, with concurrent hepatic intraarterial FUDR at a dose of 0.16 mg/kg/day for 14 days of a 28-day cycle. Both were recycled in 28-days. Dose-limiting toxicities were diarrhea and neutropenia. The response rate in this phase 1 study was 74% [23].

Toxicity of intraarterial therapy

Toxicity resulting from intraarterial hepatic chemotherapy are related to the infused drug, the pump, and vascular complications. Drug complications can be divided into regional toxicity from hepatic effects and systemic toxicity from problems with pump placement, leading to exposure of other organs or sites to high drug levels. With an appropriately placed pump, the normal liver parenchyma receives the same dose of chemotherapy as the tumor nodules within the liver. Liver toxicity with FUDR is a chemical form of hepatitis caused by high-dose chemotherapy exposure that, if allowed to progress, may result in severe biliary sclerosis with untreatable jaundice [24]. Assessment of liver function tests every 2 weeks during therapy, with appropriate dose adjustment for any increase in alkaline phosphatase level, is crucial to limiting this type of hepatic toxicity. Most patients treated with the recent phase 2 regimen experience some degree of hepatic toxicity, necessitating dose reductions during their treatment regimen [25].

A different type of toxicity relates to drug exposure of other organs to this high-dose infusion chemotherapy. One early lesson learned from the initial intraarterial FUDR trials is that the gallbladder does not tolerate such a high dose of chemotherapy [13]. The cystic artery supplying the gallbladder originates from the right hepatic artery and, if the gallbladder is not removed, receives the same dose of FUDR. Virtually all patients have severe chemical cholecystitis requiring altered therapy or removal. Based on this early experience, cholecystectomy is a standard part of placement of this intraarterial infusion pump. A second region that may receive high-dose infusion treatment is the gastric antrum or duodenum. Occasionally, small arterial branches coming from the hepatic artery to the stomach and duodenum are not ligated during the surgical procedure. After ligation of the distal gastroduodenal artery to insert the catheter and ligation of other side branches, these small branches may become dilated and have significant flow to the stomach or duodenum. Drug exposure can cause severe irritation of the stomach and duodenum that appears to be epigastric pain when chemotherapy is infused.

Pump complications include obstruction of the flow secondary to clotting of the pump. This commonly occurs within a pump that is not refilled appropriately, which allows it to become empty with clotting of the small infusion catheter. Other problems with the pump include seroma in the pump pocket in the abdominal wall and infection of the pump. When the device becomes infected, as with other mechanical devices in the body, it is virtually impossible to clear the infection without removing the device. A new pump may be placed in a different location on the abdominal wall, with the catheter spliced to the new pump and the infected pump removed. The most important vascular complication is thrombosis of the hepatic artery. This complication can be avoided by taking care to place the catheter so that the tip is not in the lumen of the hepatic artery, where it may cause turbulent flow. In experienced hands, this complication occurs less than 2% of the time.

Adjuvant intraarterial therapy after hepatic resection

For the past two decades, after introduction of the hepatic intraarterial infusion pump, virtually all clinical studies have targeted patients with extensive metastatic colorectal cancer in both lobes of the liver. Two recent trials used intraarterial infusion as adjuvant treatment after curative hepatic resection. Data from many series of hepatic resection of colorectal metastases report that between 25% and 35% of patients may have long-term disease-free survival [26]. Of the remaining patients who have recurrences, approximately half the tumors recur in the nonresected portion of the liver, and the other half recur in extrahepatic locations. Kemeny et al [27] at Memorial Sloan-Kettering Cancer Center conducted a single-institution phase 3 trial comparing intraarterial FUDR and systemic 5-FU with systemic therapy alone after curative resection of colon metastases to the liver.

Table 3
Randomized trials of adjuvant intraarterial therapy after hepatic resection for colorectal metastases

Regimen	Control arm	Intraarterial therapy arm
Memorial Sloan-Kettering Cancer Center Trial		
	5 FU 370 mg/m^2 daily	5 FU 325 mg/m^2 + Leucovorin
	× 5 q 4 wk	200 mg mg/m^2 daily × 5 q 4 wk
	Leucovorin 200 mg/m^{2}daily	FUDR 0.25 mg/kg/d + Dexamethasone
	× 5 q 4 wk	20 mg × 14 d q 4 wk
n	82	74
Actual 2-year survival	72%	86% (P =.03)
Estimated median survival	59.3 mo	72.2 mo
Hepatic 2-year disease- free survival	60%	90% (P <.001)
Overall disease-free survival	42%	57% (P =.07)
SWOG Study		
	Surgery alone	0.1–0.2 mg/kg/d × 14 d q 4 wk
		5FU 200 mg/m^2/d IV × 14 d q 4 wk
n (total)	56	53
n (assessable)	45	30
4-year overall disease- free survival	25.2%	45.7% (P =.04)
4-year hepatic disease- free survival	43%	66.9% (P =.03)
4-year overall survival	52.7%	61.5% (P =.6)

There was a significant improvement in disease-free survival, reflected almost entirely by a decrease in the number of patients with hepatic recurrences (Table 3). A similar trial conducted by Southwest Oncology Group compared systemic 5-FU and FUDR versus no adjuvant treatment after curative hepatic resection [26]. Results also demonstrate an improvement in disease-free survival in patients who undergo intraarterial therapy (see Table 3). The results of these two prospective, randomized trials suggest that it should be standard practice to place an intra-arterial infusion pump after curative hepatic resection for colorectal metastases. These improved survival rates clearly reflect the ability of intraarterial FUDR to lead to significant responses in gross disease in the liver and the ability of this regional therapy to treat micrometastases.

Chemoembolization

Chemoembolization combines hepatic artery embolization with simultaneous infusion of a concentrated dose of chemotherapeutic drugs. This technique, performed primarily by interventional radiologists, has many similarities to the intraarterial infusion pumps discussed above because both techniques use vascular delivery. Chemoembolization entails several theoretical advantages. First, embolization renders the tumor ischemic, depriving it of nutrients and oxygen. Second, tumor drug concentrations are 1 to 2 orders of magnitude higher than are achieved by infusion alone [28,29]. Third, because blood flow is arrested, the dwell time of chemotherapy is markedly prolonged, with measurable drug levels present as long as a month later [30,31]. Fourth, the ischemia induced by embolization may overcome drug resistance by causing metabolically active cell membrane pumps to fail, thereby increasing intracellular retention of the chemotherapeutic drugs [32]. Finally, because most of the drug is retained in the liver, systemic toxicity is reduced [33]. In addition, chemoembolization is a percutaneous catheter technique and does not necessitate hospitalization.

Critical to the selection of patients for regional therapy is that their tumor be confined to the liver. Patients with minimal or indolent extrahepatic disease may be candidates if liver disease is considered the dominant source of morbidity and mortality. Tolerance of hepatic artery occlusion is dependent on the presence of portal vein inflow. Compromise in portal venous blood flow is a relative contraindication to hepatic embolization. Chemoembolization can be performed safely despite portal vein tumor thrombus if hepatopetal collateral flow is present [34]. In these patients, a smaller volume of the liver should be embolized at any one time to avoid liver toxicity. When the parenchyma is diseased, the liver becomes dependent on the hepatic artery for its blood supply, and the potential complications of chemoembolization are significantly increased. A subgroup of patients has been identified who are at high risk for acute hepatic failure after hepatic artery embolization. They have a constellation of signs: more than 50% of the liver volume is replaced by tumor, lactate dehydrogenase (LDH) is greater than 425 IU/L, aspartate aminotransferase (AST) is greater than 100 IU/L, and total bilirubin is 2 mg/dL or higher [35]. Hepatic encephalopathy and jaundice are absolute contraindications to embolization. Biliary obstruction is also a contraindication. Even with a normal serum bilirubin level, the presence of dilated intrahepatic bile ducts places the patient at high risk for biliary necrosis of the obstructed segment(s) of the liver.

Procedure and periprocedural care

Pretreatment assessment

Preoperative evaluation for chemoembolization includes tissue diagnosis, cross-sectional imaging of the liver, exclusion of extrahepatic disease, and laboratory studies including complete blood count, prothrombin time, partial thromboplastin time, creatinine clearance, liver function tests, and tumor markers.

Patient education

Before embarking on this fairly arduous palliative regimen, patients should be thoroughly informed of the side effects and risks. Eighty percent to 90% of patients experience postembolization syndrome, characterized by pain, fever, nausea, and vomiting. The severity of these symptoms varies tremendously from patient to patient and can last from a few hours to several days. Other significant toxicities are rare. Serious complications occur after 5% to 7% of procedures (see below). Given the significant discomforts, hazards, and expense of this treatment, its palliative role should be clearly understood.

Procedure

Diagnostic visceral arteriography is performed to determine the arterial supply to the liver and to confirm patency of the portal vein. The origins of vessels supplying the gut, particularly the right gastric and supraduodenal arteries, are carefully noted to avoid embolization of the stomach or small bowel. The origin of the cystic artery should also be noted because chemoembolization of the gallbladder significantly worsens the intensity and duration of postembolization syndrome [35].

Once the arterial anatomy is clearly understood, a catheter is advanced selectively into the right or left hepatic artery, depending on which lobe holds the most tumor burden. The chemoembolic mixture is injected until nearly complete stasis of blood flow is achieved. In our institution, we use 100 to 150 mg cisplatin, 50 mg doxorubicin, and 10 mg mitomycin c dissolved in 10 mL radiographic contrast and emulsified with 10 mL iodized oil and 150 250 μm polyvinyl alcohol particles. The patient receives intraarterial lidocaine (30 mg boluses; up to 200 mg total) and intravenous fentanyl and morphine to alleviate pain during embolization. After the procedure, vigorous hydration (3 L/day normal saline solution), intravenous antibiotics, and antiemetic therapy (ondansetron and Decadron) are continued. Narcotics, perchlorpromazine, and acetaminophen are liberally supplied for control of pain, nausea, and fever. The patient is discharged as soon as oral intake is adequate and parenteral narcotics are not required for pain control. Approximately half the patients are discharged in 1 day, and most spend no more than 2 days in the hospital. Oral antibiotics are continued for another 5 days, as are antiemetics and oral narcotics if needed. Laboratory studies are repeated in 3 weeks, and the patient returns for a second procedure directed at the other lobe of the liver in 4 weeks. Depending on the arterial anatomy, two to four procedures are required to treat the entire liver, after which response is assessed by repeat imaging studies and tumor markers.

Complications

Major complications of hepatic embolization include hepatic insufficiency or infarction, hepatic abscess, tumor rupture, surgical cholecystitis, and nontarget embolization to the gut. With careful patient selection and scrupulous technique, the incidence of these serious events collectively is 3% to 4%. Previous biliary surgery, biliary stent, or bile duct dilation strongly predisposes a patient to the development of a hepatic abscess, despite the use of prophylactic antibiotics [36]. Oral bowel preparation and increased intensity and duration of intravenous antibiotic therapy should be considered in such patients. Other complications include periprocedural cardiac events, renal insufficiency, and anemia requiring transfusion, with incidences of less than 1% each. Thirty-day mortality rates range from 1% to 4%. Sustained deterioration in liver function rarely occurs in patients with Child class A or B cirrhosis.

Results in colorectal metastases

Phase 2 study findings of chemoembolization for metastatic colorectal cancer have been reported by several centers in the United States. Patients enrolled in these trials usually have undergone failed systemic or intraarterial infusion chemotherapy. Lang [37] used a combination of superselective segmental and selective lobar injections of a doxorubicin-iodized oil emulsion on 46 patients. Fifty-nine percent achieve stabilization or regression of disease, with 17% complete responses. Actuarial survival rates were 68% at 1 year and 37% at 2 years. At the Boston Center for Liver Cancer, 40 patients underwent chemoembolization with 5-FU, mitomycin c, oil, and gelatin sponge [38]. Sixty-three percent had partial or minor morphologic responses, and 62% had greater than a 50% decrease in carcinoembryonic antigen (CEA) level. Median survival time from first chemoembolization was 10 months. A number of prognostic factors were identified. Patients with an Eastern Cooperative Oncology Group (ECOG) performance status of 0 to 1 had a median survival of 24 months versus 3 months for those with a performance status of 2. Patients with extrahepatic disease had a median survival of 3 months versus 14 months for those without. Among patients with good performance status and no extrahepatic disease, actuarial survival rates were 73% at 1 year and 61% at 2 years. Elevation of the alkaline phosphatase of LDH levels to above 3 times normal, or elevation of the AST above normal, predicted worse survival. At Northwestern Memorial Hospital, 30 patients underwent chemoembolization with cisplatin, doxorubicin, mitomycin c (CAM), and bovine collagen [39]. Ninety-five percent had a 25% or greater decrease in CEA; 63% had a radiologic response defined as tumor necrosis or 25% or greater decrease in size. Median survival time was 8.6 months from first chemoembolization and 29 months from diagnosis. At the University of Pennsylvania, 51 patients underwent chemoembolization with CAM, iodized oil, and polyvinyl alcohol [40]. Morphologic stabilization or regression occurred in 72% of patients, and CEA stabilized or regressed in 90% of patients; median duration of response was 12 months. Actuarial survival rates from diagnosis with liver metastases was 86%, 55%, and 23% at 1, 2, and 3 years, with a median of 26 months. The results in these extensively pretreated patients are promising, but high early response rates do not necessarily improve survival. Phase 3 trials of chemoembolization are needed to determine whether a survival benefit exists. The ACR Imaging Network, or ACRIN, is funding a multicenter, randomized trial of systemic chemotherapy with or without chemoembolization for colorectal metastases to liver.

Other histologies such as primary hepatomas and neuroendocrine tumors from the gut (carcinoid tumors) or from the pancreas (islet cell tumors) have been effectively treated by chemoembolization. Hepatomas and neuroendocrine tumors are hypervascular compared with colorectal metastases, which tend to be hypovascular. Response rates for colorectal metastases using the same chemoembolization regimens are worse than in hypervascular lesions. The indolent growth pattern of neuroendocrine tumors, combined with the high response rates, make this a good target for chemoembolization.

Isolated hepatic perfusion

Two additional vascular-based treatments to the liver have been reported. These complicated procedures are isolated hepatic perfusion [41] and percutaneous isolated perfusion of the liver with extracorporal hemofiltration [42]. As opposed to isolated hepatic arterial infusion or chemoembolization, these two therapies attempt to completely isolate the liver from the systemic circulation so that high doses of chemotherapeutic agents can be delivered to the liver with the drug flushed out or filtered with essentially no systemic exposure.

Isolated hepatic perfusion is an extremely complicated, open surgical technique that completely dissects the liver from the surrounding tissues except for its vascular attachments [41]. Specifically, the inferior vena cava above and below the liver and the portal triad structures of the portal vein, hepatic artery, and bile duct are preserved, and all other attachments are divided. This surgical procedure is analogous to the more commonly used isolated limb perfusion, which treats locally advanced extremity melanoma. Isolated hepatic perfusion (IHP) was attempted in the 1960s and again in the 1980s; however, because of the complicated surgical nature of this technique and the low response rates with available drugs, it was not actively pursued. The recent addition, however, of the biologic agent tumor necrosis factor (TNF) to melphalan-isolated limb perfusion has rekindled interest in isolated hepatic perfusion. This surgical treatment was used in a series of phase 1 and 2 studies at the Surgery Branch of the National Cancer Institute and at various centers in Europe [43] using melphalan combined with TNF [41,44]. Initial trials with TNF alone produced some responses that were short-lived in patients with colorectal metastases and ocular melanoma. Phase 2 studies using TNF combined with melphalan produced objective response rates in 78% of patients with colorectal metastases [44] and 55% of patients with ocular melanoma [45]. These results are particularly impressive considering that patients in this trial were heavily pretreated and also had extensive or bulky disease.

Isolated hepatic perfusion with hemofiltration is a similar approach using a percutaneous catheter [42]. Specifically, the hepatic artery is cannulated as in chemoembolization, and a specially designed catheter is placed in the inferior vena cava to allow collection of the venous outflow of the liver. The agent is infused, and the blood from the liver is collected and externally pumped through a charcoal filter to remove the chemotherapy drug before reinfusion via insertion of a large-bore catheter in the subclavian vein. One key difference between this treatment and the surgical technique of IHP is that the portal vein flow is not controlled with the percutaneous technique. This in some ways would dilute the ability to deliver drug. In addition, heat added to the IHP technique to increase liver temperature to 39°–40° C is not possible with a percutaneous technique. Initial reports of this isolated hepatic perfusion with hemofiltration demonstrate that it is feasible, though it is a complex procedure, but they show that virtually no responses are seen in the phase 1 or 2 trials [42]. Both techniques are complicated, and specialized skills and technical apparatuses are needed. Consequently, clear benefits from these regional therapies must be demonstrated in terms of response and survival for them to be accepted as general treatment strategies. Complete isolation procedures are contrasted with intraarterial infusion and chemoembolization in Table 4.

Ablative techniques

Another category of liver-directed therapy is direct ablation or injection of individual tumor nodules. The vascular techniques described above to treat the liver target the entire organ or a large portion, such as a lobe. Ablative techniques treat each individual nodule within the liver and provide no therapy to the remaining liver. The optimal ablation technique is surgical resection. Successful removal of a hepatic metastasis with negative margins produces an immediate "complete response" for that lesion that has been removed. Advances in hepatic surgery, including the use of the argon-beam laser coagulation system, the cavitary ultrasound aspirator dissector, a tissue link dissector, and vascular stapling devices have significantly decreased the morbidity resulting from major hepatic resections in the past 10 to 15 years. Therefore, the ablative techniques described below should not be a substitute for hepatic resection in patients who are otherwise surgical candidates.

Ablative techniques can be categorized as those that use a physical device to produce extreme temperatures to lead to tissue destruction; a second category encompasses lesions ablated by injection of toxic or therapeutic agents. Injection techniques with ethanol have been used for primary hepatomas and for metastases from neuroendocrine tumors of the gut and pancreas because these lesions tend to

Table 4
Comparison of vascular techniques for regional cancer therapy

	Intraarterial pump	Chemoembolization	Isolated hepatic perfusion
Complexity of procedure	Moderate	Moderate	Significant
Days in hospital	4–7	1–2	10–14
Hepatic toxicity	Biliary sclerosis	Rarely hepatic failure	Hepatic venoocclusive disease
Systemic drug response	Minimal (in most cases)	Minimal	None
Objective response rate in colon cancer (%)	40–78	17–59	75

be soft and hypervascular and allow infusion of an agent directly. Colorectal metastases are firm and scirrhous, and it is difficult to inject in a meaningful way any agent into the tumor microenvironment at any volume. Ablative techniques using heat and cold have been used primarily to target metastatic colorectal cancer and other metastatic lesions. These techniques have no specific antitumor activity, but they rely on correct placement of the probes into the center of the tumor nodule to treat the appropriate area of the tissue.

Cryosurgery

The initial physical ablative technique was the application of cold, or cryosurgery [46]. This treatment was developed in the 1980s and was used a probe that circulated liquid nitrogen to freeze tissue. It was effective in terms of the ability to control treated lesions, but its usefulness was limited for several reasons. First, because of potential vascular and biliary complications resulting from cold temperatures, limited numbers of patients were eligible for cryosurgery. Only patients with a limited number of peripheral lesions could undergo this treatment. Often patients with limited peripheral lesions were eligible for resection either by wedge resection or combined lobar and wedge resection. Usually, patients would have evenly distributed nodules with central lesions that could not be addressed by cryosurgery because of potential vascular and biliary complications. The second problem with cryosurgery was significant operative and postoperative morbidity. During cryosurgery, a ball of ice forms in the liver, and this may lead to cracking of the tissue that could lead to bleeding as the liver thawed. In addition, the probe size used initially in cryosurgery was large and created a large tract into the surface of the substance of the liver. It was difficult to obtain hemostasis with this treatment. Postoperative complications, called post-cryo syndrome, were pain, fever, and sometimes (though rarely) multisystem organ failure [47]. A final problem with cryosurgery was the cost of the equipment, which was prohibitive and limited the use of this to a select number of institutions.

Despite these limitations, several institutions reported their series of cryosurgery treatments for metastatic cancer to the liver with long-term follow-up. In general, the recurrence rate within an individually treated lesion was between 3% and 5% at a follow-up of 2 to 5 years [46]. As may be expected, because the remainder of the liver was not treated in this patient population, there was a significant recurrence rate within the other areas of the liver.

Radiofrequency ablation

Almost all the problems associated with cryosurgery have been addressed with a relatively new technique, radiofrequency thermal ablation (RFA) (Table 5). This treatment uses heat to destroy tumor rather than cold, as in cryosurgery. Treatment is generally much safer, has application to a wider range of locations

Table 5
Advantages and disadvantages of cryosurgery and radiofrequency ablation to treat metastatic and primary liver tumors

	Cryosurgery	Radiofrequency ablation
Probe size	Moderate to large	Small
Lesion size	Large (10 cm or larger)	Limited; reliable at 4 cm, but new technology may increase this to 6–7 cm
Lesion location	Limited to more peripheral selected lesions	Able to treat more central lesions; limited by tumor adjacent to bile ducts
Efficacy	Long-term follow-up available; local recurrence rate of 3%–10% with 5-year follow-up	Short follow-up time; 3–28% recurrence rate with 1-year follow-up, particularly with larger lesions
Toxicity	Moderate (post-oryo syndrome, nausea, vomiting, fevers)	Minimal (rare abscess)
Cost	Expensive (unit price, $300,000)	Less expensive (Unit price, $30,000)

within the liver, and it is less expensive than cryosurgery. For all these reasons, RFA is more accepted during its short history than cryosurgery had been.

RFA applies high-frequency alternating current through a treatment electrode placed inside the lesion in the liver [48]. Other components of the RFA system are a dispersive electrode placed on the skin and a generating unit. In this way, RFA is similar to the standard electrocautery unit that also uses a hand-held device for cautery, a dispersive electrode, and a generator. The treatment electrode, by applying significant alternating current to the tip of the device, creates molecular friction within the surrounding tumor and hepatic tissue [49]. The electrode itself does not heat but becomes warm only as heat is created in a surrounding area. Size and shape of the thermal lesion created in the liver depend on the configuration of the treatment electrode. Initial devices were a single wire and a cylindrical region of destruction around the wire. Most currently used treatment electrodes are hollow wires with multiple tires that expand to create an array, making an ellipsoid or spherical region of destruction. Treatment is delivered based on an algorithm used by specific device manufacturers. Two different treatment strategies are used with currently available RFA devices. First, treatment may take the tissue temperature to near 100°C and then continue treatment at that energy level for a set period of time after the desired temperature is reached. A second approach is to measure impedance between opposing tines of the electrode device. As impedance increases, destruction of the tissue is reflected primarily by dessication. Final treatment is achieved by reaching a certain level of impedence.

RFA involves placement of the tip of the treatment electrode in the center of the area to be treated under ultrasound guidance. The treatment plan includes ablation of a surrounding rim of normal liver, at least 5 mm and optimally up to 1 cm in all directions, to ensure complete destruction of the nodule with an appropriate margin. For lesions larger than the cannula, overlapping thermal

Table 6
Clinical series of radiofrequency ablation for various hepatic tumors

	MD Anderson	Cleveland Clinic	John Wayne Cancer Center	Italy
No. patients	123	44	84	68
No. tumors	169	181	231	121
Tumor type	61 Colorectal (50%) 48 Hepatoma (39%) 14 Other (11%) (distribution of patients)	64 Colorectal (35%) 11 Hepatoma (6%) 79 Neuroendocrine (44%) (proportion of tumor)	37 Colorectal (44%) 11 Hepatoma (13%) 10 Melanoma (12%) 26 Other (31%)	58 Colorectal 10 Other metastatic
Operative approach	92 Open (75%) 31 Percutaneous (25%)	100% Laparoscopy	39 Open (43%) 27 Laparoscopic (11%) 25 Percutaneous (27%)	21 Open 47 Percutaneous
Median size of tumor (range)	3.4 cm (0.5–12 cm)	<1 cm to 10 cm	2 cm (0.3–9 cm)	2.0 (0.5–4.2 cm)
Median follow-up (mo)	15	12.9	9	13.7
Local recurrence rate (%)	3/109 (1.8) (2 colorectal, 1 hepatoma)	28/181 Overall (15.4) 10/64 Colorectal (28) 0/11 Hepatoma (0) 6/79 Neuroendocrine (7.5) 4/27 Other (15)	15/84 Patients (17.8)	9/100 Lesions total (9) 9/54 (17) 7/67 Percutaneous (10) 2/33 Lesions open (6)
Normalized tumor marker	76/105 (72.4%)	7/18 Colorectal (39) 3/11 Hepatoma (27) 10/29 Overall (34)	Not available	Not available
Complications	1 Hemorrhage into tissue	None	7 Complications (6%) 3 Hepatic abscesses, including 1 death 1 Hemorrhage 1 Myocardial infarct 1 Liver failure 1 Skin burn	3/68 Patients (4.4%) 2 Hepatic abscesses, 1 Bile peritoneum

spheres are created to allow treatment of a greater size. Treatment may be delivered in one of three ways. RFA may be performed by an open surgical technique using intraoperative ultrasound. Because of the accessibility of the liver, this treatment may be delivered using percutaneous ultrasound or CT. Finally, a combination of open surgical and percutaneous techniques is used comprising minimally invasive surgery, laparoscopic ultrasound, and perc- utaneous placement of catheters [50]. One limitation of RFA is the size of the thermal lesion that can be created. Initial devices created elliptical lesions with a diameter between 2 and 3.5 cm. Recent advances have led to catheters up to 5 cm in diameter and sometimes up to 7 cm. This size limitation is one of the major problems with RFA in comparison with cryosurgery, which can create an ice ball as large as 8 to 10 cm or more (see Table 5).

Initial trials of RFA have demonstrated that it is an extremely safe treatment. Again, the probe size is significantly smaller than that used for cryosurgery, and rare complications of bleeding have occurred. In addition to the small probe size, the application of heat or cautery is a well-known technique to achieve coagulation (contrast this with the freezing of cryosurgery, which may lead to significant bleeding when the frozen lesion thaws). The most common com- plication of radiofrequency ablation has been abscess formation in the treated areas. In addition, several investigators have reported treatment of more central lesions adjacent to the major hepatic veins or inferior vena cava. Only the most central regions of the bifurcation of the right and left hepatic bile ducts have been untreatable in terms of application of radiofrequency ablation.

Table 6 shows the results of recently reported trials of radiofrequency ablation. Recurrence rates of individual lesions range from 1.5% in the series by Curley [51] to between 15% and 20% [52–54] in other reported series. Bilchek [53] points out that most patients who have local recurrences of treated lesions have lesions larger than the probe size in which overlapping thermal spheres are created. This high recurrence rate of 15% to 20%, with follow-up between 1 and 1.5 years, is sig- nificantly worse than the recurrence rates recorded by the cryosurgery series. Successful control using this treatment in patients who are of the appropriate size argues that it is a useful therapy and that it is the complexity of overlapping thermal lesions that leads to failure with larger nodules.

This high rate of local recurrence, combined with relatively low morbidity, has led several investigators to combine this ablative technique with regional vascular techniques. Specifically, maximal tumor debulking or complete tumor debulking with radiofrequency ablation plus hepatic resection as needed can be coordinated with placement of an intraarterial infusion pump for patients with metastatic colorectal cancer. Furthermore, trials of adjuvant intraarterial infusion after curative hepatic resection, as discussed above, argue that the use of intraarterial therapy in conjunction with radiofrequency ablation may be advantageous for treating micrometastases not recognized in other regions of the liver. Initial reports combining these two techniques show this to be safe strategy [55]. The data, however, have to mature and undergo study in a randomized trial for assessment of the contributions of each of these therapies to be reached.

Summary

In conclusion, there are a variety of treatment approaches used by surgeons, interventional radiologists, and medical oncologists to treat metastatic cancer distributed throughout the liver. One conclusion is that the number of different techniques suggests that no single treatment has been uniformly successful to date. A second conclusion is that the number of techniques applied argues for the importance of this as a clinical problem in oncology today. The number of patients with metastatic disease to the liver and the potential for long-term survival if that disease can be controlled will lead to further combinations and refinements of these techniques in future clinical trials.

References

[1] Fraker DL. Regional therapies of cancer. In: Norton JA, Bolinger L, Change KE, et al, editors. Surgery: scientific basis and current practice. New York: Springer-Verlag; 2001. p. 1863–80.
[2] Talbot SM, Neugut AI. Epidemiological trends in colorectal cancer. In: Saltz L, editor. Colorectal cancer: multimodality management. Totowa, NJ: Humana Press.
[3] Collins JM. Pharmacologic rationale for hepatic arterial therapy. Recent Results Cancer Res 1986;100:140–7.
[4] Sigurdson ER, Ridge JA, Kemeny N, Daly JM. Tumor and liver drug uptake following hepatic artery and portal vein infusion in man. J Clin Oncol 1987;5:1836–40.
[5] Van der Eb MM, Hoeben RC, van de Velde CJ. Towards gene therapy for colorectal liver metastases. Recent Results Cancer Res 1998;147:173–86.
[6] Grem JL. 5-Fluorouracil and its biomodulation in the management of colorectal cancer. In: Saltz L, editor. Colorectal cancer: multimodality management. Totowa, NJ: Humana Press.
[7] Saltz LB. The role of irinotecan in colorectal cancer. Curr Oncol Rep 1999;1:155–60.
[8] Saltz LB, Cox JV, Blanke C, et al. Irinotecan plus fluorouracil and leucovorin for metastatic colorectal cancer. N Engl J Med 2000;343:905–14.
[9] Douillard JY, Cunningham D, Roth AD, et al. Irinotecan combined with fluorouracil compared with fluorouracil alone as first-line treatment for metastatic colorectal cancer: a multicentre randomized trial. Lancet 2000;355:1041–7.
[10] Rowinsky EK. Selected targets and rationally designed therapeutics for patients with colorectal cancer. In: Saltz L, editor. Colorectal cancer: multimodality management. Totowa, NJ: Humana Press.
[11] Curley SA, Izzo F, Delrio P, et al. Radiofrequency ablation of unresectable primary and metastatic hepatic malignancies: results in 123 patients. Ann Surg 1999;230:1–8.
[12] Ron JG, Kemeny NE, Gon B, et al. Phase 1/II study of escalating doses of systemic irinotecan (CPT-11) with hepatic arterial infusion of floxuridine (FUDR) and dexamethasone (D), with or without cryosurgery for patients with unresectable hepatic metastases from colorectal cancer. Proc ASCO 1999;18:908.
[13] Neiderhuber JE, Ensminger W, Gyves J, Thrall J, Walker S, Cozzi E. Regional chemotherapy of colorectal cancer metastatic to the liver. Cancer 1984;53:1336–43.
[14] Hohn DC, Stagg RJ, Friedman MA, et al. A randomized trial of continuous intravenous versus hepatic intra-arterial floxuridine in patients with colorectal cancer metastatic to the liver: the Northern California Oncology Group Trial. J Clin Oncol 1989;7:1646–54.
[15] Chang A, Schneider PD, Sugarbaker PH, et al. A prospective randomized trial of regional versus systemic continuous 5-fluorodeoxyuridine chemotherapy in the treatment of colorectal metastases. Ann Surg 1987;206:685–93.
[16] Kemeny N, Daly J, Reichman B, Geller N, Botet J, Oderman P. Intrahepatic or systemic infusion

of fluorodeoxyruidine in patients with liver metastases from colorectal carcinoma. Ann Intern Med 1987;107:459–65.

[17] Martin J, O'Connell M, Wieand H, et al. Intra-arterial floxuridine versus systemic fluorouracil for hepatic metastases from colorectal cancer: a randomized trial. Arch Surg 1990;125:1022–27.

[18] Rougier PH, Laplanche A, Huguier M, et al. Hepatic arterial infusion of floxuridine in patients with liver metastases from colorectal carcinoma: long-term results of a prospective randomized trial. J Clin Oncol 1992;10:1112–18.

[19] Allen-Mersh TG, Earlam S, Fordy C. Quality of life and survival with continuous hepatic artery infusion for colorectal liver metastases. Lancet 1994;344:1255–60.

[20] Patt YZ. Regional hepatic arterial chemotherapy for colorectal cancer metastatic to the liver: the controversy continues. J Clin Oncol 1993;11:815–19.

[21] Kemeny N, Conti J, Cohen A, et al. A phase 2 study of hepatic arterial FUDR, leucovorin, and dexamethasone for unresectable liver metastases from colorectal carcinoma. J Clin Oncol 1994; 12:2288–95.

[22] Stagg R, Venook A, Chase J, et al. Alternating hepatic intraarterial floxuridine and fluorouracil: a less toxic regimen for treatments of liver metastases from colorectal cancer. J Natl Cancer Inst 1991;83:423–28.

[23] Kemeny N, Gonen M, Sillivan D, et al. Phase 1 study of hepatic arterial infusion of floxuridine and dexamethasone with systemic irinotecan for unresectable hepatic metastases from colorectal cancer. J Clin Oncol 2001;19:2687–95.

[24] Venook AP, Warren RS. Regional chemotherapy approaches for primary and metastatic liver tumors. Surg Oncol Clin North Am 1996;5:411–27.

[25] Fong Y, Fortner JG, Sun R, Brennan MF, Blumgart LH. Clinical score for predicting recurrence after hepatic resection for metastatic colorectal cancer: analysis of 1001 consecutive cases. Ann Surg 1999;230:309–21.

[26] Kemeny MM, Adak S, Gray B, et al. Combined-modality treatment for resectable metastatic colorectal carcinoma to the liver: surgical resection of hepatic metastases in combination with continuous infusion of chemotherapy. An intergroup study. J Clin Oncol 2002;20:1499–505.

[27] Kemeny N, Huang Y, Cohen AM, et al. Hepatic arterial infusion of chemotherapoy after resection of hepatic metastases from colorectal cancer. N Engl J Med 1999;34:2039–48.

[28] Konno T. Targeting cancer chemotherapeutic agents by use of Lipiodol contrast medium. Cancer 1999;66:1897–903.

[29] Egawa H, Maki A, Mori K. Effects of intraarterial chemotherapy with a new lipophilic anticancer agent, estradiol-chlorambucil (KMM2210), dissolved in Lipiodol on experimental liver tumors in rats. J Surg Oncol 1990;44:109–14.

[30] Nakamura H, Hashimoto T, Oi H, et al. Transcatheter oily chemoembolization of hepatocellular carcinoma. Radiology 1989;170:783–68.

[31] Sasaki Y, Imaoka S, Kasugai H, et al. A new approach to chemoembolization therapy for hepatoma using ethiodized oil, cisplatin, and gelatin sponge. Cancer 1987;60:1194–203.

[32] Kruskal JB, Hlaty L, Hahnfeldt P, et al. In-vivo and in-vitro analysis of the effectiveness of doxorubicin combined with temporary arterial occlusion in liver tumors. J Vasc Interv Radiol 1993;4:741–48.

[33] Daniels JR, Sternlicht M, Daniels AM. Collagen chemoembolization: pharmacokinetics and tissue tolerance of cisplatin in liver and kidney. Cancer Res 1988;48:2446.

[34] Pentecost MJ, Daniels JR, Teitelbaum GP, et al. Hepatic chemoembolization: safety with portal vein thrombosis. J Vasc Interv Radiol 1993;4:347–51.

[35] Leung DA, Goin JE, Sickles C, Soulen MC. Determinants of post-embolization syndrome following hepatic chemoembolization. J Vasc Interv Radiol 2001;12:321–6.

[36] Kim W, Clark TWI, Baum RA, Soulen MC. Risk factors for liver abscess formation following hepatic chemoembolization. J Vasc Interv Radiol 2001;12:965–8.

[37] Lang EK, Brown CL Jr. Colorectal metastases to liver: selective chemoembolization. Radiology 1993;189:417–22.

[38] Sanz-Altamira PM, Spence LD, Huberman MS, et al. Selective chemoembolization in the man-

agement of hepatic metastases in refractory colorectal carcinoma. Dis Colon Rectum 1997; 40:770–5.

[39] Tellez C, Benson III AB, Lyster MY, et al. Phase 2 trial of chemoembolization for the treatment of metastatic colorectal carcinoma to the liver and review of the literature. Cancer 1998;82:1250–59.

[40] Tuite CM, Soulen MC, Baum RA, et al. Hepatic metastases from colorectal cancer treated with CAM/Ethiodol/PVA chemoembolization: evaluation of survival, biologic and morphologic response. J Vasc Interv Radiol 1999;10:260.

[41] Fraker DL, Alexander HR. Isolated limb perfusion of the liver. In: Lotze MT, Rubin JT, editors. Regional therapy of advanced cancer. Philadelphia: Lippincott-Raven; 1997. p. 141–50.

[42] Ravikumar TS, Pizzomo G, Bodden W, et al. Percutaneous hepatic vein isolation and high-dose hepatic arterial infusion chemotherapy for unresectable liver tumors. J Clin Oncol 1994;12: 2723–36.

[43] Oldhafer KJ, Lang H, Frerker M, et al. First experience and technical aspects of isolated liver perfusion for extensive liver metastases. Surgery 1998;126:622–31.

[44] Alexander HR, Bartlett DL, Libutti SK, Fraker DL, Moser T, Rosenberg SA. Isolated hepatic perfusion with tumor necrosis factor and melphalan for unresectable cancers confined to the liver. J Clin Oncol 1998;16:1479–89.

[45] Alexander HR, Libutti SK, Bartlett DL, Puhlmann M, Fraker DL, Bachenheimer LC. A phase 1–II study of isolated hepatic perfusion using melphalan with or without tumor necrosis factor for patients with ocular melanoma metastatic to the liver. Clin Cancer Res 2000;6:3062–70.

[46] Weaver ML, Atkinson D, Zemel R. Hepatic cryosurgery in treating colorectal metastases. Cancer 1995;76:210–4.

[47] Sarantou T, Bilchik A, Ramming KP. Complications of hepatic cryosurgery. Semin Surg Oncol 1998;14:156–62.

[48] McGahan JP, Dodd GD. Radiofrequency ablation of the liver: current status. AJR Am J Roentgenol 2001;176:3–16.

[49] Fraker DL. Radiofrequency ablation of colorectal metastases to the liver. In: Saltz L, editor. Colorectal cancer: multimodality management. Totowa, NJ: Humana Press.

[50] Siperstein A, Garland A, Engle K, et al. Laparoscopic radiofrequency ablation of primary and metastatic liver tumors. Surg Endosc 2000;14:400–5.

[51] Curley SA, Izzo F, Eeirio P, et al. Radiofrequency ablation of unresectable primary and metastatic hepatic malignancies. Ann Surg 1999;230:1–8.

[52] Siperstein A, Garland A, Engle K, et al. Local recurrence after laparoscopic radiofrequency thermal ablation of hepatic tumors. Ann Surg Oncol 2000;7:106–13.

[53] Wood TF, Rose DM, Chung M, Allegra DP, Foshag LI, Bilchik AJ. Radiofrequency ablation of 231 unresectable hepatic tumors: indications, limitations, and complications. Ann Surg Oncol 2000;7:593–600.

[54] deBaere T, Elias D, Dromain C, et al. Radiofrequency ablation of 100 hepatic metastases with a mean follow-up of more than 1 year. AJR Am J Roentgenol 2000;175:1619–25.

[55] Kesmodel SB, Canter RJ, Raz DJ, Bauer TW, Spitz FR, Fraker DL. Survival following regional treatment for metastatic colorectal cancer to the liver using radiofrequency ablation and hepatic artery infusion pump placement. Ann Surg Oncol 2002;9:S68.

Hematol Oncol Clin N Am
16 (2002) 969–994

HEMATOLOGY/
ONCOLOGY
CLINICS OF
NORTH AMERICA

Chemotherapy for colorectal cancer

Weijing Sun, MD*, Daniel G. Haller, MD

*Hematology/Oncology Division, University of Pennsylvania Medical Center, 16 Penn Tower,
3400 Spruce Street, Philadelphia, PA 19104-4283, USA*

Colorectal carcinoma is the most common gastrointestinal tract malignancy, and the second most common cause of cancer mortality in the United States. Based on the American Cancer Society's estimates, there will be 138,900 (68,800 in men and 70,100 in women) new cases diagnosed with colorectal cancer in 2001, and 57,200 deaths will be caused by this disease [1]. Of the new cases, nearly 60% present with lymph node involvement or metastatic disease [2]. Overall survival for colorectal cancer has improved, however, over the past several decades. This is probably because of increased screening, resulting in stage migration with more patients being diagnosed with early, localized disease. Better preoperative staging, improved surgical techniques and pathologic evaluation of resected specimens have also contributed to the improvement of the overall outcome for these patients. Survival also has been improved by the use of adjuvant chemotherapy in colon cancer and combined modality therapy with chemotherapy and radiation in rectal cancer.

Staging and prognosis

It is very important to understand the pathohistologic characteristics and the molecular markers of colorectal cancer and their relationship to the prognosis of patients. These may help physicians to select patients for adjuvant treatment, and they may also help us to predict patients' responses to treatment in the adjuvant and the advanced disease setting.

The most important factor in predicting overall survival in colorectal cancer is pathologic stage [3]. The two pathologic staging systems commonly used are the Astler-Coller modification of the original Dukes' classification [4,5] and the TNM (tumor-node-metastasis) based classification of the American Joint Committee on Cancer (AJCC) [6] (Table 1). Overall, 50–60% of patients with newly

---

* Corresponding author.
E-mail address: weijing.sun@uphs.upenn.edu (W. Sun).

Table 1
Colorectal cancer staging [4,6]

Primary tumor (T)	
TX	Primary tumor cannot be assessed
T0	No evidence of primary tumor
Tis	Carcinoma in situ; intraepithelial or invasion of lamina propria
T1	Tumor invades submucosa
T2	Tumor invades muscularis propria
T3	Tumor invades through muscularis propria into subserosa, or into nonperitonealized pericolic or perirectal tissues
T4	Tumor directly invades other organs or structures, and/or perforates visceral peritoneum

Regional lymph nodes (N)	
NX	Regional lymph nodes cannot be assessed
N0	No reginal lymph node metastasis
N1	Metastasis into $1-3$ regional lymph nodes
N2	Metastasis into $\geq$ 4 regional lymph nodes

Distant metastasis (M)	
MX	Distant metastasis cannot be assessed
M0	No distant metastasis
M1	Distant metastasis

AJCC (TNM) staging criteria		Modified Astler-Coller (Dukes')
Stage 0	Tis N0 M0	–
Stage I	T1 N0 M0	A
	T2 N0 M0	B1
Stage II	T3 N0 M0	B2
	T4 N0 M0	B3
Stage III	Any T N1 M0	C1
	Any T N2 M0	C2
Stage IV	Any T Any N M1	D

AJCC, American Joint Committee on cancer; TNM, tumor lymphnode metastasis.

diagnosed colorectal cancer will be cured with the best chance for long-term, disease-free survival in those with tumors limited to the bowel wall [7–10]. For stage I colorectal cancer, the cure rate exceeds 90% following surgery alone; however, once a tumor invades through the bowel wall (stage II), survival at 5 years decreases to 60–80%. If the pericolonic lymph nodes are found to be involved with cancer (stage III), 5-year survival falls to 30–60%, with the lower survival associated with an increasing number of lymph node metastases [3,11]. The most frequent site of metastasis for colon cancer is the liver, followed by lung and intra-abdominal sites.

Additional clinical and pathologic features that may increase the risk of recurrence include perforation, obstruction, adherence or invasion of the tumor to other organs, radial (lateral) margin involvement, lymphatic and vascular invasion, and degree of tumor differentiation [12–18]. Elevation of preoperative carcinoembryonic antigen (CEA) level may predict for prognosis, especially in patients with node-positive disease [19,20]. An elevated CEA level also may be a reflection of a more advanced colorectal carcinoma, however. Cell-cycle parameters and ploidy of tumor have been examined as prognostic factors. One retrospective study has shown that DNA aneuploidy was associated with increased recurrence rates in patients who had adjuvant chemotherapy for stage II or III colorectal cancer [21].

A number of biologic and molecular characteristics have been identified that may be of prognostic importance, although none have yet been validated in prospective clinical trials. The *p53* gene is a well-known tumor suppressor gene, which may allow the growing tumor with multiple genetic alterations to evade cell-cycle arrest and apoptosis [22]. The *p53* mutations may be important risk factors associated with poorer prognosis [23,24]. K-ras mutations may be also associated with features predictive of poor prognosis [24]. Chromosome 18q loss of heterozygosity (LOH) is seen in apporoximately 60–70% of primary colorectal cancers, and prevalence of 18q LOH rises to nearly 90–100% in liver metastases of colorectal cancer [25,26]. Several studies have reported that patients whose primary colorectal cancers have 18q LOH have an increased likelihood of distant metastasis and death from their disease [27,28]. The *DCC* (deletion in colorectal cancer) gene, cloned from the region for chromosome 18q, also has been suggested to be a candidate tumor suppressor gene [29]. Colon cancer patients with liver metastases expressed significantly lower levels of *DCC*, compared with patients without such metastases [30]. Microsatellite instability related germline mismatch repair gene mutations have also been reported to affect the prognosis of patients with colorectal cancer [31]. A recent study evaluated LOH from chromosomes 18q, 17p, and 8p; cellular levels of p53 and p21$^{WAF1/CIP1}$ proteins; and microsatellite instability as molecular predictors of outcome for stage III colon cancer after 5-fluorouracial-based adjuvant chemotherapy [32]. The result suggested that retention of 18q alleles in microsatellite stable cancers and mutation of the gene for type II receptor for transforming growth factor β1 (TGF-β1) in those patients with high levels of microsatellite instability may favor outcome. The other study suggested that high thymidylate synthase (TS), low Ki-67, and p53 positive in patients with colorectal cancer were each associated with a poor clinical outcome, which may be useful for identifying patients at high risk for relapse and death [33]. These are considered the first step toward the goal of individualized cancer treatment based on the molecular characteristics of the tumor.

Rectal cancer is similar to colon cancer biologically, but it has a somewhat different natural history, with local recurrence representing a major management issue. Rectal cancer is defined functionally as a tumor that is located either in part or entirely below the peritoneal reflection. Compared with colon cancer, a higher incidence of local failure is associated with rectal cancers, which may be associated with significant morbidity such as pain and organ obstruction. Therefore, treatment goals for rectal are somewhat different from colon cancer, mainly in the adjuvant setting.

Adjuvant treatment of colorectal cancer

The role of adjuvant therapy in colorectal cancer was unclear until the late 1980s. A meta-analysis including nearly 10,000 patients in 25 randomized trials was published in 1988 in the Journal of the American Medical Association. It reported that patients receiving adjuvant 5-fluorouracil (5-FU) may derive a small survival benefit compared with patients without postoperative treatment (odds ratio of 0.83, 95% confidence interval [CI], 0.70–0.98) [34]. The authors clarified the need for large trials to detect small but clinically meaningful benefits in specific subgroup of colorectal cancer patients with adjuvant treatment.

5-FU and levamisole

Levamisole, an antihelminthic agent, was initially tested as adjuvant therapy for colorectal cancer because of its immunomodulatory properties and its mild toxicity. A small, statistically significant survival benefit was reported in the patients treated with levamisole after surgery compared with those without further treatment [35]. An early North Central Cancer Treatment Group (NCCTG) trial showed clinic benefit from the combination of 5-FU and levamisole as adjuvant treatment for high-risk stage II and III colon cancer patients after surgery [36]. The study showed that 5-FU and levamisole reduced recurrence rate by 40% ($P = 0.02$), and increased survival in the subset of patients with node-positive disease ($P = 0.03$). To confirm these data, a large intergroup trial (INT 0035) was conducted in patients with stage II and III colon cancer [37]. The result of the study confirmed the benefit of the combination of 5-FU and levamisole in stage III patients, with a 41% reduction in the risk of recurrence ($P < 0.0001$) and a 33% reduction in mortality ($P = 0.006$), compared with patients with surgery only. The mature data from this study in 929 patients followed for more than 5 years (median follow-up, 6.5 years) showed no loss of this benefit [38]. The combination reduced the recurrence rate by 40% ($P < 0.0001$) and the death rate by 33% ($P = 0.0007$). In contrast, the study did not show a benefit from levamisole alone in reduction of either recurrence rate or death rate, which was initially suggested in the small NCCTG study. On the basis of these positive results in stage III disease, the National Cancer Institute concluded that "the therapeutic option of post-surgical observation ('no treatment' control groups) is no longer justifiable for NCI-sponsored adjuvant studies for Dukes' C patients" [39], and a Consensus Development Conference sponsored by the National Institutes of Health recommended 5-FU plus levamisole as standard therapy for patients with stage III colon cancer following surgical resection [40].

5-Fluorouracil and leucovorin

It has been demonstrated by laboratory research that the cytotoxic activity of 5-FU may be modulated by leucovorin, a reduced folate [41]. The increased antitumor activity seen is caused by an enhancement of the inhibition of thymidylate synthase by 5-FU in the presence of leucovorin. The efficacy of the combination of 5-FU plus leucovorin as adjuvant treatment for colorectal cancer has been demonstrated in the studies of the past decade [42–44]. A study of National Surgical Adjuvant Breast and Bowel Project (NSABP C-03) compared a regiment of 5-FU plus high–dose leucovorin (5-FU/LV) to a combination of 5-FU, vincristine, and semustine (MOF) in 1081 patients with Dukes' B and C colon cancer [42]. The trial was completed in 1989, prior to the NCI announcement establishing 5-FU and levamisole as the standard adjuvant treatment. The 5-year disease-free survival (DFS) rate in the 5-FU/LV group was 66% versus 54% in the MOF group ($P = 0.0004$). The 5-year survival rate was 75% in the 5-FU/LV group compared with 66% in the MOF group ($P = 0.003$). The International Multicentre Pooled Analysis of Colon Cancer Trials (IMPACT) combined data from trials of combination 5-FU and leucovorin versus surgery only in stage II and III colon cancer patients [44]. The survival rate at 3 years was 78% for the surgery alone group and 83% for the group with adjuvant 5-FU/LV treatment ($P = 0.03$). In order to determine if leucovorin-modulated 5-FU was superior to 5-FU plus levamisole in the adjuvant setting, the second intergroup study (INT-0089) was initiated in 1989. Patients with stage III/high-risk II colon cancers were randomized to standard 5-FU plus levamisole, weekly 5-FU with high dose leucovorin, 5-FU with low dose leucovorin by the Mayo Clinic technique, and a combination of 5-FU, leucovorin, and levamisole. With a median follow-up of 3.8 years, the result of the INT-0089 showed equivalent efficacy between a 5-FU/leucovorin regimen given for 7–8 months and 5-FU/levamisole given for 1 year [45] (Table 2). This resulted in the acceptance of 5-FU/LV for 7–8 months standard treatment for stage III colon cancer since approximately 1996. More mature data of the study confirmed the results [46]. The data from the NSABP C-04 study demonstrated a small but statistically significant improvement in disease-free survival (DFS) (65% versus 60%; $P = 0.04$) and a trend toward improvement in overall survival (OS) (74% versus 70%; $P = 0.07$) for patients receiving 5-FU/LV compared with 5-FU/levamisole, both given for 12 months [47]. Neither INT-0089 nor NSABP C-04 showed that the addition of levamisole to 5-FU/LV provided any additional survival benefit over treatment with 5-FU/LV alone.

Table 2
Results of INT-0089: adjuvant chemotherapy for stage II/III colon cancer

	Five-year DFS, %	Five-year OS, %
5-FU/LEV, 12 months	56	63
5-FU/LV (HD), 6 months	59	65
5-FU/LV (LD), 6 months	60	66
5-FU/LV/LEV	60	67

N = 3759
5-FU, 5-fluorouracil; LEV, levamisole; LV, leucovorin; HD, high dose; LD, low dose; DFS, disease-free survival; OS, overall survival.

The current standard adjuvant treatment for stage III colon cancer is a combination of 5-FU and leucovorin for 6–8 months. The optimal intravenous 5-FU/LV regimen remains to be determined, however, in terms of efficacy and toxicity. The more common regimens in the United States are the Roswell Park regimen (5-FU 500 mg/m^2, and LV 500 mg/m^2, weekly for 6 weeks repeated every 8 weeks for 4 cycles), and the Mayo Clinic regimen (5-FU 425 mg/m^2, and LV 20 mg/m^2, daily for 5 consecutive days, repeated every 4–5 weeks for 6 cycles). Though the schedule of 5-FU does not appear to affect efficacy, toxicities can be different, with leukopenia and stomatitis more commonly associated with the Mayo regimen. There is more grade 3 or worse diarrhea in the Roswell Park regimen, but this is usually manageable with aggressive anti-diarrheal medications. Clinicians therefore should choose a regimen best suited to their patient's individual predicted tolerance. A European study compared a monthly regimen (FUFOL), which is similar to the Mayo regimen (d,L-leucovorin 200 mg/m^2 or LV 100 mg/m^2, and 5-FU 400 mg/m^2, daily for 5 consecutive days every 28 days) to the de Gramont regiment (LV5FU2) [d,L-leucovorin 200 mg/m^2 or LV 100 mg/m^2 over 2 hours, followed by 5-FU bolus of 400 mg/m^2 and a 600 mg/m^2 5-FU 22-hour continuous infusion for 2 consecutive days every 14 days in stage II and III colon cancer patients] [48]. The incidence of maximal grade III–IV toxicities in the de Gramont (LV5FU2) regimen group were significantly lower than in the monthly (FUFOL) group (10% versus 26%; $P < 0.001$), even though patients in the bimonthly regimen group received twice the dose of 5-FU compared with those in the monthly regimen. The efficacy data will be available later in 2001.

Monoclonal antibody therapy for colorectal cancer

Edrecolomab (monoclonal antibody 17-1A, Mab 17-1A) is a murine IgG2a monoclonal antibody that recognizes the human tumor-associated antigen Ep-CAM. Ep-CAM acts as an epithelial cell adhesion molecule and is expressed on a wide variety of tumors including carcinomas of the colon, rectum, pancreas, and stomach, as well as normal epithelial tissue [49–53]. The antitumor activity of edrecolomab is proposed to be through antibody-dependent cellular cytotoxicity, complement-mediated cytolysis, and an anti-idiotype cascade, which can be accompanied by the parallel development of idiotype-reactive T cells [54–58]. A randomized phase III trial of edrecolomab as adjuvant treatment for Dukes' C (stage III) colorectal cancer was performed in Germany. The primary endpoints were overall survival and disease-free survival. One hundred and eighty-nine patients were randomized to receive a total of 900 mg edrecolomab (500 mg postoperatively followed by four doses of 100 mg at monthly intervals, n = 99), or to observation (n = 90). The data from the study were reported after 5-year and 7-year follow-ups [59,60]. The results showed that edrecolomab reduced the relative risk of recurrence (52% versus 68%; hazard ratio, 0.66; $P = 0.04$) and overall mortality (43% versus 63%; hazard ratio, 0.57; $P < 0.01$) with 7-year follow-up. In order to confirm the efficacy of edrecolomab as adjuvant treatment for colorectal cancer after surgical resection, 4 phase III studies of edrecolomab for either stage II or III colon or rectal cancer have been conducted (157-001, and 157-002: edrecolomab and 5-FU/LV versus 5-FU/LV following resection of stage III colon cancer; 157-003: edrecolomab versus no adjuvant therapy following resection of stage II colon cancer; and 157-004: edrecolomab and 5-FU/LV versus 5-FU/LV in patients with stage II/III operable rectal carcinoma) [61]. The preliminary results of 157-002, which was conducted in Europe with the primary endpoint of overall survival (OS) and the secondary endpoint of disease-free survival (DFS), has been reported recently [62]. Two thousand seven hundred and sixty-one stage III colon cancer patients postsurgery were randomly allocated to three arms (Arm 1: 900 mg edrecolomab with an initial 500 mg infusion followed four 100 mg infusion every 4 weeks, and 5-FU/LV [Mayo regimen] for 6 cycles, n = 912; Arm 2: 5-FU/LV [Mayo regimen], n = 927; and Arm 3: edrecolomab only [as above], n = 922). The median follow-up time was 26 months. There was no additional benefit of adding edrecolomab to 5FU/LV in adjuvant treatment for stage III colon cancer, either in OS (74.7% versus 76.1%; hazard ratio 0.936; 95% CI 0.763–1.149; $P = 0.528$) or DFS (63.8% versus 65.5%; hazard ratio 0.901. 95% CI 0.763–1.064; $P = 0.220$). Edrecolomab montherapy was associated with significantly shorter OS and DFS compared with 5FU/LV (3-year OS: 76.1% versus 70.1%; hazard ratio 0.821; 95% CI, 0.674–1.000; $P = 0.050$; and 3-year DFS: 65.5% versus 53.0%, hazard ratio 0.623, 95% CI, 0.533–0.729; $P < 0.001$). These data do not support the antitumor activity suggested in the earlier Reithmuller trial [59,60]. Recruitment to study 157-001 has also been completed, and results are pending. If this trial also shows no additive benefit from edrecolomab, this avenue of therapy will likely not be pursued.

Adjuvant treatment for stage II colon cancer

Though the evidence for the use of adjuvant chemotherapy in stage III (Dukes' C) colorectal cancer is clear, the role of adjuvant chemotherapy for localized, node-negative disease (stage II or Dukes' B) is still controversial. Subset analyses have been performed for many of the large trials of adjuvant chemotherapy. A comparative analysis of patients with Dukes' B versus Dukes' C colon cancer who were enrolled in four separate NSABP studies was published recently [63]. Each of these studies had different treatment and control arms, which made any direct comparison impossible. Furthermore, none of the studies compared standard 5-FU/leucovorin chemotherapy with surgery alone. The authors concluded that there were relative improvements in DFS and OS with adjuvant therapy for patients with Dukes' B colon cancer similar to that seen for Dukes' C patients. This conclusion was not supported by the IMPACT analyses, however [8,64]. A pooled analysis of five separate trials compared 1016 patients randomized to 5-FU/leucovorin (n = 507) versus observation (n = 509) after potentially curative resection with a median follow-up time of 5.75 years. This meta-analysis had the advantage of comparing similar adjuvant regimens to the same control arm of observation. The results showed no significant difference in 5-year OS between adjuvant treatment and observation (82% versus 80%) in Dukes' B2 colon cancer. There was also no significant increase in 5-year event-free survival for patients receiving 5-FU/LV compared with no treatment (76% versus 73%, hazard ratio, 0.83, 90% CI 0.72–1.07; $P = 0.137$). The investigators concluded that "The IMPACT 2 did not support the use of 5-FU/LV as a standard adjuvant treatment for all patients with Dukes' B2 colon cancer," though there was a trend toward a small effect of treatment, it was not significant. The consensus from the 4th International Conference on Colorectal Cancer in Paris suggested that "The relative effect of chemotherapy is the same in Dukes' C (stage III) and in Dukes' B (stage II) colon cancers; whereas the absolute survival benefit is smaller in patients with Dukes' B cancer because their risk of death is smaller" [65].

To investigate the impact of controversy regarding the role of adjuvant chemotherapy for stage II colon cancer, a group of researchers examined "real life" (SEER-Medicare) medical records of 3,725 patients who had resection of stage II colon cancer [66]. The study found that a substantial minority of patients with stage II colon cancer (31%) received adjuvant chemotherapy, and there appeared to be no significant survival benefit for those treated with adjuvant therapy (5-year survival: 74% versus 72%; hazard ratio 0.93; 95% CI 0.81–1.07). Among 448 patients with a poor prognostic feature (T4 tumor, obstruction, perforation), 38% received chemotherapy and the 5-year survival was 62% for treated and 60% for untreated patients (hazard ratio 0.91 (95% CI = 0.66–1.26). The investigators of the study suggested that "Clinicians should feel reassured about enrolling patients in randomized clinical trials with a no treatment control arm." It is not doubted that a more accurate characterization of node negative colon cancers is needed. Clinical trials and biologic research must be encouraged to define better which patients require or benefit the most from adjuvant therapy.

Adjuvant treatment of rectal cancer

The goal of adjuvant therapy in rectal cancer is to decrease the risk of both distant metastases and the incidence of local recurrence, as locoregional failure occurs in 25–50% of patients undergoing curative surgery for carcinoma of the rectum [67–69]. Radiation therapy may reduce locoregional failure [70–72]. The impact of radiation on OS was uncertain until the Swedish Rectal Cancer Trial [73]. Between 1987 and 1990, 1168 patients with resectable rectal cancer were randomized to undergo preoperative irradiation (25 Gy in 5 fractions in 1 week) followed by surgery within 1 week, or to surgery alone. After a 5-year follow-up, there was not only a significant difference in local recurrence (11% versus 27%, $P < 0.001$), but also an overall 5-year survival rate (58% versus 48%, $P = 0.004$), all favoring the radiation arm. The trial was criticized for irradiating patients with only stage I disease and for a higher than expected recurrence rate in stage I patients [74]. A meta-analysis showed improvement of OS and cancer-specific survival in resectable rectal cancer patients with combination of preoperative radiation and surgery compared with those having surgery alone [75]. Because surgical technique plays a key role in success of tumor control of rectal cancer, standardization of surgery is important for comparing combination therapy versus surgery alone. The Dutch Colorectal Cancer Group performed a prospective, randomized trial to investigate the efficacy of preoperative radiation with standardized total mesorectal excision in patients with resectable rectal cancer. From 1/1996 to 12/1999, 1861 patients were randomized to either preoperative radiation (5 Gy on each of five days) followed by surgery (n = 924) or surgery alone (n = 937) [76]. The preliminary results showed that the 2-year local recurrent rate was 2.4% in the combined modality group, and 8.2% in the surgery-alone group ($P < 0.001$).

Early studies using combined modality treatment of postoperative pelvic radiation and 5-FU-based chemotherapy showed a significant survival advantage compared with surgery alone [77,78]. The first intergroup rectal cancer trial addressed the issue of whether administration of protracted venous infusion (PVI) of 5-FU was advantageous compared with bolus 5-FU as the chemosensitizing regimen in conjunction with radiation. The result demonstrated that PVI of 5-FU (225 mg/m^2 per day) during pelvic radiation significantly decreased the risk of distant metastatic recurrence compared with bolus 5-FU, with an absolute improvement in overall survival of 10% [79]. This study also showed no difference in survival between single-agent 5-FU and combination chemotherapy 5-FU and semustine.

Paralleling the INT-0089 trial, the effect of biochemical modulation of 5-FU with leucovorin and levamisole was similarly investigated in rectal cancer. The preliminary data from this intergroup trial (INT-0114) showed no survival advantage with the addition of leucovorin or levamisole to bolus 5-FU alone [80]. The final report of INT 0114 was reported in the 2001 American Society of Clinical Oncology (ASCO) meeting with 1,696 patients evaluable, and median follow-up of 7.6 years [81]. No significant differences were found in OS and DFS rates among treatment groups, but those rates did differ significantly according to disease stage (lower risk: T1-2, N+ and T3N0 versus higher risk: T3N+ and T4, any N). Local recurrence rate was 9% for patients at lower risk and 18% for those at higher risk (RR 2.2, $P < 0.0001$). The most recent intergroup adjuvant trial, INT-0144, completed accrual in August 2000 and compared bolus 5-FU with continuous infusion 5-FU before, during, and after pelvic radiation.

Though postoperative chemoradiation is more standard in the United States, other countries employ neoadjuvant chemoradiation or preoperative radiation alone. The European Organization for Research and Treatment of Cancer (EORTC) is currently investigating the role of preoperative and postoperative chemotherapy in patients receiving preoperative radiation for resectable rectal cancer. The NSABP R-03 trial compared preoperative neoadjuvant with postoperative adjuvant chemoradiation [82]. Over a period of 6 years, only 130 patients were randomized to preoperative treatment and 130 patients to postoperative treatment. The endpoints of the study were identified as response rate, sphincter-saving surgery (SSS), and DFS. One year after randomization, more patients who received preoperative therapy had SSS and no evidence of disease (NED) compared with those w2ho received postoperative therapy. Disease-free survival at 1 year was higher in the preoperative group (83% versus 78%, $P = 0.29$), but toxicity was greater in the preoperative group ($P = 0.07$). A larger, more definitive trial of preoperative versus postoperative therapy is being completed by a German multicenter group. This may further delineate the relative benefits of preoperative and postoperative therapy.

Other adjuvant treatment-related issues

NSABP C-02 demonstrated that perioperative portal venous infusion of 5-FU resulted in an improvement in DFS (69% versus 60% at 5 years, $P = 0.02$) and an OS advantage (78% versus 70% at 5 years, $P = 0.07$) compared with surgery alone in stage II/III colon cancer [83]. Because of recent progress in systemic chemotherapy, portal vein infusion 5-FU is not considered as a standard approach to adjuvant treatment of colon cancer.

There is no benefit advantage of adding interferon alfa-2a (IFN) to 5-FU/LV as adjuvant treatment for stage II/III colon cancer patients from the NSABP C-03 trial [84].

Oral fluoropyrimidines have recently been extensively studied in metastatic colorectal cancer in order to replace intravenous chemotherapy by an entirely ambulatory treatment. Capecitabine has been approved by the United States Food and Drug Administration (FDA) for advanced colorectal cancer, and UFT (uracil/tegafur) also is available in Japan and Europe. The NSABP has conducted a trial comparing 5-FU/LV (Roswell Park regimen) with UFT/LV in stage II/III colon cancer patients [85]. The final results will not be available before 2003. Capecitabine is currently being studied as an adjuvant treatment for patients with recently resected Dukes' C colon cancer. One thousand nine hundred patients 18–75 years old are to be randomized to two arms (capecitabine 2,500 mg/m^2/day orally for 2 weeks followed by 1 week of rest for 8 cycles versus 6 cycles of Mayo regimen 5-FU/LV). Efficacy and safety data are also expected to be available in 2003 [86].

With the clear activity of new agents such as irinotecan and oxaliplatin in treatment of advanced colorectal cancer, ongoing adjuvant studies are aiming to compare the standard 5-FU/LV regimen with 5-FU/LV plus irinotecan (C89803) or oxaliplatin (NSABP C-07) in North America. In Europe, the EORTC is also comparing infusion 5FU/LV, with or without irinotecan, in stage II colon cancer. The ACCORD trial is comparing the same regimens, limiting accrual to high-risk stage III patients (obstruction and N2), which will allow for the earliest assessment of efficacy of combination therapy in the adjuvant setting. There is also a European trial, similar to NSABP C-07, in which infusional 5FU/LV is compared with infusional 5FU/LV with oxaliplatin.

Treatment of advanced colorectal cancer

Surgical resection is the treatment choice for locally recurrent colorectal cancer, such as in the anastomotic site or surgical bed, when it is suitable. If potentially curative surgery for localized disease is performed, then prognosis is similar to primary colorectal tumors. The liver is the most common site of distal metastases for colorectal cancer [87]. Over the past 2 decades, resection of liver metastases has been shown to be safe and potentially curative in selected patients. Prognostic factors, which correlate with long-term survival after resection of hepatic metastases have been evaluated [88]. If two or more of these factors are present, the 5-year survival is considered substantially decreased (Table 3). It has been shown that the addition of postoperative systemic adjuvant chemotherapy plus hepatic artery infusion (HAI) may improve survival compared with post-operative systemic chemotherapy alone [89]. It has also suggested that systemic chemotherapy may also increase the resectability for those initially considered not as candidates for hepatic lesion resection [90]. There are other hepatic-directed treatments of colorectal cancer metastases, including radiofrequency ablation (RFA) [91], hepatic artery chemoembolization (HACE) [92], and percutaneous ethanol injection [93]. All these procedures have their limits, and no survival benefits have been proved, compared with standard surgical resection. For those colorectal cancer patients with extrahepatic metastasis, or who are not candidates for metastectomy, systemic chemotherapy is the treatment.

Fluorouracil

The utility of chemotherapy in the management of metastatic colorectal cancer has been demonstrated by many studies in the past 2–3 decades [94–96]. Fluorouracil (5-FU) remained the mainstay of treatment of advanced colorectal cancer for over 40 years until recently. Unfortunately, only about 20 percent of patients who receive 5-FU demonstrate objective response by standard criteria. Tremendous efforts have been undertaken to improve the efficacy of 5-FU in the past 25 years. Protracted intravenous infusion results in a marginally higher rate of response, compared with bolus administration and is also associated with reduced toxicity [97,98]. Biochemical modulators (eg, leucovorin, methotrexate, and interferon alfa) have also been explored to increase antitumor activity of 5-FU, with leucovorin as the most extensively used biochemical modulator. In a meta-analysis of 9 randomized clinical trials of advanced cancer comparing

Table 3
Survival after resection of hepatic metastases

Clinical risk score (points)	Five-year OS, %
0 – 1	52
2 – 3	23
4 – 5	11

OS = overall survival.
Presence of each of the following factors is assigned one point:
- The largest tumor > 5 cm
- The disease-free interval < 12 months
- Number of tumors in liver > 1
- Node-positive in the primary tumor
- CEA > 200 ng/mL

5-FU alone with 5-FU plus leucovorin, a significant improvement in response rate was shown in patients who received 5-FU and leucovorin [99]. This level of improvement in response rate failed to translate, however, into a significant survival advantage. Although there were some early studies indicating the benefit of interferon-α in combination with 5FU in the treatment of advanced colorectal cancer [100,101], this was not confirmed by large randomized phase III studies, and there was far more toxicity in the interferon and 5-FU combination [102,103].

Irinotecan

A camptothecin derivative, irinotecan (CPT-11), is a topoisomerase I inhibitor that traps the topo-I/DNA cleavable complex following cleavage of single-strand DNA [104]. Collision of the replication fork converts this single-strand break into a double-strand break, thus inducing cell death [105]. Based on trials reviewed by the FDA [106], irinotecan was approved in 1996 as a second-line agent for treating patients with colorectal cancer whose disease had progressed on 5-FU based therapy. Initial approval was based on tumor response alone comparable with that seen with 5-FU as first-line treatment. Two phase III randomized studies conducted in Europe on colorectal cancer refractory to bolus 5-FU also showed a survival benefit from irinotecan as a second-line treatment, leading to a full approval of this drug in the United States [107,108].

The survival benefit of irinotecan combined with 5-FU with leucovorin as first-line treatment for advanced colorectal cancer has been shown recently by two phase III randomized clinical studies. The first trial compared weekly irinotecan plus weekly 5-FU/leucovorin (IFL regimen) to 5-FU/leucovorin (Mayo regimen) or to weekly irinotecan [109]. Objective response rates were noted in 50% of patients receiving the three-drug combination versus 28% of patients received 5-FU/leucovorin (confirmed response rate 39% versus 21%, p < 0.001). Median survival for the IFL arm was 14.8 months versus 12.6 months for the 5-FU/leucovorin arm (p = 0.04). Grade 3 (severe) diarrhea was more common during treatment with irinotecan/5-FU/leucovorin, but the incidence of grade 4 (life-threatening) diarrhea was similar in the two groups. The other trial, conducted in Europe, also found a significant advantage in favor of the combination of irinotecan/5-FU/leucovorin vs. infusional 5-FU/leucovorin in terms of median overall survival (17.4 months versus 14.1 months, $P = 0.035$), progression-free survival (6.7 months versus 4.4 months, $P < 0.001$) and confirmed objective response (35% versus 22%, $P < 0.005$) [110]. All these endpoints demonstrated a slight yet definite superiority of the combination of irinotecan, 5-FU, and leucovorin. As exciting as these data are, after many years of clinical trials in colorectal cancer, several issues are still uncertain. The data from the European trials suggest that infusional 5-FU in combination therapy might be a better approach, both in terms of activity and toxicity. The recent data from clinical studies of N9741 (a study comparing weekly 5FU/LV/irinotecan [IFL] versus 5-FU/LV/oxaliplatin versus irinotecan/oxaliplatin as the first-line treatment for metastatic colorectal cancer) and C89803 (a adjuvant treatment trial by comparing current standard 5-FU/LV versus 5-FU/LV and irinotecan for stage III and high-risk stage II colorectal cancer patients) showed more death on the IFL arms, indicating that further investigation may be needed for the weekly bolus 5-FU/LV and irinotecan regimen regarding toxicity issues [111]. Whether sequential instead of concomitant administration of these drugs could achieve similar effect but less toxicity is still somewhat uncertain, although the retrospective data from the combination trials suggest that survival benefit is maintained, even when the majority of patients initially assigned to single agent therapy subsequently received second-line chemotherapy or other salvage treatments. Whether the combination of irinotecan, 5-FU, and leucovorin should be considered as the first line treatment in a subgroup of patients with poor performance status (≥ ECOG 2), or with abnormal organ system function for survival, toxicity and clinical benefit is unknown. Ultimately, biologic markers that may predict response or toxicity from standard chemotherapy drugs may help to determine which patients should be considered for choosing irinotecan, 5-FU, and leucovorin as the first-line treatment or not.

Oxaliplatin

Oxaliplatin (Eloxatin, L-OHP), a diaminocyclohexane (DACH) platin, inhibits DNA replication and transcription through the formation of intra- and interstrand DNA adducts. A member of the platinum family, the antitumor spectrum of oxaliplatin is different from that of cisplatin and carboplatin, with significant activity in colon cancer cell lines [112]. Compared with cisplatin and carboplatin, the toxicity of oxaliplatin is also different, with a reversible, cold-related sensory neuropathy predominating [113]. It has demonstrated synergistic antitumor activity in combination with 5-FU and leucovorin both in vitro and in vivo [114,115]. As a first-line or second-line therapy, oxaliplatin monotherapy has been shown in phase II trials to be similar in clinical activity to single-agent irinotecan [116]. Phase II trials evaluating the combination of oxaliplatin and 5-FU/leucovorin as initial therapy for patients with metastatic colorectal cancer by using chronomodulated drug administration schedules suggested increased cytotoxicity, manifested by encouraging response rates, progression-free survival, and overall survival [117,118].

Based on these encouraging data, two randomized trials of oxaliplatin with 5-FU and leucovorin as first-line chemotherapy in patients with metastatic colorectal cancer were conducted in Europe (EFC 2961 and EFC 2962) to evaluate oxaliplatin combined with 5FU/leucovorin versus 5-FU and leucovorin [119,120]. The results of both trials showed statistically significant benefit for oxaliplatin in objective response rate (53% versus 16% with 2961, and of 50.7% versus 22.3% with 2962), and in progression-free survival (8.7 versus 6.1 months, p = 0.048 in the 2961; and 9.0 versus 6.2 months, p = 0.0003 in the 2962). Although a trend toward longer median survival was identified in the oxaliplatin-treated group, the difference did not achieve statistical significance in either study (16.2 versus 14.7 months with p = 0.12, in the 2962 trial; and 19.4 versus 19.9 months in the 2961 trial). Because of the lack of detectable impact of front-line oxaliplatin on prolonging overall survival, oxaliplatin has not been approved by the FDA for treatment of advanced colorectal cancer.

It is not clear why significant differences in response rate (RR) and progress free survival (PFS) did not translate into a statistically significant survival benefit. The differences in baseline patient characters could have obscured the assessment of the impact of oxaliplatin on survival. The OS benefit of adding oxalipatin was suggested by the subanalysis when the baseline differences were taken into account by Cox regression analysis in the EFC 2962 study ($P = 0.0001$) [119]. It is also possible that the effects of oxaliplatin are too transient to have an impact on overall survival, or the use of other salvage therapies (eg, surgery or irinotecan) influenced survival results. Both studies had an unusually good survival among patients on the control arms, which could be explained as that infusional 5-FU/LV was more active than bolus 5FU/LV. The relatively small sample size of both studies may also be a reason no statistically significant survival benefit was demonstrated in these two trials.

Studies in the second-line setting of the combination of oxaliplatin and 5-FU/LV have shown encouraging results [121]. Several important questions need to be answered, including the impact of retreatment with alternative methodologies of 5-FU/leucovorin in the combination. As a second-line therapy, it is necessary to clarify that the improvement of activity is caused by oxaliplatin rather than secondary to the change of 5-FU/leucovorin dose or schedule. In the United States, a pivotal trial is ongoing in order to answer these questions. Patients with advanced colorectal cancer progressing after irinotecan/5FU/leucovorin treatment are randomized to one of three arms: a control arm of bolus plus infusion 5-FU and leucovorin (de Gramont regimen), or oxaliplatin as a single-agent every 2 weeks, or a combination of 5-FU, leucovorin, and oxaliplatin. (Update: On August 12, 2002, FDA announced the approval of oxaliplatin for use in combination with infusional 5-FU and leucovorin as the second-line treatment for patients with colorectal cancer through 'Fast Track'.)

Oral fluoropyrimidines

The development of oral fluoropyrimidine is based on the principle of providing an alternative to intravenous delivery of fluorouracil, thereby potentially improving the quality of life of patients. Dihydropyrimidine dehydrogenase (DPD) is the initial rate-limiting enzymatic step in the catabolism of 5-FU [122,123] and is widely distributed in many tissues, including the liver, lung, gastrointestinal tract, kidney, and many tumors [124]. DPD in the gastrointestinal (GI) tract is largely responsible for the poor oral absorption of 5FU. There also is a broad variation in DPD activity from person to person, which is partly responsible for great variation in the $t_{1/2}$ and bioavailability of 5-FU.

Capecitabine

Capecitabine is a tumor-activated and tumor-selective fluoropyrimidine carbamate. Capecitabine is readily absorbed through the intestinal mucosa as an intact molecule and metabolized in the liver by carboxylesterase to 5′-deoxy-5-fluorocytidine (5′-DFCR), which is then converted to doxifluridine (5′-DFUR) by cytidine deaminase in liver and tumor tissue (Fig.1). Doxifluridine is finally metabolized to 5-FU in tumor tissue by thymidine phosphorylase [125,126]. Preclinical data showed tumor selectivity of capecitabine and activity in both 5-FU-sensitive and -resistant tumors [127]. In xenograft models, the concentration of 5-FU was found to be higher in tumor than in plasma and healthy tissue (127-fold higher than in plasma and 22-fold higher than in muscle). Tumor selectivity of capecitabine was also demonstrated in a clinical study [128]. Nineteen colorectal cancer patients requiring surgical resection of primary tumors or/and liver metastasis received capecitabine twice daily for 5–7days prior surgery. Concentration of 5-FU in primary tumor was 2.5 times more than adjacent healthy tissues and 1.17 times more in liver metastasis than in noncancer liver tissues. 5-FU concentration is fourteenfold greater in primary tumor than in plasma and eightfold higher in liver metastasis than in plasma.

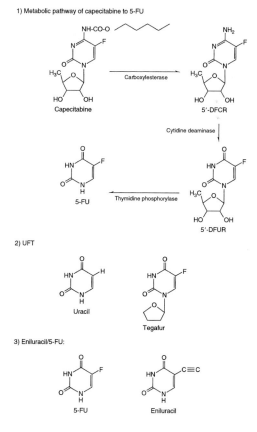

Fig. 1. Oral fluoropyrimidines.

Side effects of oral capecitabine in phase I clinical trials were similar to those observed with infusional 5-FU, including nausea, vomiting, diarrhea, and palmar-plantar erythrodysesthesia (hand-foot syndrome) [129]. A large multinational, randomized, open-label phase II trial evaluated three schedules of capecitabine in metastatic colorectal cancer: continuous, intermittent, and intermittent with leucovorin. The response rates for these arms were 21%, 24%, and 23%, with complete responses (CRs) in each group. The media times to progression (TTP) in three arms were 107, 230, and 165 days. The addition of leucovorin showed no improved activity, but increased the incidence of toxic effects [130]. Two phase III studies have been reported in Europe and the United States [131,132]. In the European trial, 602 untreated metastatic colorectal cancer patients were randomized to receive either capecitabine or 5-FU/leucovorin (Mayo regimen). A higher response rate was reported in the capecitabine arm (26.6% versus 17.9%, p = 0.013), but there was no difference in response duration, progression free survival, or overall survival. A similar phase III study was conducted in the United States. The response rate was 24.8% in the capecitabine arm and 15.5% in the IV 5-FU/leucovorin arm ($P = 0.005$), and there were no differences in TTP and OS. Based on these data, capecitabine has been recently approved by the FDA for patients with metastatic colorectal cancer as first-line treatment.

UFT

UFT contains two components, tegafur and uracil, with a 1:4 molar ratio (equivalent to 100 mg tegafur and 224 mg uracil). Tegafur is a pro-drug that is hydroxylated and converted to 5-FU by hepatic microsomal enzymes. Uracil competitively inhibits DPD, leading to increased and sustained levels of 5-FU after tegafur ingestion. Both uracil and tegafur are rapidly and completely absorbed into the systemic circulation after oral UFT administration. Clinical trials in Japan demonstrated the antitumor activity of UFT in breast, colorectal, gastric, bladder, and head and neck cancer [133]. Clinical development of UFT in the United States began in 1990. Phase I trials evaluated UFT as a single agent in 5-day and 28-day schedules, divided dose t.i.d. The dose-limiting toxicities were neutropenia and diarrhea. From 1993, several phase II trials of UFT (tegafur/uracil) and leucovorin were studied in the United States. All patients enrolled in these trials had measurable disease and no prior chemotherapy for metastatic colorectal cancer. The combination of UFT and leucovorin was well tolerated, and toxicity was proportional to administered dose. There was evidence of moderate activity in each of these trials (RR, 23–59%) [134–137]. Based on these results from phase II trials, two large phase III trials of UFT/leucovorin (Orzel[R] Bristol-Myero Squibb, Princeton, NJ) as first-line treatment for metastatic colorectal cancer have been completed [138,139]. Study 011 was performed in the United States, Canada, and Europe, and Study 012 in Europe. These trials compared oral UFT plus leucovorin versus a 5-day intravenous bolus regimen of 5-FU (425 mg/m^2/day) and leucovorin (20 mg/m^2/day) every 4–5 weeks (Mayo Clinic regimen, every 4 weeks for trial 011 and every 5 weeks for trial 012). In

011 trial, 816 patients were accrued with 409 in the UFT/leucovorin arm, and 407 in the 5-FU/leucovorin arm. The median survival was 12.4 months (95% CI, 11.2–13.6 months) in the UFT/leucovorin arm and 13.4 (95% CI, 11.6–15.4 months) in the 5-FU/leucovorin arm (pc = 0.65). The overall response rate was 12% (48/409) in the UFT/leucovorin arm and 15% (59/407) in the 5-FU/leucovorin arm (p = 0.232). In the 012 study, 380 patients were accrued (with 190 patients in each arm). The median survival was 12.3 months (95% CI, 10.4–13.8 months) in the oral UFT plus leucovorin arm and 10.3 months (8.2–13.0 months) in the IV 5-FU/leucovorin arm. The overall response rate was 11% (20/190) in the UFT/LV arm and 9% (17/190) in the 5-FU/leucovorin arm (p = 0.593). Both large phase III trials appeared to demonstrate that oral UFT plus leucovorin as an initial treatment for metastatic colorectal cancer produces equivalent survival to intravenous 5-FU and leucovorin (Mayo Clinic regimen). But UFT/LV was not approved by the FDA, as the noninferiority of UFT/LV to the Mayo Clinic regimen could not be proven.

Eniluracil/5-fluorouracil

Eniluracil (Ethynyluracil, GW776C85) is a potent irreversible inactivator of DPD in vitro and in vivo [140,141]. Eniluracil is a synthetic pyrimidine with an ethynyl substituent at the 5′ position, and a structure similar to that of both uracil and 5-FU. Preclinical studies showed that eniluracil inhibits >99% activity of DPD and is relatively nontoxic itself. The combination of eniluracil and 5-FU demonstrates the improved effectiveness of 5-FU in vitro and in vivo [142]. The dose-limiting neurotoxicity seen with 5-FU alone did not occur with the enciluracil/5-FU combination. With eniluracil, oral bioavailability of 5-FU was demonstrated to be approximately 100%, and its antitumor index increased by sixfold [143]. The improvement of antitumor efficacy, oral bioavailability of 5-FU by combination of eniluracil, and 5-FU has been confirmed by several phase I and phase II studies [144]. Eniluracil/5-FU is Eniluracil mixed with 5-FU in a 10:1 ratio. The response rates in a study with oral administration of a 10:1 ratio of eniluracil/5-FU BID for 28 days of a 5-week course for treatment of colorectal cancer compare favorably with those obtained in trials of intravenous 5-FU and leucovorin. The response rates were 25% and 29% for the 1.0 and 1.15 mg/m^2 dose groups, respectively [145–147]. But two large multi-center, randomized trials showed inferiority in OS of oral eniluracil/5FU to 5-FU/LV [148,149].

Molecular biological characteristics of colorectal cancer and other novel agents

Recent studies suggest that resistance to 5-FU-based therapy can in part be explained by overexpression of thymidylate synthase (TS), thymidine phospha-rylase (TP), or DPD [150,151]. Testing of tumor specimens for expression of these enzymes may help medical oncologists to select treatment plans for patients. For those patients whose tumor with overexpression of TS, irinotecan might be the initial treatment choice, whereas those with TP overexpression in their tumor cells might receive more benefit from capecitabine.

With better understanding of the molecular biologic characteristics of colorectal cancer, including angiogenesis and signal transduction, new "target-oriented" agents are under investigation. The preliminary data from some of them are very encouraging.

Cetuximab

Cetuximab (IMC-C225) is a chimeric monoclonal antibody selectively against the epidermal growth factor receptor (EGFR). By blocking the ligand and receptor binding, with tyrosine kinase kept inactive, cetuximab inhibits tumor growth. A phase II study of combination of cetuximab with irinotecan was given to 121 metastatic colorectal cancer patients, who failed on both 5-FU and inotecan and whose tumors tested positive for EGFR [152]. The result showed that 17% (21 points) had a partial response and 31% (37 points) had stable disease or minor response. Further study of a combination of cetuximab with 5-FU/LV/irinotecan for chemotherapy-naive metastatic colorectal cancer patients is ongoing.

Bevacizumab

Bevacizumab (RhuMAb VEGF) is a recombinant humanized monoclonal antibody against vascular endothelial growth factor (VEGF). Preliminary results of a randomized phase II trial compared the combination of bevacizumab (low and high doses)/5-FU/LV with 5-FU/LV in metastatic colorectal cancer patients having chemonaive disease or in those who had only adjuvant treatment [153]. An improvement in response rate and time to tumor progression was reported in the arms with bevacizumab/5-FU/LV. At 17.3 months of following when the data was presented, the median survival was 13.8 in the 5-FU/LV arm and 16.1 months in the high-dose bevacizumab arm. The median survival had not yet been reached in the low-dose bevacizumab arm. A large randomized phase III trial is being conducted in the United States for comparing irinotecan/5-FU/LV with and without bevacizumab as first-line treatment for patients with metastatic colorectal cancer.

Summary

With effective chemotherapy as adjuvant treatment, the survival benefit is clearly achieved for certain (stage III) colorectal cancer patients, though there still exist many unsettled issues including the controversies in the treatment of stage II disease. Advances in the development of a new generation of cytotoxic agents in the past several years have allowed us to move forward from the "fluorouracil-only era" in the treatment of advanced/metastatic colorectal cancer. It is still not very clear how best to minimize toxicity without compromising efficacy of the ombination therapy with newer agents, or how to maximize the benefit of chemotherapy (concurrent versus sequential). There are many current ongoing clinical trials designed to address these issues. With better understanding of the signal transduction and molecular biology character-istics of colorectal cancer, and the development of biologic and molecular target agents, the outcomes of patients with colorectal cancer will be improved further. Future clinical trials should be focused on optimizing and individu-alizing therapy for patients based on their molecular profiles to achieve maxi-mal clinical benefit.

References

[1] Greenlee RT, Hill-Harmon MB, Murray T, et al. Cancer Statistics, 2001. CA Cancer J Clin 2001;51:15–36.
[2] Ries LA, Eisner MP, Kosary CL, et al, editors. SEER Cancer statistic review, 1973–1997. Bethesda, MD: National Cancer Institute; 2000.
[3] Macdonald JS. Adjuvant therapy of colon cancer. CA Cancer J Clin 1999;49(4):202–19.
[4] Astler WB, Coller FA. The prognostic significance of direct extension of carcinoma of the colon and rectum. Ann Surg 1954;139:846–51.
[5] Dukes CE. The classification of cancer of the rectum. J Pathol Bacteriol 1940;50:527–39.
[6] American Joint Committee on Cancer, Colon and Rectum. In: AJCC Cancer Staging Manual. 5th edition. Philadelphia: Lippincott-Raven Publishers; 1997. p. 83–8.
[7] International Multicentre Pooled Analysis of B2 Colon Cancer Trials (IMPACT) Investigators. Efficacy of adjuvant fluorouracil and folinic acid in colon cancer. Lancet 1995;345:939–44.
[8] International Multicentre Pooled Analysis of B2 Colon Cancer Trials (IMPACT B2) Inves-tigators. Efficacy of adjuvant fluorouracil and folinic acid in colon cancer. J Cli Oncol 1999; 17(5):1356–63.
[9] Wolmark N, Rockette H, Mamounas E, et al. Clinical trial to assess the relative efficacy of fluorouracil and levamisole, and fluorouracil, leucovorin, and levamisole in patients with Dukes' B and C carcinoma of the colon: results from National Surgical Adjuvant Breast and Bowel Project C-04. J Clin Oncol 1999;17:3553–9.
[10] Haller D, Catalano P, Macdonald J, et al. Fluorouracil (FU), leucovorin (LV) and levamisole (LEV) adjuvant therapy for colon cancer: five year final report of INT-0089. Proc Am Soc Clin Oncol 1998;17:256a.
[11] Bokey EL, Ojerskog B, Cahpuis PH, et al. Local recurrence after curative excision of the rectum for cancer without adjuvant therapy: role of total anatomical dissection. Br J Surg 1999;86(9):1164–70.
[12] Griffin MR, Bergstralh EJ, Coffey RJ, et al. Predictors of survival after curative resection of carcinoma of the colon and rectum. Cancer 1987;60:2318.
[13] Eldar S, Kemeney MM, Terz JJ. Extended resections for carcinoma of the colon and rectum. Surg Gynecol Obstet 1986;1:996.
[14] Minsky BD, Mies C, Rich TA, et al. Potentially curative surgery of colon cancer. The influence of blood vessel invasion. J Cli Oncol 1988;6:119.
[15] Haas-Kock DFM, Baeten CGMI, Jager JJ, et al. Prognostic significance of radial margins of clearance in rectal cancer. Br J Surg 1996;83:781.
[16] Wiggers T, Arends JW, Schutte B, et al. A multivariate analysis of pathologic prognostic indicators in large bowel cancer. Cancer 1988;61:386.
[17] Krasna MJ, Flancbaum L, Cody RP, et al. Vascular and neural invasion in colorectal carcinoma. Incidence and prognostic significance. Cancer 1988;61:1018.
[18] Peethambaram P, Weiss M, Loprinzi CL, et al. Am evaluation of postoperative follow-up tests in colon cancer patients treated for cure. Oncology 1997;54:287.

[19] Wanebo CD, Rao B, Pinsky CM, et al. Preoperative carcinoembryonic antigen level as a prognostic indicator in colorectal cancer. N Engl J Med 1978;299:448–51.

[20] Harrison LE, Guillem JG, Paty P, et al. Preoperative carcinoembryonic antigen predicts outcomes in node-nective colon cancer patients: a multivaraiate analysis of 572 patients. J Am Coll Surg 1997;185:55.

[21] Witzig TE, Loprinzi CL, Gonchoroff NJ, et al. DNA ploidy and cell kinetic measurements as predictors of reurrence and survival in stages B2 and colorectal adenocarcinoma. Cancer 1991; 68:879.

[22] Gryfe R, Swallow C, Bapat B, et al. Molecular biology of colorectal cancer. Curr Probl Cancer 1997;21:233.

[23] Pricolo VE, Finkelstein SD, Hansen K, et al. Mutated p53 gene is an independent adverse predictor of survival in colon carcinoma. Arch Surg 1997;132:371.

[24] Ahnen DJ, Feigl P, Quan G, et al. Ki-ras mutation and p53 overexpression predict the clinic behavior of colorectal cancer: a Southwest Oncology Group study. Cancer Res 1998;58:1149.

[25] Vogelstein B, Fearon ER, Hamilton S, et al. Genetic alterations during colorectal-tumor development. N Engl J Med 1988;319:525.

[26] Ookawa K, Sakamoto M, Hirohshi S, et al. Concordant p53 and DCC alterations and allelic losses on chromosome 13q and 14q associated with liver metastases of colorectal carcinoma. Int J Cancer 1993;53:385.

[27] Jen J, Kim H, Piantadosi S, et al. Allelic loss pf chromosome 18Q and prognosis in colorectal cancer. N Engl J Med 1994;331:213.

[28] Ogunbiyi OA, Goodfellow BJ, Herfarth K, et al. confirmation that chromosome 18q allelic loss in colon cancer is a prognostic indicator. J Clin Oncol 1998;16:427.

[29] Cho KR, Fearon ER. DCC-linking tumour suppressor genes and altered cell surface interactions in cancer. Curr Poin Genet Dev 1995;5:525.

[30] Saito M, Yamaguchi A. Goi T, et al: Expression of DCC protein in colorectal tumors and its relationship to tumor progression and metastasis. Oncology 1999;56:134.

[31] Genurdi M, Viel A, Bonora D, et al. Characterization of MLH1 and MSH2 alternative splicing and its relevance to molecular testing of colorectal cancer susceptibility. Genet 1998;102:15.

[32] Watanabe T, Wu T-T, Catalano PL, et al. Molecular predictors of survival after adjuvant chemotherapy for colon cancer. N Engl J Med 2001;344:1196–206.

[33] Allegra CJ, Paik S, Parr A, et al. Prognostic value of thymidylate synthase (TS), Ki-67 and p53 in patients (Pts) withDukes' B & C colon cancer. Proc Am Soc Clin Oncol 2001;20:124a.

[34] Buyse M, Zeleniuch-Jaquitte A, Chalmers T, et al. Adjuvant therapy of colorectal cancer: why we still don't know. JAMA 1988;259:3571–8.

[35] Verhaegen H, DeCree J, DeCock W, et al. Levaminsole therapy in patients with colorectal cancer. In: Terry W, Rosenburg S, editors. Immunotherapy of human cancer. New York: Elsevier; 1982. p. 225–9.

[36] Laurie JA, Moertel CG, Fleming TR, et al: Surgical adjuvant therapy of large bowel carcinoma: an evaluation of levamisole and the combination of levamisole and 5-fluorouracil. J Clin Oncol 1989;7:1447–56.

[37] Moertel CG, Fleming TR, Macdonald JS, et al: Levamisole and fluorouracil for adjuvant therapy of resected colon carcinoma. N Engl J Med 1990;322:352–8.

[38] Moertel CG, Fleming TR, Macdonald JS, et al. Fluorouracil plus levamisole as effective adjuvant therapy after resection of stage III colon carcinoma: a final report. Ann Intern Med 1995;122:321–6.

[39] The efficacy of the group C status of levamisole and 5-FU for patients with the Dukes' C colon cancer. National Cancer Institute Update, October 1989.

[40] National Institute of Health Consensus Conference. Adjuvant therapy for patients with colon and rectal cancer. JAMA 1990;264:1444–50.

[41] Rustum YM. Modulation of fluoropyrimidines by leucovorin: rationale and status. J Surg Oncol Suppl 1991;2:116–23.

[42] Wolmark N, Rockette H, Fisher B, et al. The benefit of leucovorin-modulated fluorouracil as

postoperative adjuvant therapy for primary colon cancer: results from National Surgical Adjuvant Breast and Bowel Project Protocol C-03. J Clin Oncol 1993;11:1879–87.

[43] Francin G, Petrioli R, Lorenzini L, et al. Folinic acid and 5-fluorouracil as adjuvant chemotherapy in colon cancer. Gastroenterology 1994;106:899–906.

[44] International Multicentre Pooled Analysis of Colon Cancer Trials (IMPACT). Efficacy of adjuvant fluorouracil and folinic acid in colon cancer. Lancet 1995;345:939–44.

[45] Haller DG, Catalano PJ, Macdonald JS, et al. Fluorouracil (FU), leucovorin (LV), and levamisole (LEV) adjuvant therapy for colon cancer: preliminary results of INT-0089. Proc Am Soc Clin Oncol 1996;15:211.

[46] Haller DG, Catalano PJ, Macdonald JS, et al. Fluorouracil, leucovorin, and levamisole adjuvant therapy for colon cancer: five-year final report of INT-0089. Proc Am Soc Clin Oncol 1998;17:265a.

[47] Wolmark N, Rockette H, Mamounas E, et al. Clinical trial to assess the relative efficacy of fluorouracil and leucovorin, fluorouracil and levamisole, and fluorouracil, leucovorin, and levamisole in patients with Dukes' B and C carcinoma of the colon: results from the National Surgical Adjuvant Breast and Bowel Project C-04. J Clin Oncol 1999;17:3553–9.

[48] Andre T, Colin P, Louvet C, et al. Randomized adjuvant study comparing two schemes of 5-fluorouracil and leucovorin in stage B2 and C colon adenocarcinoma:study design and preliminary safety results. Semin Oncol 2001;28(suppl 1):35–40.

[49] Balzar M, Winter J, de Boer CJ, et al. The biology of the 17–1A antigen (Ep-CAM). J Mol Med 1999;17:699–712.

[50] Shen J-W, Atkinson B, Koprowski H, et al. Binding of murine immunoglobulin to human tissues after immunotherapy with anticolorectal carcinoma monoclonal antibody. Int J Cancer 1984;33:465–8.

[51] Gottlinger HG, Funke I, Johnson JP, et al. The epithelial cell surface antigen 17–1A, a target for antibody-mediated tumor therapy: its biochemical nature, tissue distribution and recognition by different monocolonal antibodies. Int J Cancer 1986;38:47–53.

[52] Shetye J, Frodin J-E, Christenssen B, et al. Immunohistochemical monitoring of metastatic colorectal carcinoma in patients treated with monocolonal antibodies (Mab 17–1A). Cancer Immunol Immunother 1988;27:154–62.

[53] Goodwin RA, Tuttle SE, Bucci DM, et al. Tumor-associated antigen expression of primary and metastatic colorectal carcinomas detected by monoclonal antibody 17–1A. Am J Clin Pathol 1987;88:462–7.

[54] Steplewski Z, Lubeck MD, Koprowski H, et al. Human macrophages armed with murine immunoglobulin G2a antibodies to tumors destroy human cancer cell lines. Science 1983; 221:865–7.

[55] Liesveld JL, Frediani KE, Winslow JM, et al. Cytokine effects and role of adhesive proteins and Fc receptors in human macrophage-mediated antibody dependent cellular cyto toxicity. J Cell Biochem 1991;45:381–90.

[56] Fogler We, Kinger MR, Abraham KG, et al. Enhanced cytotoxicity against colon carcinoma by combination of non-competing monoclonal antibodies to the 17–1A antigen. Cancer Res 1988; 48:6303–8.

[57] Herlyn D, Sears H, Iliopoilos D, et al. Anti-idiotype antibodies to monoclonal antibody CO17–1A. Hybridoma 1986;5:S51–8.

[58] Fagerberg J, Hjelm A-L, Ragnhammar P, et al. Tumoral regression in monoclonal antibody-treated patients correlates with the presence of anti-idiotype reactive T-lymphocytes. Cancer Res 1995;55:1824–7.

[59] Riethmuller G, Scheider-Gadicke E, Schlimok G, et al. Randomised trial of monoclonal antibody for adjuvant therapy of resected Dukes' C colorectal carcinoma. Lancet 1994;343: 1177–83.

[60] Riethmuller G, Holz E, Schlimok G, et al. Monoclonal antibody therapy for resected Dukes's C colorectal carcinoma: seven year outcome of a multicenter randomized trial. J Clin Oncol 1998; 16:1788–94.

[61] Haller DG. Update of clinical trials with edrecolomab: a monoclonal antibody therapy for colorectal cancer. Semin Oncol 2001;28(suppl 1):25–30.

[62] Punt CJ, Nagy J, Douillard A, et al. Edrecolomab (17–1A antibody) alone or in combination with 5-fluorouracil based chemotherapy in the adjuvant treatment of stage III colon cancer: results of a phase III study. Pro Am Soc Clin Oncol 2001;20:123a.

[63] Mamounas E, Wieand S, Wolmark N, et al. Comparative efficacy of adjuvant chemotherapy in patients with Dukes' B versus Dukes' C colon cancer: results from four National Surgical Adjuvant Breast and Bowel Project adjuvant studies (C-01, C-02, C-03, and C-04). J Clin Oncol 1999;17:1349–55.

[64] Marsoni S for IMPACT investigators. Efficacy of adjuvant fluorouracil and leucovorin in stage B2 and C colon cancer. Semin Onocl 2001;28(suppl 1):14–9.

[65] Piedbois P. Introduction, 4th International Conference on Colorectal Cancer in Paris. Semin Oncol 2001;28(suppl 1):1–3.

[66] Schrag D, Gelfand S, Bach P, et al: Adjuvant chemotherapy for stage II colon cancer: Insight from a SEER-medicare cohort. Proc Am Soc Clin Oncol 2001;20:123a.

[67] Mendenhall MW, Million RR, Pfaff WW. Patterns of recurrence in adenocarcinoma of the rectum and rectosigmoid treated with surgery alone: implications in treatment planning with adjuvant radiation therapy. Int J Radiat Oncol 1983;9:977–85.

[68] Rao AR, Kagan AR, Chan PM, et al. Patterns of recurrence following curative resection alone for adenocarcinoma of the rectum and sigmoid colon. Cancer 1981;48:1492–5.

[69] Pilipshen SJ, Hielweil M, Quan SHQ, et al. Patterns of pelvic recurrence following definitive resections of colorectal cancer. Cancer 1984;53:1354–62.

[70] Higgins GA, Humphrey EW, Dwight RW, et al. Preoperative radiation and surgery for cancer of the rectum. Veterans Administration Surgerical Oncology Group Trial II. Cancer 1986;58:352–9.

[71] Bentzen SM, Balstev I, Penderson M, et al. A regression analysis of prognostic factors after resection of Dukes' B and C carcinoma of the rectum and rectosigmoid. Does postoperative radiotherapy change the prognosis? Br J Cancer 1988;58:195–201.

[72] Fisher B, Wolmark N, Rockette H, et al. Postoperative adjuvant chemotherapy or radiation therapy for rectal cancer: results from NSABP protocol R-01. J Natl Cancer Inst 1988;80:21–9.

[73] Swedish Rectal Cancer Trial. Improved survival with preoperative radiotherapy in resectable rectal cancer. N Eng J Med 1997;336:980–7.

[74] Lavery IC, Fazio VW, Lopez-Kostner F. Radiotherapy for rectal cancer. N Engl J Med 1997;337:346–8.

[75] Camma C, Giunta M, Fiorica F, et al. Preoperative radiotherapy for respectable rectal cancer: a meta-analysis. JAMA 2000;284:1008–15.

[76] Kapitijin E, Marijnen CAM, Magtegaal ID, et al. Preoperative radiotherapy combined with total mesorectal excision for respectable rectal cancer. N Engl J Med 2001;345:638–46.

[77] Douglass Jr HO, Moertel CG, Mayer RJ, et al. Survival after postoperative combination treatment of rectal cancer. N Engl J Med 1986;315(20):1294–5.

[78] Krook JE, Moertel CG, Gunderson LL, et al. Effective surgical adjuvant therapy for high-risk rectal carcinoma. N Engl J Med 1991;324(11):709–15.

[79] O'Connell MJ, Martenson JA, Weiand HS, et al. Improving adjuvant therapy for rectal cancer by combining protracted-infusion fluorouracil with radiation therapy after curative surgery. N Engl J Med 1994;331(8):502–7.

[80] Tepper JE, O'Connell MJ, Petroni GR, et al. Adjuvant postoperative fluorouracil-modulated chemotherapy combined with pelvic radiation therapy for rectal cancer: initial results of intergroup 0114. J Clin Onc 1997;15(5):2030–9.

[81] Tepper JE, O'Connell MJ, Niedzwiecki D, et al. Final Report of INT 0114–adjuvant therapy in rectal cancer: analysis by treatment, stage and gender. Proc Am Soc Clin Oncol 2001;20:123a.

[82] Roh MS, Petrelli N, Wieand S, et al. Phase III randomized trial of preoperative versus postoperative multimodality therapy in patients with carcinoma of rectum (NSABP R-03). Proc Am Soc Clin Oncol 2001;20:123a.

[83] Wolmark N, Rockette H, Wickerham D, et al. Adjuvant therapy of Dukes' A, B, and C adenocarcinoma of the colon with portal-vein fluorouracil hepatic infusion: preliminary results of National Surgical Adjuvant Breast and Bowel Project protocol C-02. J Clin Oncol 1990;8: 1466–75.

[84] Wolmark N, Bryant J, Smith R, et al. Adjuvant 5-fluorouracil and leucovorin with and without interferon alfa-2a in colon carcinoma: National Surgical Adjuvant Breast and Bowel Project Protocol C-05. J Natl Cancer Inst 1998;90:1810–6.

[85] Wolmark N, Colangelo L, Wieand S. National Surgical Adjuvant Breast and Bowel Project trials in colon cancer. Semin Oncol 2001;28(suppl 1):9–13.

[86] Seitz J-F. 5-fluorouracil/leucovorin versus capecitabine in patients with stage III colon cancer. Semin Oncol 2001;28(suppl 1):41–4.

[87] Fong Y. Surgical therapy of hepatic colorectal metastasis. CA Cancer J Clin 1999;49(4):231–55.

[88] Fong Y, Cohen AM, Fortner JG, et al. Liver resection for colorectal metastases. J Clin Oncol 1997;15:938–46.

[89] Kemeny N, Huang Y, Cohen AM, et al. Hepatic arterial infusion of chemotherapy after re-section of hepatic metastases from colorectal cancer. N Engl J Med 1999;341:2039–48.

[90] Giacchetti S, Itzhaki M, Gruia G, et al. Long-term survival of patients with unresectable colorectal cancer liver metastases following infusional chemotherapy with 5-flurouracial, leu-covorin, oxaliplatin and surgeey. Ann Oncol 1999;10:663–9.

[91] Sanz-Altamira PM, Spence LD, Huberman MS, et al. Selective chemoembolization in the management of hepatic metastases in refractory colorectal carcinoma: a phase II trial. Dis Colon Rectum 1997;40:770–5.

[92] Leichman CG, Jacobson J, Modiano M, et al. Hepatic chemoembolization combined with systemic infusion of 5-fluorouracil and bolus leucovorin for patients with metastatic colorectal carcinoma: a Southwest Oncology Group pilot trial. Cancer 1999;86:775–81.

[93] Giovannini M, Seitz JF. Ultrasound-guided percutaneous alcohol injection of small liver meta-stases. Result in 40 patients. Cancer 1994;73:294–7.

[94] Poon MA, O'Connell MJ, Moertel CG, et al. Biochemical modulation of fluorouracil: evidence of significant improvement of survival and quality of life in patients with advanced colorectal carcinoma. J Clin Oncol 1989;7:1407–18.

[95] Buroker TR, O'Connell MJ, Wieand HS, et al. Randomized comparison of two schedules of fluorouracil and leucovorin in the treatment of advanced colorectal cancer. J Clin Oncol 1994; 12:14–20.

[96] Leichman CG, Fleming TR, Muggia FM, et al. Phase II study of fluorouracil and its modu-lation in advanced colorectal cancer: a Southwest Oncology Group study. J Clin Oncol 1995; 13:1303–11.

[97] Lokich JJ, Ahlgren JD, Gullo JJ, et al. A prospective randomized comparison of continuous infusion fluorouracil with a conventional bolus schedule in metastatic colorectal carcinoma: A Mid-Atlantic Oncology Program Study. J Clin Oncol 1989;7:425–32.

[98] The Meta-analysis Group in Cancer. Efficacy of intravenous continuous infusion of fluoro-uracil compared with bolus administration in advanced colorectal cancer. J Clin Oncol 1998; 16:301–8.

[99] Advanced Colorectal Meta-Analysis Project. Modulation of fluorouracil by leucovorin in pa-tients with advanced colorectal cancer: evidence in terms of response rate. J Clin Oncol 1992; 10:896–903.

[100] Wadler S, Wiernik PH. Clinic update on the role of fluorouracil and recombinant interferon alfa-2a in the treatment of colorectal carcinoma. Semin Oncol 1990;17:16–21.

[101] Wadler S, Lembersky B, Atkins M, et al. Phase II trial of fluorouracil and recombinant inter-feron alfa-2a in patients with advanced colorectal carcinoma: an Eastern Cooperative Oncology Group study. J Clin Oncol 1991;9:1806–10.

[102] Hill M, Norman A, Cunningham D, et al. Royal Marsden phase III trial of fluorouracil with or without interferon alfa-2b in advanced colorectal cancer. J Clin Oncol 1995;13:1297–1302.

[103] Corfu-A Study Group. Phase III randomized study of two fluorouracil combination with

either interferon alfa-2a or leucovorin for advanced colorectal cancer. J Clin Oncol 1995; 13:921–8.

[104] Hsiang YH, Liu LF. Identification of mammalian DNA topoisomerase I as an intracellular target of the anticancer drug camptothecin. Cancer Res 1988;48:1722–6.

[105] Pommier Y, Tanizawa A, Kohn KW. Mechanisms of topoisomerase I inhibition by anticancer drugs. In: Liu LF, editor. Advances in pharmacology. New York: Academic Press; 1994. p. 29B:73–92.

[106] Pitot HC. US pivotal studies of irinotecan in colorectal carcinoma. Oncology 1998;12(suppl 6): 48–53.

[107] Cunningham D, Pyrhonen S, James RP, et al. Randomised trial of irinotecan plus supportive care verse supportive care alone after fluorouracil failure for patients with metastatic colorectal cancer. Lancet 1998;352:1413–8.

[108] Rougier P, Van Cutsem E, Bajetta E, et al. Randomized trial of irinotecan versus fluorouracil by continuous infusion after fluorouracil failure in patients with metastatic colorectal cancer. Lancet 1998;352:1407–12.

[109] Saltz LB, Cox JV, Blanke CB, et al. Irinotecan plus fluorouracil and leucovorin for metastatic colorectal cancer. N Engl J Med 2000;343:905–14.

[110] Douillard JY, Cunningham D, Roth AD, et al. Irinotecan combined with fluorouracil compared with fluorouracil alone as first-line treatment for metastatic colorectal cancer: a multicenter randomized trial. Lancet 2000;355:1041–7.

[111] Sargent D, Niedzwiecki D, O'Connell MJ, et al. Recommendation for caution with irinotecan, fluorouracil, and leucovorin for colorectal cancer. N Engl J Med 2001;345:144–6.

[112] Raymond E, Buquet-Fagot C, Djelloul S, et al. Antitumor activity of oxaliplatin in combination with 5-fluorouracil and the thymidylate synthase inhibitor AG337 in human colon, breast, and ovarian cancers. Anticancer Drugs 1997;8:876–85.

[113] Extra JM, Espie M, Calvo F, et al. Phase I study of oxaliplatin in patients with advanced cancer. Cancer Chemother Pharmacol 1990;25:299–303.

[114] Raymond E, Chaney SG, Taamma A, et al. Oxaliplatin: a review of preclinical and clinical studies. Ann Oncol 1998;9:1053–71.

[115] De Braud F, Munzone E, Nole F, et al. Synergistic activity of oxaliplatin and 5-fluorouracil in patients with metastatic colorectal cancer with progressive disease while on or after 5-fluorouracil. Am J Clin Oncol 1998;21:279–83.

[116] Becouarn Y, Rougier P. Clinical efficacy of oxaliplatin monotherapy: phase II trials in advanced colorectal cancer. Semin Oncol 1998;25(supp 5):23–31.

[117] Levi F, Misset JL, Brienz S, et al. A chronopharmacologic phase II clinical trial with fluorouracil, folinic acid, and oxaliplatin using an ambulatory multichannel programmable pump. High antitumor effectiveness against metastatic colorectal cancer. Cancer 1992;69: 893–900.

[118] Levi F, Zidani R, Brienza S, et al. A multicenter evaluation of intensified, ambulatory, chronomodulated chemotherapy with oxaliplatin, fluorouracil, and leucovorin as initial treatment of patients with metastatic colorectal carcinoma. Cancer 1999;85:2532–40.

[119] De Gramont A, Figer A, Seymour M, et al. Leucovorin and fluorouracil with or without oxaliplatin as first-line treatment in advanced colorectal cancer. J Clin Oncol 2000;18:2938–47.

[120] Giacchetti S, Perpoint B, Zidani R, et al. Phase III multicenter randomized trials of oxaliplatin added to chronomodulated fluorouracil-leucovorin as first-line treatment of metastatic colorectal cancer. J Clin Oncol 2000;18:136–47.

[121] Andre T, Bensmaine MA, Louvet C, et al. Multicenter phase II study of bimonthly high-dose leucovorin. Fluorouracil infusion and oxaliplation for metastatic colorectal cancer resistant to the same leucovorin and fluorouracil regimin. J Clin Oncol 1999;17:3560–8.

[122] Diasio RB, Harris BE. Clinical pharmacology of 5-fluorouracil. Clin Pharmacokinet 1989;16: 215–37.

[123] Naguib FNM, El-Kouni MH, Sha S. Enzymes of uracil catabolism in normal and neoplastic human tissues. Cancer Res 1985;45:5402–12.

[124] Lu Z, Zhang R, Diasio RB. Dihydropyrimidine dehydrogenase activity in human liver: population characteristics and clinical implication in 5-FU chemotherapy. Clin Pharmacol Ther 1995;58:512–22.

[125] Ishitsuka H, Miwa M, Ishikawa T, et al. Capecitabine: an oral available fluoropyrimidine with tumor selective activity. Proc Am Assoc Cancer Res 1995;36:A407.

[126] Ishitasaka T, Utoh M, Sawada N, et al. Xeloda (capecitabine), an oral available tumor-selective fluoro-pyrimidine carbamate. Proc Am Soc Clin Oncol 1997;16:A208.

[127] Cao S, Lu K, Ishtsuka H, et al. Antitumor activity of capecitabine against fluorouracil sensitive and resistant tumors. Proc Am Soc Clin Oncol 1997;16:A226.

[128] Schuller J, Cassidy J, Reigner B, et al. Tumor selectivity of Xeloda™ in colorectal cancer patients. Proc Am Soc Clin Oncol 1997;16:A227.

[129] Mackean M, Planting A, Twelves C, et al. Phase I and pharmaclogic study of interminttent twice-daily oral therapy with capecitabine in patients with advanced and/or metastatic cancer. J Clin Oncol 1998;16:2977–85.

[130] Van Cutsem E, Findlay M, Osterwalder B, et al. Capecitabine, an oral fluoropyrimidine carbamate with substantial activity in advanced colorectal cancer: results of a randomized phase II study. J Clin Oncol 2000;18:1337–45.

[131] Twelves C, Harper P, Van Cutsem E, et al. A phase III trial (SO14796) of Xeloda™ (capecitabine) in previously untreated advaced/metastatic colorectal cancer. Proc Am Soc Clin Oncol 1999;18:263a.

[132] Hoff PM, Ansari R, Batist G, Cox J, et al. Comparison of oral capecitabine versus intravenous fluorouracil plus leucovorin as first-line treatment in 605 patients with metastatic colorectal cancer: results of a randomized phase III study. J Clin Oncol 2001;19:2282–92.

[133] Taguchi T. Experience with UFT in Japan. Oncology (Huntingt) 1997;11(Suppl 10):30–4.

[134] Saltz L, Leichman C, Young C, et al. A fixed-ratio combination of uracil and ftorafur (UFT) with low dose leucovorin: an active oral regimen for advanced colorectal cancer. Cancer 1995; 75:782–5.

[135] Pazdur R, Lessere Y, Phodes V, et al. Phase II trials of uracil and tegafur plus oral leucovorin: an effective oral regimen in the treatment of metastatic colorectal carcinoma. J Clin Oncol 1994; 12:2296–300.

[136] Priest D, Schmitz J, Banni M, et al. Pharmacokinetics of LV metabolites in human plasma as a function of dose administration orally and intravenously. J Natl Cancer Inst 1991;83:1806–12.

[137] Gonzalez-Baron M, Felin J, de la Gandara I, et al. Efficacy of oral tegafur modulation by uracil and leucovorin in advanced colorectal cancer. A phase II study. Eur J Cancer 1995;31A:2215–9.

[138] Pazdur R, Douillard JY, Shilling JR, et al: Multicenter phase III study of 5-fluorouracil (5-FU) or UFT in combination with leucovorin (LV) in patients with metastatic colorectal cancer. Proc Am Soc Clin Oncol 1999;18:263a.

[139] Carmichael J, Popiela T, Radstone D, et al. Randomized comparative study of ORZEL (oral uracil/tegafur [UFT] plus leucovorin [LV]) versus parenteral 5-fluorouracil (5-FU) plus LV in patients with metastatic colorectal cancer. Proc Am Soc Clin Oncol 1999;18:264a.

[140] Spector T, Harrington JA, Porter DJ. 5-ethynyluracil (776C85): inactivation of dihydropyrimidine dehydrogenase in vivo. Biochem Pharmacol 1993;46:2243–8.

[141] Porter DJT, Chestnut WG, Merrill BM, et al. Mechanism-based inactivation of dihydropyrimidine dehydrogenase by 5-ethynyluracil. J Biol Chem 1992;267:5236–42.

[142] Diasio RB. Improving 5-FU with a novel dihydropyrimidine dehydrogenase inactivator. Oncology 1998;12(Suppl 4):51–6.

[143] Baccanari DP, Davis ST, Knick VC, et al. 5-ethynyluracil: effects on the pharmacokinetics and antitumor activity of 5-fluorouracil. Proc Natl Acad Sci USA 1993;90:11064–8.

[144] Hohneker JA. Clinical development of eniluracil. Current Status. Oncology 1998;12(Suppl 7): 52–6.

[145] Mani S, Beck T, Chevlen E, et al. A phase II open-label study to evaluate a 28-day regimen oral 5-fluorouracil (5-FU) plus 776C85 for the treatment of patients with previously untreated metastatic colorectal cancer (CRC). Proc Am Soc Clin Oncol 1998;17:281A.

W. Sun, D.G. Haller / Hematol Oncol Clin N Am 16 (2002) 969–994

[146] Leichman CG, Fleming TR, Muggia FM, et al. Phase II study of fluorouracil and is modulation in advanced colorectal cancer. A Southwest Oncology Group Study. J Clin Oncol 1995;13: 1303–11.
[147] Buroker TR, O'Connell MJ, Wieand HS, et al. Randomized comparison of two schedules of fluorouracil and leucovorin in the treatment of advanced colorectal cancer. J Clin Oncol 1994; 12:14–20.
[148] Levin J, Schilsky R, Burris H, et al. North American phase III study of oral eniluracil (EU) plus oral 5-fluorouracil (5-FU) versus intravenous (IV) 5-FU plus leucovorin (LV) in the treatment of advanced colorectal cancer (ACC). Proc Am Soc Clin Oncol 2001;20:132a.
[149] Van Cutsen E, Sorensen J, Cassidy J, et al. International phase III study of oral eniluracil (EU) plus 5-fluorouracil (5-FU) versus intravenous (IV) 5-FU plus leucovorin (LV) in the treatment of advanced colorectal cancer (ACC). Proc Am Soc Clin Oncol 2001;20:132a.
[150] Gorlick R, Bertino JR. Drug resistance in colon cancers. Semin Oncol 1999;26:606–11.
[151] Ishikawa T, Sekiguchi F, Fukase Y, et al. Positive correlation between the efficacy of capecitabine and doxifluridine and the ratio of thymidine phosphorylase to dihydropyrimidine dehydrogenase activities in tumors in human cancer xenografts. Cancer Res 1998;58:685–90.
[152] Saltz L, Rubin M, Hochster H, et al. Cetuximab (IMC-C225) plus irinotecan (CP-11) is active in CPT-11 refractory colorectal cancer (CRC) that expresses epidermamal growth factor receptor (EGFR). Prp Am Soc Clin Oncol 2001;20:3a.
[153] Bergsland E, Hurwitz H, Fehrenbacher L, et al. A randomized phase II trial comparing rhuMAb VEGF (recombinant humanized monoclonal antibody to vascular endothelial cell growth factor) plus 5-fluorouracil/Leucovorin (FU/LV) to FU/LV alone in patients with metastatic colorectal cancer. Proc Am Clin Oncol 2000;19:242a.

Hematol Oncol Clin N Am
16 (2002) 995–1014

HEMATOLOGY/
ONCOLOGY
CLINICS OF
NORTH AMERICA

Chemoradiotherapy in the treatment of rectal cancer

Roberto J. Santiago, MD*, James M. Metz, MD,
Stephen Hanh, MD

*Department of Radiation Oncology, Division of Hematology Oncology, Department of Medicine,
University of Pennsylvania School of Medicine, 2 Donner, 3400 Spruce Street, Philadelphia,
PA 19104, USA*

The integration of radiotherapy to the adjuvant treatment of rectal cancer was prompted by the predominance of locoregional failures after curative surgery [1,2]. This characteristic in the pattern of failure is one of the main reasons adjuvant radiotherapy plays a greater role in rectal cancer than in colon cancer. Local failure rates at 5 years for selected patients with stage II and stage III rectal cancer treated with conventional surgery alone are approximately 30% and 50%, respectively [1,2]. These rates are higher when the margins of resection are positive [2,3]. It has been demonstrated that local failure rates after surgery alone for rectal cancer are strongly dependent on the degree of bowel wall invasion, lymph node involvement, and margins of resection [1,2]. These same locoregional factors are also predictive of distant metastasis and survival. In addition, local failure is associated with devastating symptoms that severely affect the quality of life of patients. For these reasons, locoregional control remains a major issue in the treatment of rectal cancer.

Studies comparing postoperative pelvic radiotherapy to surgery alone in patients with stage II-III rectal cancer found that radiotherapy conferred an advantage in locoregional control but no improvement in survival [4–6]. These results prompted researchers to investigate the addition of chemotherapy to postoperative radiotherapy with the hope of decreasing the rate of distant failures and improving the effectiveness of pelvic irradiation on local control. A number of randomized trials evaluating postoperative 5-fluorouracil (5-FU)–based chemoradiotherapy have demonstrated that this modality yields superior local control, disease-free survival, and overall survival compared to surgery

---

* Corresponding author.
  E-mail address: Santiago@xrt.upenn.edu (R.J. Santiago).

alone or surgery plus radiotherapy in patients with stage II-III rectal cancer [7–10].

The delivery of therapy before surgery has some potential advantages compared with postoperative therapy. Possible benefits of preoperative treatment in rectal cancer are downstaging of the tumor, decrease in acute complications, and less tumor hypoperfusion/hypoxia. Preoperative radiotherapy alone has been shown to improve local control and survival for patients with resectable stage II-III rectal cancer [11]. Furthermore, numerous phase 2 studies demonstrate encouraging results with the use of preoperative chemoradiotherapy in patients with marginally resectable or unresectable rectal cancer. Extrapolating from these findings, ongoing phase 3 trials are comparing preoperative chemoradiotherapy with preoperative radiotherapy or with postoperative chemoradiotherapy.

Radical resection alone remains the standard treatment for patients with stage I disease. Selected patients with early disease and tumor characteristics associated with a low-risk for locoregional extension are candidates for sphincter-conservative treatment based on local excision or endocavitary irradiation. Some patients within this group are at increased risk for relapse and benefit from treatment with supplemental external irradiation or chemoradiation [12,13].

Local recurrence in the pelvis affects 10% to 25% of patients after initial combined modality therapy for rectal cancer [7–15]. Local failure is associated with decreased survival and symptoms that severely affect the quality of life of patients [16]. Resection of recurrent disease, though difficult, is paramount in the salvage of these patients [17,18]. Chemoradiotherapy can improve the resectability and local control of recurrent disease and thus improves the probability of salvage [18].

Chemoradiotherapy is associated with higher rates of complications than either chemotherapy or radiotherapy alone. Inadequate radiotherapy techniques and selection of chemotherapy regimens increase the toxicity associated with chemoradiotherapy. Conceivably, the increased toxicity observed in some of the early studies worsened the therapeutic ratio of chemoradiotherapy and masked its potential benefit. Better radiotherapy techniques and adjustments in chemotherapy agents, doses, and routes of delivery have improved the toxicity profile of combined modality.

This article summarizes the evidence that has established chemoradiotherapy as part of the standard of care for rectal cancer and the techniques used for its delivery.

Postoperative chemoradiotherapy

Postoperative chemoradiotherapy is a commonly used approach in the treatment of rectal cancer. A postoperative approach permits detailed staging information to be gathered from surgery. This information is valuable for accurately estimating the patient's prognosis and for making treatment choices. Furthermore, surgical staging may identify a group of patients with early disease in whom chemoradiotherapy may not be necessary. Another advantage of a postoperative approach is that surgical clips often help define the tumor bed and areas at high risk for relapse, which is useful in guiding radiotherapy techniques. In addition, normal structures such as the small bowel can be mobilized during surgery to minimize their presence in the field to be radiated.

A number of randomized trials evaluating postoperative 5-FU–based chemoradiotherapy have demonstrated that this modality yields superior local control, disease-free survival, and overall survival compared to surgery alone or surgery plus radiotherapy in patients with stage II-III rectal cancer [7–10] (Table 1). These trials evaluated different radiotherapy techniques, chemotherapy combinations, and treatment delivery techniques. The results of the following studies have established postoperative chemoradiotherapy as a standard approach for patients with stage II-III resected rectal cancer.

In 1985 and 1986, the Gastrointestinal Tumor Study Group (GITSG) published the results of Trial 7175 [7,8], which examined the effects of postoperative chemoradiotherapy on patients with fully resected rectal cancer (MAC stages B2-C). Patients were randomly assigned to 1 of 4 treatment groups:

No adjuvant therapy (58 patients)
Postoperative radiotherapy with 40 to 48 Gy (50 patients)
Postoperative chemotherapy with 5-FU and methylCCNU (MeCCNU)
 (48 patients)
Combination of radiotherapy (40–44 Gy) and chemotherapy (46 patients)

The trial demonstrated a significant advantage in 5-year disease-free (67% versus 45%, $P = 0.009$) and overall (58% versus 45%, $P = 0.07$) survival rates and in 7-year overall (57% versus 33%, $P = 0.005$) survival rates for the chemoradiotherapy arm when compared to the surgery alone arm. In addition, locoregional control at 5 years was greatest with the chemoradiotherapy arm (89%) than with surgery (76%), postoperative radiotherapy (80%), or postoperative chemotherapy (73%). One patient who received MeCCNU chemotherapy acquired acute myeloid leukemia. These results supported the use of postoperative chemoradiotherapy for patients with cancer involving the perirectal fat or regional lymph nodes (MAC stages B2-C).

GITSG Trial 7175 is recognized as an important study but is not without criticism. First, a number of patients did not complete or receive the treatments to which they were randomized, and they were excluded from the study rather than included based on intent to treat. Second, the AP/PA radiation technique used is associated with higher toxicity, which likely contributed to poor compliance or interruptions of the study protocol guidelines. Third, 50% of the patients in the radiotherapy arms received less than 42 Gy and approximately 20% received more than 46 Gy.

Although postoperative chemoradiotherapy was found to be superior to surgery alone, many thought postoperative radiotherapy alone would be a more appropriate control for comparison. The North Central Cancer Treatment Group

Table 1
Treatment techniques in randomized trials of postoperative chemoradiation for rectal cancer

Study	Treatment	RT dose (Gv)	RT tecnique	Chemotherapy (mg/m^2)
GITSG 7175	Surgery			
	Surgery + RT	40–48/ 1.8–2.0/fx	AP-PA	
	Surgery + CT			8 Cycles MeCCNU (130) d 1, 5 FU (325) d 1–5, and 5 FU (375) d 36–40
	Surgery + CRT	40–44/ 1.8–2.0/fx	AP-PA	5 FU first 3 and last 3 d of RT, then same as surgery + CT
NCCTG 79-47-51	Surgery + RT	45–50.4/ 1.8 fx	4 field	
	Surgery + CRT	45–50.4/ 1.8/fx	4 field	With RT: 5 FU (500) d 1–3 and 29–31 Pre/post RT: MeCCNU (130/100) d 1, and 5 FU (300)d 1–5, and 5 FU (400) d 36–40
GITSG 7180	Surgery + CRT + 12 mo 5 FU and MeCCNU	41.4/1.8/fx	3–4 fields	5 FU (500) first 3 and last 3 d of RT, then 8 cycles of MeCCNU (130) d 1, 5 FU (325) d 1–5, and 5 FU (375) d 36–40
	Surgery + CRT + 6 mo escalating 5 FU	41.4/1.8/fx	3–4 fields	5 FU (500) first 3 and last 3 d of RT, then 6 cycles of 5 FU on d 1–5 and d 36–40 up to 500 mg/m^2
NCCTG 86-47-51	Surgery + bolus 5 FU CRT preceded and followed by 5 FU and MeCCNU	45–54/1.8/fx starting on day 64	3–4 fields	With RT: 5 FU (500) d 1–3 and 36–38 Pre/post RT: MeCCNU (130/100) d 1, 5 FU (500)d 1–5, and 5 FU (450) d 36–40
	Surgery + PVI CRT preceded and followed by 5 FU and MeCCNU	45–54/1.8/fx starting on day 64	3–4 fields	With RT: PVI 225 mg/m^2/d Pre/post RT: MeCCNU (130/100) d 1, 5 FU (500)d 1–5, and 5 FU (450) d 36–40
	Surgery + bolus 5 FU CRT preceded and followed by 5 FU alone	45–54/1.8/fx starting on day 64	3–4 fields	With RT: 5 FU (500) d 1–3 and 36–38 Pre/post RT: 5 FU (500)d 1–5 and 5 FU (450) d 36–40
	Surgery + PVI CRT preceded and followed by 5 FU alone	45–54/1.8/fx starting on day 64	3–4 fields	With RT: PVI 225 mg/m^2/d Pre/post RT: 5 FU (500)d 1–5 and 5 FU (450) d 35–40
INT 0114	Surgery + 5 FU alone CRT	50.4–54/1.8/fx	3–4 fields	Pre/during RT/post RT: 5 FU = 500/500/450

(continued on next page)

Table 1 (*continued*)

Study	Treatment	RT dose (Gv)	RT tecnique	Chemotherapy (mg/m^2)
	Surgery + 5 FU/LV CRT	50.4–54/1.8/fx	3–4 fields	Pre/during RT/post RT: 5 FU + LV = 425 + 20/400 + 20/380 + 20
	Surgery + 5 FU/LM CRT	50.4–54/1.8/fx	3–4 fields	Pre/during RT/post RT: 5 FU + LM = 450 + 150+/500 + 150/400 + 150
	Surgery + 5 FU/ LV/LM CRT	50.4–54/1.8/fx	3–4 fields	Pre/during RT/post RT: 5 FU + LV + LM = 425 + 20 + 150/ 400 + 20 + 150/380 + 20 + 150
Norwegian ARCPG	Surgery			
	Surgery + CRT	46/2/fx	3 field	5 FU (500 if < 1.75, 750 if > 1.75 m^2) on days 1, 2, 11, 12, 21, and 22 of RT

RT, radiotherapy; GITSG, Gastrointestinal Tumor Study Group; CT, chemotherapy; NCCTG, North Central Cancer Treatment Group; CRT, chemoradiotherapy; MeCCNU, methylCCNU; PVI, protracted venous infusion; INT, intergroup; ARCPG, Adjuvant Rectal Cancer Project Group.

(NCCTG) trial 79-47-51 demonstrated that postoperative chemoradiotherapy improved survival in patients with deeply invasive or regional lymph node-positive rectal cancer when compared with adjuvant radiotherapy alone [9]. In this trial, patients were randomly assigned to one of two treatments:

Postoperative radiotherapy with 45 to 50.4 Gy (100 patients)
Postoperative radiotherapy plus concurrent bolus 5-FU, preceded and followed by bolus 5-FU plus MeCCNU (104 patients)

The chemoradiotherapy arm in this trial yielded a significant reduction in local recurrence (13.5% versus 25%, $P = 0.036$) and distant metastases (28.8% versus 46%, $P = 0.011$). Significant improvement in 5-year disease-free (58% versus 38%, $P = 0.0016$) and overall (58% versus 48%, $P = 0.04$) survival rates was observed in the chemoradiotherapy arm. The advantage in overall survival remained significant at 7 years ($P = 0.025$). Acute toxicities were more prevalent in the chemoradiotherapy arm. Twelve of the patients had secondary malignancies (6 in each group), though no cases of leukemia were reported.

Concern about the late sequelae associated with MeCCNU, including the development of leukemia and renal insufficiency, led the GITSG to evaluate the contribution of MeCCNU to adjuvant chemoradiotherapy for rectal cancer [14]. GITSG Trial 7180 randomized 210 patients with fully resected MAC stage B2 through C disease to 1 of 2 treatments:

Postoperative chemoradiotherapy with 5-FU plus 12 months of additional 5-FU with MeCCNU
Postoperative chemoradiotherapy with 5-FU plus 6 months of escalating 5-FU

The incidence of toxic effects was similar between the two therapy groups; approximately 50% of the patients in each treatment arm experienced severe or worse toxicity episodes as defined by the GITSG toxicity scale. There was one treatment-related death in each arm. No episodes of leukemia were reported during the relatively short follow-up time. The 3-year disease-free survival rate was 54% in the MeCCNU arm and 68% in the escalating 5-FU arm. The 3-year overall survival rate was 66% in the MeCCNU arm and 75% in the escalating 5-FU arm. These differences were not statistically significant (in fact, there was a trend toward superior outcome with 5-FU alone); therefore, the investigators concluded that MeCCNU was not an essential component of effective post-operative chemoradiotherapy for rectal cancer.

The use of MeCCNU and the efficacy of administering 5-FU through a protracted venous infusion (PVI) regimen throughout radiotherapy was addressed by NCCTG Trial 86-47-51 [15]. Six hundred sixty patients with stage II-III rectal cancer were randomized to 1 of 4 treatment groups:

- 5-FU and MeCCNU, followed by chemoradiotherapy with bolus 5-FU, followed by additional 5-FU and MeCCNU
- 5-FU and MeCCNU, followed by chemoradiotherapy with PVI, followed by additional 5-FU and MeCCNU
- 5-FU, followed by chemoradiotherapy with bolus 5-FU, followed by additional 5-FU
- 5-FU, followed by chemoradiotherapy with PVI, followed by additional 5-FU

Patients who received PVI had significantly increased rates of 4-year disease-free (63% versus 53%, $P = 0.01$) and overall (70% versus 60%, $P = 0.005$) survival compared with those who received bolus 5-FU. There was also a significant decrease in distant metastases in those who received PVI compared with bolus 5-FU ($P = 0.03$) and a decrease in local recurrence that did not reach statistical significance ($P = 0.11$). Overall, the incidence of severe reactions was low. The incidence of severe diarrhea was significantly higher among patients who received PVI; and the incidence of severe leukopenia was significantly higher among those who received bolus 5-FU. Comparing single-agent 5-FU to 5-FU plus MeCCNU, the incidence of severe diarrhea, stomatitis, and leukopenia was significantly higher among patients who received 5-FU alone, and the incidence of severe thrombocytopenia was significantly higher among those who received 5-FU plus MeCCNU. In addition, one patient who received 5-FU alone developed acute leukemia not otherwise specified. There was no significant difference in survival or local control between those who received MeCCNU and those who did not. These data confirmed the GITSG data and led to the conclusion that the addition of MeCCNU to 5-FU does not provide an advantage over a higher dose of 5-FU given alone and thus is not an essential component of chemoradiotherapy for rectal cancer. The authors also concluded that PVI plus postoperative pelvic irradiation was well tolerated and could improve the outcome of patients with high-risk rectal cancer compared with bolus 5-FU–based chemoradiotherapy.

In the late 1980s and early 1990s several trials investigated 5-FU modulation with either leucovorin (LV) or levamisole (LM). Leucovorin enhances the 5-FU–induced inhibition of thymidylate synthase by covalently binding to the active derivative of 5-FU and to the enzyme, forming a ternary complex. The action of LM is thought to derive from enhancement of the host immune response to the tumor. A number of these trials showed an improvement in outcome with these agents when compared with bolus 5-FU in patients with advanced and metastatic colorectal cancer. These findings prompted Intergroup Adjuvant Trial 0114, designed to evaluate the efficacy of postoperative 5-FU–based chemoradiotherapy modulated by the addition of LV or LM in stage II-III rectal cancer [19]. The trial randomized 1696 patients to 1 of 4 treatment schemes:

Two cycles of bolus 5-FU, followed by chemoradiotherapy with bolus 5-FU, followed by two more cycles of bolus 5-FU

Two cycles of bolus 5-FU plus LV, followed by chemoradiotherapy with bolus 5-FU plus LV, followed by two more cycles of bolus 5-FU plus LV

Two cycles of bolus 5-FU plus LM, followed by chemoradiotherapy with bolus 5-FU plus LM, followed by two more cycles of bolus 5-FU plus LM

Two cycles of bolus 5-FU plus LV and LM, followed by chemoradiotherapy with bolus 5-FU plus LV and LM, followed by two more cycles of bolus 5-FU plus LV and LM

There was evidence of increased gastrointestinal toxicity with the three-drug combination compared with bolus 5-FU alone. Toxic reactions were significantly more common in females. One percent of the patients died of treatment-related causes. Despite a trend for increased disease-free survival in the LV arm, there was no significant advantage in local control, disease-free survival, or overall survival to any of the treatment regimens compared with bolus 5-FU alone. The authors concluded that the addition of LM or LV plus LM was unlikely to yield a benefit over chemoradiotherapy with 5-FU alone. Thus, these regimens were not recommended outside of clinical trials. Although this trial had some statistical power limitations, the trend for increased disease-free survival with 5-FU plus LV suggested that this regimen deserved further investigation.

The Norwegian Adjuvant Rectal Cancer Project Group conducted a study to investigate whether a regimen of postoperative radiotherapy combined with short-term, single-agent 5-FU, could improve the local control and survival in 144 patients with Dukes B and C rectal cancer [10]. This study differed from the previously discussed trials in two significant aspects. First, chemotherapy was given exclusively during the radiotherapy period without a maintenance course after radiotherapy. In addition, this trial used 5-FU alone instead of 5-FU combinations with MeCCNU, LM, or LV. These differences were expected to achieve a decrease in the toxicity of chemotherapy without significantly affecting its effectiveness. Patients in the adjuvant treatment group had a cumulative local recurrence rate of 12% compared with 30% in the group that had surgery only ($P = 0.01$). Five-year recurrence-free survival and overall survival rates in the chemoradiotherapy group were 64% compared with 46% ($P = 0.01$) and 50% ($P = 0.05$) in the surgery group. No treatment deaths were observed. World Health Organization grade 3 acute toxicity was seen in only three patients (all skin reactions). Only 4% of patients required surgical intervention for late small bowel complications; two were from the surgery alone arm.

Based on these trials, the postoperative combination of radiotherapy with 5-FU–based chemotherapy has been accepted as a standard treatment for patients with rectal carcinoma that extends through the bowel wall or involves regional lymph nodes (stage II-III). Some investigators have pointed to a lack of evidence in support of radiotherapy as an essential component to the postoperative treatment of rectal cancer because postoperative radiotherapy alone had not been associated with improvement in survival. This view was further supported by the fact that a substantial portion of the long-term complications of postoperative chemoradiotherapy was attributed to radiotherapy and by the encouraging results of adjuvant chemotherapy in patients with high-risk colon cancer. NSABP protocol R-01, comparing surgery alone with postoperative chemotherapy (MeCCNU, vincristine, and 5-FU) or with postoperative radiotherapy, demonstrated a disease-free ($P = 0.006$) and an overall survival ($P = 0.05$) advantage for the chemotherapy arm [4]. Despite a nearly significant reduction in locoregional relapse with radiotherapy ($P = 0.06$), this did not translate to a survival advantage. Interestingly, subgroup analyses revealed that the benefit in disease-free and overall survival observed with chemotherapy was limited to males and patients younger than 65. In fact, females treated with chemotherapy had poorer survival than patients receiving surgery alone did.

NSABP protocol R-02 was carried out to address whether the addition of radiotherapy to chemotherapy affects survival and to determine whether 5-FU plus LV was superior to the combination of MeCCNU, vincristine, and 5-FU (MOF) in men [20]. Six hundred ninety-four patients with Dukes B or C carcinoma of the rectum were stratified according to sex, number of positive lymph nodes, age, and institution. Male patients (total, 407) were randomly assigned to receive 1 of 4 treatment groups:

Five cycles of postoperative MOF (n = 103)
Postoperative MOF plus radiotherapy (n = 104)
Six cycles of postoperative 5-FU plus LV (n = 102)
Postoperative 5-FU plus LV plus radiotherapy (n = 98)

Although the contrasting response to therapy in men and women who participated in Protocol R-01 could not be conclusively explained, it was decided that the randomization of female patients (n = 287) would be limited to 1 of 2 treatments:

Six cycles of postoperative 5-FU plus LV (n = 143)
Postoperative 5-FU plus LV plus radiotherapy (n = 144)

Overall, 348 patients received adjuvant chemotherapy alone, and 346 received chemotherapy plus postoperative radiotherapy. Radiotherapy was initiated 3 to 5 weeks after the completion of cycle 1 of chemotherapy and consisted of 45 Gy to the pelvis followed by a boost, for a total tumor dose of 54 Gy. Radiotherapy was delivered in fractions of 1.8 Gy using a four-field technique. Bolus 5-FU was delivered on the first 3 and the last 3 days of radiotherapy. The addition of postoperative radiotherapy did not increase relapse-free ($P = 0.38$), disease-free ($P = 0.90$), or overall ($P = 0.89$) survival, regardless of which chemotherapy was used. Additionally, radiotherapy did not alter the incidence of distant disease. Nonetheless, the addition of radiotherapy was found to significantly reduce the 5-year locoregional relapse rate from 13% to 8% ($P = 0.02$). In the cohort of male patients, 5-FU plus LV demonstrated a benefit in 5-year relapse-free (61% versus 55%; $P = 0.046$) and disease-free (55% versus 47%; $P = 0.009$) survival rates when compared with MOF, but it demonstrated no significant difference in 5-year overall survival (65% versus 62%; $P = 0.17$). Men appeared to tolerate the 5-FU plus LV regimen better than women, especially when comparing the nonirradiated group. Radiotherapy was associated with more skin reactions and leukopenia, but there was no difference in the rate of diarrhea.

The lack of survival benefit with the addition of radiotherapy to chemotherapy in Protocol R-02 supports the findings of Protocol R-01 in that radiotherapy alone affects locoregional control but not survival. Presumably, this stems from the lack of impact of radiotherapy in distant disease. Still, these findings suggest that a subgroup of patients at high risk for locoregional failure (large T3, T4, or N2 disease) benefit from adding postoperative radiotherapy to adjuvant chemotherapy [21].

Postoperative conclusions

In conclusion, postoperative combined-modality therapy with 5-FU and radiotherapy is an accepted treatment for rectal cancers at high risk for local recurrence. Postoperative pelvic radiotherapy alone improves locoregional control but is not associated with an improvement in survival. MeCCNU does not improve on the local control or the survival provided by 5-FU alone. Protracted infusional 5-FU has been associated with decreased tumor recurrence and improved survival when combined with postoperative adjuvant pelvic radiotherapy. Although there may be an advantage to the combination of 5-FU and LV, the addition of LM alone or LV plus LM has not yielded a benefit over chemoradiotherapy with 5-FU alone.

We recommend postoperative chemoradiotherapy as follows:

For patients with stage III and high-risk stage II resectable rectal cancer (T3, node-positive disease, or positive margins of resection)
Radiation to 45 Gy over 5 weeks to the whole pelvis plus a 5.4 to 9 Gy boost to areas at high risk

Use of 1.8 to 2.0 Gy fractions 5 days a week delivered with a high-energy photon beam from a linear accelerator

Use of a three-or four-field technique with treatment of all fields each day

Use of prone positioning, belly board, bladder distention, oral contrast for visualization of the small bowel, and a three-dimensional/comparative treatment planning

Inclusion of the perineal scar in the initial pelvic fields for patients who have undergone APR

Use of bolus 5-FU during the first and fifth weeks of radiation or protracted infusional 5-FU throughout irradiation

Use of surgical clips to assist in the definition of the tumor volume to be treated

Participation in a clinical trial whenever possible

Preoperative chemoradiotherapy

The advantages of preoperative chemoradiotherapy include downstaging the tumor, which means decreasing the size of the primary tumor volume and regional nodal disease, potentially converting patients initially deemed unresectable to resectable status. This reduction in the burden of disease may also permit patients with distal tumors who are candidates for APR to become candidates for sphincter-conserving surgery. Physiologically, the intact preoperative tissues are better perfused, potentially providing for improved availability of cytotoxic drugs and oxygen. Furthermore, neoadjuvant therapy may also sterilize microscopic foci of tumor, thus reducing the probability of spilling viable tumor cells during surgery. On the other hand, preoperative therapy can suppress details of the initial stage of disease and thereby limit the prognostic information from the surgical staging. In addition, preoperative treatment may delay postsurgical wound healing, especially when surgery is performed less than 4 weeks from the completion of radiotherapy or when high doses per fraction (>2 Gy) are used.

Preoperative radiotherapy in resectable rectal cancer

Postoperative radiation alone and preoperative radiotherapy alone have been shown to improve local control, but only preoperative radiotherapy has been shown to improve survival. The Swedish Rectal Cancer Trial demonstrated a survival advantage for preoperative radiotherapy when compared to surgery alone [11]. This trial randomized 1168 patients with Dukes stage A-C resectable rectal cancer to surgery alone or to a 1-week regimen of preoperative radiotherapy (25 Gy in five fractions over 5 days) followed by surgery within 1 week. After 5 years of follow-up, patients in the preoperative radiotherapy arm were found to have substantially improved local control (89% versus 73%; $P < 0.001$) and overall survival (58% versus 48%; $P = 0.004$). The improvement in local control benefited every stage subgroup, and preoperative radiotherapy was also associated with a disease-specific survival advantage. Metaanalysis of 14 randomized trials of preoperative radiotherapy for rectal cancer confirmed a reduction in local recurrence (odds ratio [OR], 0.49; $P < 0.001$), overall mortality (OR, 0.84; $P = 0.03$), and cancer-related mortality (OR, 0.71; $P < 0.001$) [22].

Preoperative chemoradiotherapy in locally advanced rectal cancer

Often, disease-free margins cannot be obtained by primary surgery in clinical T3-4 rectal carcinoma. Even when complete resection is accomplished in these patients, local failure remains high (30–50%) with surgery alone [1–3]. Preoperative therapy improves resectability and, in some patients, can induce a complete pathologic response. Sometimes a short distance between the lower pole of the tumor and the anorectal ring (<2 cm) deems patients ineligible for sphincter-preserving surgery. The downstaging observed with preoperative therapy facilitates sphincter preservation, which can have an impact on the quality of life of patients. Results of numerous phase 2 studies using preoperative chemoradiotherapy for locally advanced or distal tumors are encouraging. Ongoing phase 3 trials compare preoperative chemoradiotherapy to preoperative radiotherapy alone or to postoperative chemoradiotherapy.

In 1984, the EORTC evaluated preoperative chemoradiotherapy in patients with potentially operable rectal cancer [23]. Two hundred forty-seven patients were randomized to radiotherapy alone or radiotherapy plus 5-FU. The chemoradiotherapy arm yielded a trend toward superior control of distant metastases to the liver ($P = 0.07$) when compared with radiotherapy alone. On the other hand, the 5-year survival rate was superior in the radiotherapy alone arm than in the chemoradiotherapy arm (59% versus 46%, $P = 0.06$). The incidence of death from malignancy was higher in the radiotherapy-alone group, whereas nonmalignant and treatment-related deaths were higher in the chemoradiotherapy group. In fact, censorship of deaths not attributable to rectal cancer from the analysis yielded no significant difference in survival between the treatment arms. The resectability rate was high and equivalent in both groups despite the higher incidence of T4 tumors in the chemoradiotherapy arm. In addition, there were twice as many complete responders in the chemoradiotherapy arm. In conclusion, this trial did not show a survival benefit from chemoradiotherapy. The improvement in distant control and in disease-specific mortality observed with chemoradiotherapy suggested that an increase in survival could be achieved if complications were reduced.

These results and those observed with postoperative chemoradiotherapy prompted increased interest in neoadjuvant chemoradiotherapy in the United States. Memorial Sloan-Kettering (MSK) conducted several phase 1 trials to evaluate preoperative chemoradiotherapy in patients with unresectable tumors [24–27]. All trials used 2 cycles of bolus 5-FU plus LV and pelvic radiotherapy (50.4 Gy) followed by surgery (with or without intraoperative brachytherapy) and postoperative bolus 5-FU/LV.

The first trial investigated sequential preoperative chemoradiotherapy with bolus 5-FU plus high-dose LV (200 mg/m^2) in 20 patients (7 with recurrent disease) [24]. Chemotherapy was started on day 1 and radiotherapy on day 8. The second cycle of LV–5-FU was given concurrently during the fourth week of radiotherapy. Resection with negative margins was achieved in 89% of patients, and the pathologic complete response rate was 20%. The 3-year actuarial local failure, disease-free survival, and overall survival rates were 29%, 64%, and 69%, respectively. Subsequent trials explored the tolerability and efficacy of low-dose LV (20 mg/m^2) preoperative regimens. One trial studied radiotherapy starting concurrently on day 1with bolus 5-FU plus low-dose LV in 24 patients [25]. The resectability rate with negative margins was 100%. The clinical complete response rate (cCR) was 30%, with 13% attaining a pathologic complete response. The recommended dose of 5-FU for preoperative chemoradiotherapy was 325 mg/m^2. Another trial examined a sequential regimen with low-dose LV in 12 patients [26]. Chemotherapy began on day 1 and radiation on day 8. The resectability rate with negative margins was 91%, and the pathologic complete response rate was 9% (20% cCR). When both low-dose LV trials are considered together, the 4-year actuarial disease-free, overall survival, and local failure rates were 67%, 76%, and 30%, respectively [27]. There was a trend for lower rates of local relapse in patients who achieved pathologic complete response. Because the toxicity data from the sequential regimen with low-dose LV suggested that the dose of 5-FU should be lower than 325 mg/m^2, concern for a potential compromise in systemic control led the investigators not to endorse that regimen. The concurrent regimen with 5-FU plus low dose LV was preferred.

Chemoradiotherapy for unresectable rectal cancer has also been evaluated in several European studies. The EORTC conducted three consecutive phase 2 trials using 2 cycles of bolus 5-FU plus low-dose LV during pelvic irradiation (45 Gy, 25 fractions) [28]. The trials included 37 patients with unresectable primary tumors, 13 with local recurrence, 15 with gross residual after resection, and 20 with potentially resectable disease. None had received previous radiotherapy, and 22 patients had coexisting distant metastases. The three trials differed only in 5-FU dose. After a mean of 8 weeks following chemoradiotherapy, half the patients underwent surgery. Ninety-five percent had complete resections, 29% were downstaged, and 15% had pathologic complete response. Analysis identified 350 mg/m^2/d 5-FU as the most efficacious dose.

In 1998, a group from Canada led by Videtic et al [29] reported their experience with preoperative PVI chemoradiotherapy in patients with unresectable rectal cancer. Twenty-nine patients with clinical stage T4 rectal cancer were treated with preoperative PVI (225 mg/m^2/day) and concurrent radiotherapy (median dose, 54 Gy/28 fractions). Seventy-nine percent of the patients underwent surgery. Of the 23 patients who underwent surgery, 78% had a complete resection. Thirteen percent of the entire group had complete response, and 90% were clinically downstaged. With a median follow-up of 28 months, 83% of the patients who had a complete resection were free of disease.

Preoperative chemoradiotherapy in resectable rectal cancer

After studying the efficacy of preoperative combined modality regimens on unresectable disease, investigators became interested in evaluating resectable tumors. The group at MSK tested the concurrent chemoradiotherapy regimen using 5-FU plus low-dose LV in patients with resectable T3 rectal cancer [30]. Chemoradiotherapy was followed by total mesorectal excision and 4 cycles of postoperative 5-FU plus LV. The pathologic complete response rate was 13% (22% cCR). Eighty-nine percent of the patients, judged by their surgeons to require APR, were able to undergo sphincter-preserving surgery. Total grade 3+ toxicity was 28%. The 3-year pattern of failure reflected an effective local control (2% local, 8% abdominal, and 13% distant). The 3-year actuarial survival rate was 95%.

Similarly, the M. D. Anderson Cancer Center reported their experience with preoperative chemoradiotherapy using infusional 5-FU in patients with resectable rectal cancer [31]. Seventy-seven patients with clinical stage T3 rectal cancer received infusional 5-FU (300 mg/m^2/d) concurrently with radiotherapy (45 Gy/ 25 fractions). Sixty-eight percent of the surgeries were sphincter preserving, and 29% revealed no evidence of tumor. Local tumor control was 96%. Patients with pathologic complete response were more likely to be alive 3 years after therapy. The 3-year actuarial survival rate was 83%.

Two Italian studies by Valentini et al [32,33] explored the use of different chemotherapeutic combinations in the treatment of resectable rectal cancer. In the first study, 83 patients received preoperative radiotherapy (37.8 Gy) concurrently with continuous-infusion 5-FU (1000 mg/m^2/day, days 1–4) and bolus mitomycin c (10 mg/m^2 on day 1). Nine percent of the patients had complete pathologic response. Fifty-seven percent of the patients experienced tumor downstaging and nodal downstaging. Seventy-eight percent of the patients underwent sphincter-saving surgery, including 44% of those initially judged to require APR. The second trial used a higher preoperative radiotherapy dose (45 Gy + 5.4 Gy boost) concurrently with continuous-infusion 5-FU (1000 mg/m^2/day, days 1–4 and days 29–32) and slow infusion of cisplatin (60 mg/m^2/day on days 1 and 29). Radical resection was attained in all patients. Twenty-three percent of the patients had complete pathologic response (33% cCR). Tumor downstaging was observed in 68%. Eighty-five percent of the patients underwent sphincter-saving surgery, including 40% of those judged to require APR. The investigators concluded the addition of c-DDP to 5-FU improved the pathologic locoregional rate in comparison with their previous experience with mitomycin c and recommend further investigation of this regimen.

Preoperative conclusions

Studies have shown that preoperative chemoradiotherapy improves resectability and, in some patients, induces a complete pathological response. Complete pathologic responses after preoperative therapy are associated with higher local control rates than those achieved with surgery alone. Moreover, it appears that the rate of complete pathologic response with concurrent preoperative chemoradiotherapy is approximately twice that observed with preoperative radiotherapy alone (20% versus 10%). Ongoing phase 3 trials comparing preoperative chemoradiotherapy with preoperative irradiation alone or postoperative chemoradiotherapy should validate the efficacy of this approach and provide valuable survival data.

In conclusion, data from several small phase 1 and 2 trials suggest that preoperative chemoradiotherapy:

Converts a substantial fraction of patients with unresectable tumors to candidates for resection

Improves the probability of attaining negative margins of resection

Induces complete pathological response in approximately 20% of patients

Converts a substantial fraction of patients deemed to require APR to candidates for sphincter-saving surgical procedures

Is tolerable of, and is of at least comparable effectiveness as, preoperative radiotherapy and postoperative chemoradiotherapy

We would consider preoperative chemoradiotherapy under the following conditions:

- In the setting of recurrent disease, locally advanced "marginally resectable" tumors, and distal tumors deemed to require an APR
- For resectable stage III and high-risk stage II through participation in a clinical trial
- Participation in a clinical trial whenever possible
- Radiation to 45 Gy over 5 weeks to the whole pelvis with consideration of a 5.4-Gy boost to regions of gross disease
- Use of 1.8-to 2.0-Gy fractions 5 days a week delivered with a high-energy photon beam from a linear accelerator
- Use of a three-or four-field technique with treatment of all fields each day
- Use of prone positioning, belly board, bladder distention, oral contrast for visualization of the small bowel, and three-dimensional/comparative treatment planning
- Use of bolus 5-FU during the first and fifth weeks of radiation or protracted infusional 5-FU throughout irradiation
- A 4-to 6-week interval between the completion of chemoradiotherapy and surgery to allow for tumor downstaging and recovery of normal tissues

Comparative studies of postoperative versus preoperative therapy

National Surgical Adjuvant Breast and Bowel Project (NSABP) Protocol R-03 was designed to compare a preoperative chemoradiotherapy regimen with identical postoperative chemoradiotherapy in patients with operable rectal cancer. In 1997, the NSABP published a progress report on Protocol R-03 [34]. At the time of the report, 59 patients had been randomized to preoperative chemoradiotherapy and 57 patients to postoperative chemoradiotherapy. All patients received seven cycles of 5-FU plus LV chemotherapy. Cycles 2 and 3 consisted of bolus 5-FU with low-dose LV given during the first and fifth weeks of radiotherapy (50.4 Gy). The rest of the cycles used 5-FU plus high-dose LV. In the preoperative arm, the first three cycles of chemotherapy and radiotherapy were delivered before surgery. In the postoperative arm, all therapy was delivered after surgery. No patient was deemed inoperable because of local disease progression. At randomization, sphincter-saving surgery was intended in 31% of patients in the preoperative arm and 33% of patients in the postoperative arm. Such surgery was actually performed in 50% of the patients in the preoperative arm and in 33% of the patients in the postoperative arm. Predictably, the higher rate of sphincter preservation was associated with a tendency toward tumor downstaging in the preoperative arm. Eight percent of the patients treated before surgery had pathologic complete response. Overall, the frequency of treatment-related toxicities and perioperative complications was similar in both groups. We await the final results of this study

Chemoradiotherapy with local excision for limited disease

Although surgical resection remains the standard treatment for patients with stage I disease, there is increasing interest in the use of sphincter-sparing, local therapies for selected early rectal cancers. The objective of these treatments is to preserve sphincter function and to achieve adequate local tumor control. Candidates should have tumor characteristics associated with a low risk for locoregional extension—among them, 4 cm or smaller, mobile, not poorly differentiated or mucinous, and no evidence of nodal or perirectal tissue involvement. Some patients within this group are at increased risk for local relapse after excision alone because of tumor features such as T2 primary, close margins of resection, or lymphovascular invasion. This subgroup of patients is thought to benefit from treatment with adjuvant external radiotherapy or chemoradiotherapy. Transmural (T3) tumors have approximately 30% risk for local recurrence with this technique and are treated more effectively with standard surgery plus preoperative or postoperative therapy. Conservative therapy is an alternative in patients with contraindications to major surgery who have T3 or smaller tumors with suboptimal tumor characteristics.

In 1999, Cancer and Leukemia Group B published their experience with anal sphincter preservation in patients with clinically favorable distal rectal cancer [12]. Clinically favorable cancer was defined as T1/T2 adenocarcinoma 4 cm or smaller in diameter, encompassing 40% or less of the bowel circumference, and located 10 cm or less from the dentate line. Of the 177 patients enrolled, 59 had T1 tumors, 51 had T2 tumors, and 67 were ruled ineligible. Patients with T1 tumors were treated with full-thickness local excision alone. Those with T2 tumors received external radiotherapy (pelvis, 45 Gy/25 fractions + 9 Gy/5 fractions) with bolus 5-FU (500 mg/m^2 on days 1–3 and 29–31) after local excision. The 6-year overall and disease-free survival rates for the whole group were 85% and 78%, respectively. The 6-year overall survival rates for T1 and T2 tumors were 87% and 85%, respectively. The 6-year disease-free survival rates for T1 and T2 tumors were 83% and 71%, respectively. Two patients with T1 and seven with T2 tumors experienced isolated local recurrences; all underwent salvage APR. Of the 9 patients with recurrences, 5 remained free of disease. The investigators concluded that local excision followed by chemoradiotherapy was an effective way of preserving the sphincter in patients with favorable T2 tumors. Salvage APR appeared to control local recurrence effectively in the patients who had local recurrences.

Radiation Therapy Oncology Group Protocol 89-02 also assessed the concept of functional preservation of the rectal sphincter in patients with clinically mobile, distal rectal cancers [13]. Patients were eligible for this protocol if they had rectal tumors that measured 4 cm or less in diameter, occupied 40% or less of the rectal circumference, and were medically unfit for sphincter conservation through anterior resection. Primary tumors were excised by en bloc, full-thickness resection through a transanal, transcoccygeal, or transsacral approach. Fourteen patients with T1 tumors, grade 1-2, without lymphovascular invasion, and margins of resection uninvolved for more than 3 mm were treated with local excision alone. Fifty-one patients with T2-3 tumors, high grade, or lymphovascular invasion were treated with local excision followed by external radiotherapy (50-56 Gy or 59.4-65 Gy if margins measured less than 3 mm) with 2 cycles of bolus 5-FU. The 5-year freedom from pelvic relapse rate was 88% for the entire study group and 86% for patients treated with chemoradiotherapy. Five-year disease-free survival rates were 86% for patients treated with local excision alone and 82% for patients treated with chemoradiotherapy. A correlation between the locoregional failure rate and the percentage of rectal circumference involved with cancer was identified. If 20% or less of the circumference was involved, the locoregional failure rate was 6%; if 21% to 40% of the circumference was involved, the rate was 18%. The locoregional failure was also related to T-stage: T1, 4%; T2, 16%; and T3, 23%. The distant relapse rate was found to increase with increasing T-stage as well (31% of T3 failed distally). Sixty-three percent of local-regional recurrences were salvaged with subsequent interventions.

Together, these trials support the use of chemoradiotherapy after local excision of early, distal rectal cancers at high risk for locoregional failure. Chemoradiation reduces the risk for locoregional recurrence in high-risk subgroups to a rate similar to that observed in the low-risk group treated with excision alone. In general, radiotherapy is given after surgery and concurrently with 5-FU–based chemotherapy. Pelvic irradiation makes use of a dose of approximately 45 Gy, followed by a 5.4- to 9.0-Gy boost to the primary tumor bed. Salvage surgery appears to be successful in at least half the patients who experience local failure. It is important to bear in mind that these results are the product of a highly selected cohort of patients and that information from large prospective studies is still needed to determine whether this approach will have local control and survival rates similar to those of standard surgery.

Chemoradiotherapy for locally recurrent disease

Local recurrence in the pelvis affects 10% to 25% of patients in the first 5 years after initial combined modality therapy for stage II-III rectal cancer [4–15,19]. Local failure is associated with a decrease in survival and is associated with symptoms such as pelvic pain, bone pain, incontinence, and obstruction. Resection of recurrent disease, though difficult, remains paramount in the salvage of these patients. The role of preoperative chemoradiotherapy in the treatment of recurrent rectal cancer has been partially addressed in some studies of neo-adjuvant therapy in patients with locally advanced disease [24–28].

Mohiuddin et al [18] assessed the role of chemoradiotherapy followed by resection of residual disease for recurrent rectal cancer. The study excluded patients with distant metastases, obvious lateral pelvic wall invasion, or sacral involvement. Thirty-nine patients previously irradiated (median, 50.4 Gy) were treated with radiotherapy (median dose, 36 Gy; range, 20.0–49.2 Gy) with concurrent infusional 5-FU. Eighteen percent of patients required a treatment break during reirradiation, and 13% required early termination of treatment because of diarrhea, moist desquamation, or mucositis. Seventy-nine percent of patients underwent gross total resection of disease. No surgical deaths were observed. The median survival time was 45 months, with a 5-year actuarial survival rate of 24%. The 5-year actuarial local failure and distant metastases rates were 55% and 17%, respectively. The most common late complications were small bowel obstruction (6/39 patients) and bowel fistula (3/39 patients).

Gunderson et al [16,17] reported the use of intraoperative electron irradiation (IOERT) with or without 5-FU for locally recurrent, previously unirradiated rectal cancer. IOERT was used to supplement external beam irradiation (EBRT) and resection. In one series, 123 patients received EBRT (45 Gy + 5.4- to 9.0-Gy boost, 1.8 Gy per fraction) with or without concomitant 5-FU–based chemotherapy after surgery [16]. IOERT doses ranged from 10 to 20 Gy. Median survival was 28 months, with an overall survival rate at 5 years of 20%. The actuarial 5-year failure rate within the IOERT field was 26%, and within the EBRT field it was 37%. The actuarial 5-year distant failure rate was 72%. The high distant relapse rates observed prompted the authors to recommend consistent use of 5-FU with EBRT and the addition of maintenance chemotherapy.

In conclusion, selected patients with locally recurrent rectal cancer after previous adjuvant therapy can be treated successfully with salvage therapy. Chemoradiotherapy and resection play key roles in the successful control of recurrent disease.

Future directions

Randomized trials are in progress to determine the ideal chemotherapeutic agents and their optimal doses and routes of administration in combination with radiotherapy. A Southwest Oncology Group study (SWOG 9403, INT 0144) is comparing postoperative radiotherapy given concurrently with 5-FU by PVI versus radiotherapy given concurrently with 5-FU plus LV by bolus injections in patients with rectal cancer MAC stages B2, B3, and C. In the concurrent bolus 5-FU plus LV arm, radiotherapy is preceded and followed by 5-FU plus LV plus LM chemotherapy. In the concurrent PVI arm, patients are further randomized to either a regimen of bolus 5-FU versus a regimen of PVI before and after concurrent PVI chemoradiotherapy. The NSABP is currently evaluating (protocol R-03) whether the administration of preoperative chemotherapy (5-FU + LV) and radiotherapy, followed by postoperative chemotherapy, is more effective than the administration of postoperative chemotherapy and radiotherapy in improving the survival of patients with operable carcinoma of the rectum. Unfortunately, a study (RTOG 9401, INT 0147) designed to compare the efficacy of preoperative versus postoperative chemoradiotherapy closed because of low accrual. More recently, the RTOG opened a randomized trial (R-0012) comparing preoperative continuous 5-FU plus twice-daily radiotherapy versus continuous 5-FU plus CPT-11 plus conventional radiotherapy for distal T3-T4 rectal cancers. Meanwhile, a number of phase 1 and 2 studies are evaluating the incorporation of altered fractionation schedules and new chemotherapy agents. In conclusion, the combined modality treatment of rectal cancer has and will advance through the continued effort and collaboration of specialists in multiple fields of the clinical and basic sciences. To optimize the treatment outcomes of patients with rectal cancer, accurate pretreatment staging is required, and the same degree of diligence and collaboration among surgical, medical, and radiation oncologist is essential.

References

[1] Mendenhall WM, Million RR, Pfaff WW. Patterns of recurrence in adenocarcinoma of the rectum and rectosigmoid treated with surgery alone: implications in treatment planning with adjuvant radiation therapy. Int J Radiat Oncol Biol Phys. 1983;9:977–85.
[2] Rich T, Gunderson LL, Lew R, Galdibini JJ, Cohen AM, Donaldson G. Patterns of recurrence of rectal cancer after potentially curative surgery. Cancer. 1983;52:1317–29.
[3] Quirke P, Durdey P, Dixon MF, Williams NS. Local recurrence of rectal adenocarcinoma due to inadequate surgical resection: histopathological study of lateral tumor spread and surgical excision. Lancet. 1986;2:996–9.
[4] Fisher B, Wolmark N, Rockette H, et al. Postoperative adjuvant chemotherapy or radiation therapy for rectal cancer: results from NSABP protocol R-01. J Natl Cancer Inst. 1988;80:21–9.
[5] Treurniet-Donker AD, van Putten WL, Wereldsma JC, et al. Postoperative radiation therapy for rectal cancer: an interim analysis of a prospective, randomized multicenter trial in The Netherlands. Cancer. 1991;67:2042–8.
[6] Medical Research Council Rectal Cancer Working Party. Randomized trial of surgery alone versus surgery followed by radiotherapy for mobile cancer of the rectum. Lancet. 1996;348: 1610–4.
[7] Gastrointestinal Tumor Study Group. Prolongation of the disease-free interval in surgically treated rectal carcinoma. N Engl J Med. 1985;312:1465–72.
[8] Douglass HO Jr, Moertel CG, Mayer R, et al. Survival after postoperative combination treatment of rectal cancer. N Engl J Med. 1986;315:1294–5.

[9] Krook JE, Moertel CG, Gunderson LL, et al. Effective surgical adjuvant therapy for high-risk rectal carcinoma. N Engl J Med. 1991;324:709–15.

[10] Tveit KM, Guldvog I, Hagen S, et al. Randomized controlled trial of postoperative radiotherapy and short-term time-scheduled 5-fluorouracil against surgery alone in the treatment of Dukes B and C rectal cancer: Norwegian Adjuvant Rectal Cancer Project Group. Br J Surg. 1997; 84:1130–5.

[11] Improved survival with preoperative radiotherapy in resectable rectal cancer: Swedish Rectal Cancer Trial. N Engl J Med. 1997;336:980–7.

[12] Steele GD Jr, Herndon JE, Bleday R, et al. Sphincter-sparing treatment for distal rectal adenocarcinoma. Ann Surg Oncol. 1999;6:433–41.

[13] Russell AH, Harris J, Rosenberg PJ, et al. Anal sphincter conservation for patients with adenocarcinoma of the distal rectum: long-term results of radiation therapy oncology group protocol 89–02. Int J Radiat Oncol Biol Phys. 2000;46:313–22.

[14] Gastrointestinal Tumor Study Group. Radiation therapy and fluorouracil with or without semustine for the treatment of patients with surgical adjuvant adenocarcinoma of the rectum. J Clin Oncol. 1992;10:549–57.

[15] O'Connell MJ, Martenson JA, Wieand HS, et al. Improving adjuvant therapy for rectal cancer by combining protracted-infusional fluorouracil with radiation therapy after curative surgery. N Engl J Med. 1994;331:502–7.

[16] Gunderson LL, Nelson H, Martenson JA, et al. Intraoperative electron and external beam irradiation with or without 5-fluorouracil and maximum surgical resection for previously unirradiated, locally recurrent colorectal cancer. Dis Colon Rectum. 1996;39:1379–95.

[17] Gunderson LL, Nelson H, Martenson JA, et al. Locally advanced primary colorectal cancer: intraoperative electron and external beam irradiation +/− 5-FU. Int J Radiat Oncol Biol Phys. 1997;37:601–14.

[18] Mohiuddin M, Marks GM, Lingareddy V, Marks J. Curative surgical resection following reirradiation for recurrent rectal cancer. Int J Radiat Oncol Biol Phys. 1997;39:643–9.

[19] Tepper JE, O'Connell MJ, Petroni GR, et al. Adjuvant postoperative fluorouracil-modulated chemotherapy combined with pelvic radiation therapy for rectal cancer: initial results of intergroup 0114. J Clin Oncol. 1997;15:2030–9.

[20] Wolmark N, Wieand HS, Hyams DM, et al. Randomized trial of postoperative adjuvant chemotherapy with or without radiotherapy for carcinoma of the rectum: National Surgical Adjuvant Breast and Bowel Project Protocol R-02. J Natl Cancer Inst. 2000;92:388–96.

[21] Haller DG. Defining the optimal therapy for rectal cancer. J Natl Cancer Inst. 2000;92:361–2.

[22] Camma C, Giunta M, Fiorica F, Pagliaro L, Craxi A, Cottone M. Preoperative radiotherapy for resectable rectal cancer: a meta-analysis. JAMA. 2000;284:1008–15.

[23] Hyams DM, Mamounas EP, Petrelli N, et al. A clinical trial to evaluate the worth of preoperative multimodality therapy in patients with operable carcinoma of the rectum: a progress report of National Surgical Breast and Bowel Project Protocol R-03. Dis Colon Rectum. 1997;40:131–9.

[24] Videtic GM, Fisher BJ, Perera FE, et al. Preoperative radiation with concurrent 5-fluorouracil continuous infusional for locally advanced unresectable rectal cancer. Int J Radiat Oncol Biol Phys. 1998;42:319–24.

[25] Minsky BD, Cohen AM, Enker WE, et al. Preoperative 5-FU, low-dose leucovorin, and radiation therapy for locally advanced and unresectable rectal cancer. Int J Radiat Oncol Biol Phys. 1997;37:289–95.

[26] Minsky B, Cohen A, Enker W, et al. Preoperative 5-fluorouracil, low-dose leucovorin, and concurrent radiation therapy for rectal cancer. Cancer. 1994;73:273–80.

[27] Valentini V, Coco C, Cellini N, et al. Preoperative chemoradiation with cisplatin and 5-fluorouracil for extraperitoneal T3 rectal cancer: acute toxicity, tumor response, sphincter preservation. Int J Radiat Oncol Biol Phys. 1999;45:1175–84.

[28] Valentini V, Coco C, Cellini N, et al. Preoperative chemoradiation for extraperitoneal T3 rectal cancer: acute toxicity, tumor response, and sphincter preservation. Int J Radiat Oncol Biol Phys. 1998;40:1067–75.

[29] Boulis-Wassif S, Gerard A, Loygue J, Camelot D, Buyse M, Duez N. Final results of a random-ized trial on the treatment of rectal cancer with preoperative radiotherapy alone or in combination with 5-fluorouracil, followed by radical surgery: Trial of the European Organization on Research and Treatment of Cancer Gastrointestinal Tract Cancer Cooperative Group. Cancer. 1984;53: 1811–8.

[30] Minsky BD, Cohen AM, Kemeny N, et al. The efficacy of preoperative 5-fluorouracil, high-dose leucovorin, and sequential radiation therapy for unresectable rectal cancer. Cancer. 1993; 71:3486–92.

[31] Minsky BD, Cohen AM, Kemeny N, et al. Pre-operative combined 5-FU, low dose leucovorin, and sequential radiation therapy for unresectable rectal cancer. Int J Radiat Oncol Biol Phys. 1993;25:821–7.

[32] Grann A, Feng C, Wong D, et al. Preoperative combined modality therapy for clinically resect-able uT3 rectal adenocarcinoma. Int J Radiat Oncol Biol Phys. 2001;49:987–95.

[33] Bosset JF, Pavy JJ, Hamers HP, et al. Determination of the optimal dose of 5-fluorouracil when combined with low dose D,L-leucovorin and irradiation in rectal cancer: results of three con-secutive phase II studies: EORTC Radiotherapy Group. Eur J Cancer. 1993;29A:1406–10.

[34] Rich TA, Skibber JM, Ajani JA, et al. Preoperative infusional chemoradiation therapy for stage T3 rectal cancer. Int J Radiat Oncol Biol Phys. 1995;32:1025–9.

Hematol Oncol Clin N Am
16 (2002) 1015–1029

HEMATOLOGY/
ONCOLOGY
CLINICS OF
NORTH AMERICA

Endoscopic palliation of colorectal cancer

Douglas G. Adler, MD, Todd H. Baron, MD, FACP*

*Department of Medicine, Division of Gastroenterology and Hepatology, Mayo Medical Center,
200 First Street Southwest, Eisenberg 8A, Rochester, MN 55905, USA*

Gastrointestinal endoscopy has experienced tremendous growth and technical advancement over the past decade. Many of the largest gains have been in the ability to palliate advanced malignancies and malignant obstructions throughout the gastrointestinal tract. This has been achieved mainly through advances in self-expanding metallic stent (SEMS) technology. Although once seen as revolutionary, the use of SEMS to relieve malignant esophageal, gastroduodenal, and, most frequently, biliary obstruction is now commonplace. The idea that a SEMS could be placed in the colon was once thought to be both impractical and unsafe, mainly for technical reasons. Over time, and with the development of dedicated devices for use in the colon, the practice of colonic stenting is now proving itself to be a valid and sometimes lifesaving technique. Colonic stents can now obviate palliative surgeries in many patients with advanced malignancies who were otherwise high-risk surgical candidates. This article focuses on the palliative use of expandable metal stents in the colon, with emphasis on their indications, use risks, and benefits. The use of laser therapy to palliate colorectal cancer also is discussed, both as a therapy in and of itself and in conjunction with the use of colonic SEMS.

Colorectal cancer and colonic obstruction

Colon cancer remains widely prevalent. Each year, more than 150,000 deaths worldwide result from colorectal cancer. Despite aggressive screening and surveillance incentives in the United States and abroad, total or near-total colonic obstruction is still a very common presentation of colorectal cancer, especially in nations that do not practice aggressive screening. Between 8% and 29% of patients will have subtotal or complete colonic obstruction at the time of presentation [1]. Colonic obstruction secondary to malignancy is the number one cause for emer-

---

* Corresponding author.
E-mail address: baron.todd@mayo.edu (T.H. Baron).

gency large bowel surgery, accounting for as much as 85% of such procedures [2,3]. Approximately one half of all patients with splenic flexure tumors and one quarter of all patients with left sided tumors present with obstruction [1]. Tumors of the distal colon and rectosigmoid, the most common subtype, present with obstruction in only 6% of cases. This is largely thought to be caused by the wider endoluminal diameter in this region, making obstruction less likely [1]. Although primary colorectal malignancy is the most common cause of obstruction, metastatic lesions can occasionally invade the colon and cause obstruction. Metastatic tumors from genitourinary cancers can extrinsically compress the colon resulting in large bowel obstruction with an identical clinical presentation.

As would be expected, patients with malignant large bowel obstruction are quite ill. Severe dehydration is common. Those with obstruction from malignancy frequently are malnourished as well because of their underlying disease state [4]. Patients with primary colorectal cancer presenting with obstruction frequently harbor advanced malignancies. Almost all of these patients will be found to have Duke's stage C or D disease [5], and nearly all of these patients lack adequate bowel preparation for surgery. Colonic mucosa proximal to the obstruction is dilated and extremely friable and is a poor substrate for surgical constructions such as internal anastomoses [4]. Patients demonstrating this constellation of characteristics desperately need surgical intervention as well as clinical decompression. Overall, patients with malignant large bowel obstruction are extremely poor surgical candidates, and surgical mortality for these patients can range up to 15% [1].

Surgical management

Historically, surgical management of colonic obstruction from colorectal cancer was performed via a "three-stage" operation. According to this schema, a decompressing colostomy was constructed in the first surgery. At the time of the second operation, resection of the primary lesion was accomplished. Even patients with incurable disease could benefit from these two surgeries, and the combination of decompressing colostomy and subsequent resection offered good surgical palliation and often could be accomplished during one extended stay. A third surgery, to internalize the large bowel via anastomosis, took place weeks to months later and usually was reserved for patients being treated with a curative intent. Patients following this course of treatment often stayed in the hospital up to 30 days. A large number of these patients never completed all three stages of the series, usually because of severe illness or death. Mortality from this three-stage approach was as high, and the 5-year survival for those who completed all three operations was only 19–38% [1].

Given the difficulty caregivers and patients faced in the three-stage surgical process, it should come as no surprise that a two-stage surgical approach was rapidly accepted after its development. Hartman's procedure, as it came to be known, combined the decompressing tumor and resecting surgeries into one procedure and was used in patients being treated either curatively or palliatively.

Later, if indicated and appropriate, a second procedure could be performed to internalize the anastomosis. Two-stage procedures resulted in shorter hospital stays and were at least as effective, if not more so, than the three-stage approach.

One-stage surgical procedures for colonic obstruction have been in use for some time now. The procedure consists of a primary tumor resection and anastomosis formation at the same time. Unprepared bowel is cleansed in an on-table fashion via colonic lavage. This lavaging can significantly increase the length of the surgery, and anastomoses formed at a one-stage procedure are at an increased risk for postoperative leakage [1]. Still, some researchers have concluded that, in the proper hands, a one-stage surgery is as safe as a two-stage surgery and carries no greater risk: both surgeries have an approximate 30-day mortality rate of 1% [1]. Additionally, the mean length of hospitalization after a one-stage surgery for malignant obstruction has not been shown to be significantly different from that of a two-stage surgery. Other surgical options, such as subtotal colectomy with ileocolic anastomosis, also can be done in one procedure.

Endoscopic options in the management and palliation of colorectal cancer

Decompression tubes for relief of acute obstructive symptoms

Long before the invention of SEMS for use in the colon, endoscopically placed decompression tubes have been employed as a temporizing measure to acutely relieve large bowel malignant obstruction. These tubes decompress distended bowel and decrease the risk of perforation—as well as allow an attempt at preoperative bowel cleansing. Decompression tubes are placed by manual advancement over an endoscopically or fluoroscopically placed guidewire.

Advantages of decompression tubes include wide availability, low cost, and the potential to provide patient stabilization while obviating one or more surgical procedures, typically the decompressing colostomy.

Disadvantages include the time-consuming nature of the procedure and the fact that these tubes are, at best, a temporary solution. Additionally, the risks of the procedure itself include perforation and bleeding. Also, these tubes offer little to patients with widespread disease who will remain poor surgical candidates even if adequate decompression is achieved. Tube placement can sometimes be problematic, especially in cases where the tube needs to be advanced through completely obstructing lesions. Other problems include difficulties in reaching proximal tumors and in advancing decompression tubes in patients with tortuous sigmoid colons.

Despite these difficulties, a variety of methods [6–8] of placing these tubes have met with varying degrees of success, and the technique remains widely applied. Recent attempts to increase the success rate of such procedures has led to the use of an endoscopic overtube to facilitate tube placement through the rectosigmoid, and a recently published series of nine patients in Japan undergoing this procedure all had good outcomes and one-stage surgical procedures [9]. More commonly, however, after successful placement of the tube, decompression of colonic gas is seen, but adequate stool removal and bowel cleansing are difficult to obtain. Still, the benefits of gaseous decompression even in the absence of stool decompression often make colonic decompression tubes worthwhile.

Laser therapy

Palliative endoscopic therapy of inoperable or advanced colorectal cancers with Neodymium: Yttrium Aluminum Garnet (Nd: YAG) lasers has been performed for well over a decade with good results. Laser therapy is primarily applied to recanalize obstructed large bowel in patients with bulky tumors. Laser therapy treats only intrinsic lesions of the colon. It is contraindicated for the treatment of extrinsically compressing tumors.

The application of laser therapy to the colon followed the successful used of the Nd: YAG laser for similar purposes in patients with obstructing esophageal carcinomas, where obstruction and dysphagia were relieved by simple laser ablation of obstructing tissue [10–13]. Studies of large numbers of patients who had received laser therapy for colonic lesions began appearing in the early 1990s. Advantages of laser therapy include the ability to treat bulky, exophytic tumors under direct vision and the fact that the technique relies on widely available technology with which many endoscopists are familiar. The main disadvantage of the technique is that it is technically difficult in the proximal large bowel and rarely used to treat tumors above sigmoid colon.

One early study [14] of 49 patients with distal colorectal cancers who were considered unsuitable for surgical intervention found that if the tumor was less than 3 cm in diameter (n = 7), symptomatic improvement from obstructive symptoms was universal, and, in very rare cases, complete tumor eradication could be achieved. The remaining 42 patients in this study, all of whom had large tumors, underwent a mean of 3.4 sessions of laser therapy over a mean of 19 weeks. Thirty-one of these 42 remaining patients (75%) had good symptomatic improvement. The 11 patients who failed to respond to treatment all had extensive tumors that could not be sufficiently treated with the laser. Other studies of similar size [15–17] had similar results, with success rates in the 80–90% range. An average of approximately three procedures was required to achieve sufficient and lasting relief of obstructive symptoms. Serious complications (bleeding perforation and severe pain) developed in 10–15% of patients.

The largest series of patients undergoing laser therapy for colorectal cancers was published in 1995 and represents the 14-year experience of a group from France [18]. This study included 272 patients undergoing palliative therapy for rectosigmoid cancers. This study had both a high immediate success rate in treating obstructive symptoms (85%) and a low major complication rate of (2%), both of which are likely a reflection of the large experience of the treating endoscopists.

Overall, laser therapy is effective in treating obstructive lesions of the distal colon, but its use is limited in proximal lesions. Multiple treatment sessions are often required to achieve significant and ongoing relief of obstructive symptoms, and the risk of severe complications, including perforation, can undermine patient outcome. Laser therapy does not appear to prolong life.

Colonic self-expanding metal stents

Colonic stents represent the latest development in endoscopic palliation of colorectal cancer. The placement of such devices in patients suffering from malignant large bowel obstruction allows relatively rapid bowel decompression and patient stabilization. Once obstruction is relieved, patients can undergo a more thorough evaluation, including a full assessment of the stage of their disease, in a nonemergent fashion [19]. The other key advantage is that, in contrast with colon decompression tubes, stents have the potential to dilate the obstructed portion of the colon to a near-normal diameter, allowing the patient to pass both stool and gas quickly.

If patients with malignant obstruction are found to have extensive or widespread disease at presentation or are considered poor operative candidates based on comorbid illnesses, the placement of a stent in the large bowel may be the only treatment required. Of course, if a patient with an indewlling colonic stent is deemed a candidate for a curative or palliative surgery, the decompressed bowel can be prepared in a more traditional fashion, and the patient can undergo surgery in a nonemergent fashion. At the time of surgery, the tumor and the stent can be removed en bloc.

For the most part, the placement of a colonic stent requires minimal sedation, no more than is used for a routine screening colonoscopy. The majority of patients do not require endoscopic dilation of the stricture site before stent deployment, as this does not increase the success rate of the procedure and can increase the risk of complications such as tumor fracture or perforation. If the patient has a subtotal obstruction and has had a standard bowel preparation prior to the procedure, stent placement can be done on an outpatient basis, thus avoiding a hospitalization [20].

Other advantages to endoscopic stenting of large bowel obstructions include the ability to place the devices across comparatively long lesions. If the stricture is longer than any single available stent, the devices can be overlapped in a stent-within-stent fashion [4].

Prior to the development and United States Food and Drug Administration (FDA) approval of dedicated colonic stents, earlier investigators used biliary, esophageal, tracheo-bronchial, or even vascular stents to treat malignant large bowel obstruction. Currently, the FDA has approved three stents for use in the large bowel. Each of these stents is constructed of metal wire mesh but varies from the others in the type of lattice-work woven into the metal wires. Although silicon coatings designed to prevent tumor ingrowth through the stent interstices are common in esophageal stents, all three FDA-approved colon stents are uncoated.

Microvasive Corporation (Natick, MA) manufactures SEMS that are approved for use both within the small bowel (most commonly to relieve malignant gastric outlet obstruction) and the colon, and the devices are collectively referred to by the manufacturer as "enteral stents." The Microvasive product is available in 60 and 90 mm lengths and with internal diameters of 20 and 22 mm. In contrast with the other stents available for use in the colon, the Microvasive stent uses "through-the-scope" or "TTS" technology. The entire stent/delivery system complex can pass through the working channel of the endoscope. Thus, the stent can be deployed under direct vision without having to reinsert the endoscope alongside the delivery system to visualize deployment. The ability to advance the undeployed stent through the endoscope greatly simplifies the use of the device in the ascending or transverse colon. With this system, a stent can be placed in any portion of the colon that can be reached by the endoscope. In addition, the Microvasive product is reconstrainable as long as approximately 10% of the stent is still contained in the delivery system. This allows recapture on repositioning and redeployment if the initial position of the stent is deemed suboptimal.

C.R. Bard (Billerica, MA) manufactures a dedicated colonic SEMS made of nitinol wire. When deployed, the device is 30 mm wide and comes in 60, 80, and 100 mm lengths. The device comes preconstrained on a delivery system that employs a "pistol-grip" operating system to control stepwise deployment of the stent. The device is too wide to pass through the working channel of an endoscope. Once deployment has begun, the stent cannot be reconstrained if the position appears suboptimal.

Wilson-Cook (Winston-Salem, NC) also manufactures a dedicated colonic SEMS (the "colonic Z-stent," so named because of its Z-shaped wire configuration). The device has flared ends to decrease the risk of postdeployment migration. The device is 35 mm wide at the ends and 25 mm wide in the center and is available in 40-, 60-, 80-, 100-,or 120-mm lengths. Like the Bard device, the Wilson-Cook stent comes constrained on a long delivery catheter that is too wide to pass through the working channel of an endoscope and, it too, is not reconstrainable once deployment has begun. Both the Bard and Wilson-Cook products are placed over a guidewire under fluoroscopy, although a colonoscope or flexible sigmoidoscope can be placed alongside the delivery system to observe the deployment directly.

All of these SEMS are deployed over a guidewire under endoscopic guidance, fluoroscopic guidance, or a combination thereof (Fig. 1). Interventional radiologists have placed colon stents under fluoroscopic guidance alone, but the stents are limited, for the most part, to treating obstructions in the distal colon. More commonly, however, colon stents are placed by gastrointestinal endocopists using colonoscopes or flexible sigmoidoscopes with the aid of fluoroscopy (Fig. 2). Although most gastroenterologists should be able to place a colon stent, we have found that knowledge of interventional endoscopy techniques (Endoscopic Retrograde Cholangiopancreatography [ERCP], etc) is extremely helpful in learning to deploy these devices effectively.

Clinical studies of colonic stenting for large bowel obstruction

Many studies on the use of stents within the large bowel have been published in recent years, and a review of all these studies is beyond the scope of this article. This review will focus on some of the largest and most relevant publications on colonic stenting.

The largest series published to date was performed by Camunez et al [21], and represents a retrospective analysis of 80 patients who underwent placement of

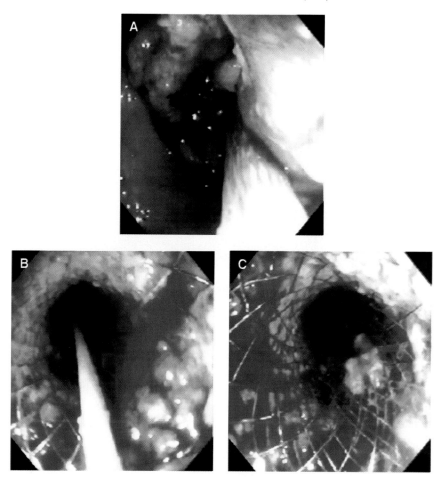

Fig. 1. (A) Endoscopic photo of a predeployed stent advanced over guidewire across site of malignant obstruction. (B) Successfully deployed stent with recanalized lumen; guidewire is still in place. (C) Endoscopic view of deployed stent after delivery system withdrawn. Note widely patent endoluminal diameter.

colon stents for malignant large bowel obstruction over a 3-year period in Spain. All of the patients in this series had left-sided disease. Esophageal Wallstents (Schneider, Bullach, Switzerland) were used in all patients. Successful stent placement (technical success) was achieved in 70 out of 80 patients (87.5%), and 67 of those patients (96%) who received stents had satisfactory clinical decompression. Complications were notable for two perforations, one of which resulted in death. Total luminal obstruction resulted in 9 of 10 patients following failed procedures. In 35 patients, the placement of the stent was purely for palliation, and 28 of these patients still had patent stents at a mean of 138 days (range, 36–334 days) after implantation. The remaining 7 patients in the palliative

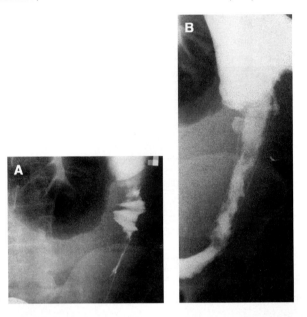

Fig. 2. (A) Contrast injection performed at the time of endoscopy in a patient with clinical malignant large bowel obstruction. A long, high-grade stricture is seen in the descending colon. (B) Water-soluble contrast enema radiographic study of same patient 24 hours after placement of colonic self-expanding metal stent. Note free passage of contrast through stent lumen and decompression of proximal bowel.

group developed re-obstruction, stent migration resulting in stent expulsion, or intractable tenesmus. Long-term survival in the palliative group was 55% at 3 months, 44% at 6 months, and 25% at 9 months.

The second largest study of this kind, also from Spain, is by Mainar et al [22], and presents the results of a multi-center retrospective analysis of 71 patients with acute large bowel obstruction, all of whom had primary colorectal cancer. Of these, 70 had left-sided disease and 1 patient had obstruction of the transverse colon. Of note, Mainar et al performed the procedures with fluoroscopy alone and without the aid of endoscopy. This group achieved technical success in 64 out of 71 patients (90%). Ninety-three percent of those who received stents developed clinical and radiographic signs of decompression and stool passage. Unlike the study by Camunez, Mainar predominately looked at the use of colonic stents in patients with operable disease. Sixty-five patients in this study underwent elective single-stage surgery with partial large bowel resection and primary anastomosis.

Baron et al [2] reported results in 25 patients with large bowel obstruction over a 30-month period. Baron reported on the use of stents both as a precursor to surgery or as a primary palliative procedure. Patients were considered for treatment if they had clinical symptoms of obstruction for greater than 2 days and had a confirmatory contrast study. Twenty-two of 25 patients were obstructed because of primary or recurrent colon cancers or metastatic cancers, whereas the remaining 3 patients were obstructed because of diverticulitis. All of the obstructions were located either in or beyond the distal transverse colon, with the majority (13) being in the sigmoid colon. Eight of the patients presented without an underlying diagnosis, and all would have been treated with emergency surgery. As was typical before the development of dedicated colonic stents, Baron used coiled and meshed esophageal stents as well as meshed tracheobronchial stents when it was deemed feasible. Nine of 10 (90%) patients in the operative group were successfully decompressed. Fourteen of 17 (82%) patients treated with palliative intent were successfully decompressed. (Two patients initially treated in the preoperative group were found to have inoperable disease and were thus also included in the palliative group.)

Complications of note included sepsis in one patient and distal migration of the stent in two patients who had diverticulitis causing obstruction. The migrated stents migrated to the rectum and had to be removed at sigmoidcoscopy with biopsy forceps. No reobstruction occurred, and both underwent uneventful elective resection of the involved large bowel.

Among those in the palliative group, the mean duration of stent placement was 17.3 weeks, and 10 of 17 patients died without the need for reintervention. Four perforations occurred among the palliative patients, and two patients required restenting.

Law et al [23] reported from Hong Kong on 24 patients with acute left-sided obstruction who underwent stent placement performed by colorectal surgeons. Thirteen patients had primary colorectal cancer, whereas the remainder had either recurrent colorectal cancers or tumors that had metastasized to the colon. Stent placement was successful in all patients and resulted in clinical decompression in all but one patient. Law used an Uncovered Esophageal Wallstent (then manufactured by Schneider USA, Inc, Plymouth, MA) in all but one patient. Among the 13 patients with primary colorectal cancer, six were deemed operative candidates and underwent surgery with a curative intent, and all had internal anastomoses created at the time of the primary surgery.

As of this writing, the literature contains other reports on almost 300 patients treated with stents for large bowel obstruction, and many more patients have undergone the procedure. A review of colonic stenting published in 2000 catalogued the findings of 12 studies available at that time, representing a total of 234 patients [24]. This retrospective included the results of small and large studies and found that the overall technical success rate was 93%, and the overall clinical success rate was 90%.

Many of the published case series on colon stents include only a small number of patients. Still, some of these smaller studies highlight interesting aspects of the technique and merit special attention.

Binkert et al [25] reported a series of 19 patients treated with SEMS for large bowel obstruction of either benign or malignant origin and were able to relieve obstruction in 17 patients (88%). Binkert placed the devices with endoscopic guidance, fluoroscopic guidance, or a combination thereof. Although reporting similar findings to the aforementioned studies, this study is notable for the observation that although obstruction was clinically relieved (in most patients) within 12 hours, abdominal films could be suggestive of obstruction for up to 4 days after stent placement.

Wholey et al [26] reported results of 10 patients with left-sided lesions who were treated with tracheo-bronchial stents. The procedures were done under fluoroscopic guidance and without endoscopy. Wholey documented technical success in all patients and clinical success in 9 patients, which is somewhat surprising as tracheo-bronchial stents are, for the most part, narrower then stents designed for use in the esophagus or colon. Three patients had migration of the devices to the rectum causing painful spasm and requiring removal with an anoscope.

The larger studies of colonic stenting have all reported overall success rates in excess of 85%. Some smaller studies, such as the one by Soonwalla et al [27], have reported similar success rates in this situation. But smaller case series [4,28,29] have been seen to report lower success rates, often in the 70% range, probably because of inadequate study population size for statistical interpretation, inadequate clinical experience with a technically challenging procedure, or both.

Cost effectiveness

Despite almost a decade of experience with stenting of the large bowel, cost effectiveness has not been thoroughly evaluated. To date, only Binkert [30] has evaluated cost-effectiveness in this setting, and only on a group of 13 patients. Nine of these were operative candidates, whereas the other four were considered for palliative therapy only. Stents were successfully placed in 12 of 13 patients, and all 12 of those patients clinically decompressed. Eight of nine patients treated in the preoperative group went on to have one-stage surgical procedures. Binkert compared the costs of stenting (the stent itself, colonoscopy, fluoroscopy, and a semiprivate hospital room, as well as surgical, anesthesiology, and professional fees) with the cost of 13 control patients who underwent surgical treatment alone for large bowel obstruction at the same hospital.

In a study performed in Switzerland, Binkert found that average costs in the stented group were 19.7% lower than in the control group. For patients initially treated with stents, the mean length of hospital stay was 6 days shorter (27 days versus 33.1 days), fewer surgical procedures were performed, and the average number of days in the ICU was dramatically shorter (0 days versus 2.3 days). When the subset of patients (7/13) with primary colon cancer was analyzed, the overall costs were 28.8% less than those of control patients.

Complications of colonic stenting

The placement of a SEMS in the colon differs from the placement of such a device in the biliary tree or esophagus. The colon is tortuous, has prominent folds, lacks fixation to nearby organs, undergoes active peristalsis, and does not have the assistance of gravity to pass contents through its lumen. In addition, stool in the large bowel is frequently viscous, with a greater potential to clog a stent.

At the time of delivery, stents can be malpositioned despite endoscopic and fluoroscopic guidance. This is usually caused by slippage of the stent at the time of deployment. Malpositioned devices sometimes can be removed immediately, but they can be unretrievable, especially if they are placed proximal to the sigmoid colon. In some instances, malpositioned stents can be left in place as long as they do not threaten to perforate the bowel or obstruct the lumen. Stents can also migrate at the time of deployment or afterwards. Stents can at times pass in the stool uneventfully, or they may lodge in the rectum, where they can cause pain or tenesmus and require removal [26]. The authors have also noted that stents placed at the splenic flexure may have a higher rate of migration caused by the acute angulation of the bowel.

Stent migrations have been seen to occur primarily in the setting of benign diseases (most commonly caused by diverticulitis). In this setting, obstruction is typically secondary to inflammation, and when the primary process causing the inflammation resolves, the stent cannot adequately anchor itself [26]. Uncovered stents placed within an obstructing malignancy rarely migrate unless the tumor itself undergoes some significant change, usually as a result of treatment, as in the case of tumor regression from radiation therapy [2].

Both tumor ingrowth (through the stent interstices) or tumor overgrowth (beyond the ends of a stent) have been documented to cause partial or complete obstruction of previously placed stents. Currently, all FDA approved colon stents available in the United States are uncoated, but it seems logical that eventually colon stents with a silicon coating (to prevent tumor ingrowth but not overgrowth) will become commercially available.

Perforation can occur either at the time of deployment or afterward, although it is most likely during deployment caused by the rapid expansion of the device and the relative friability of the colonic mucosa in patients with obstruction. Perforation at the time of deployment, especially in patients with obstruction, almost invariably mandates surgery. Somewhat counterintuitively, predeployment dilation of the stricture itself is rarely warranted and was shown to increase the risk of perforation and tumor fracture in one study [2]. The inherent expansile force of the stent itself is enough to dilate the stricture in a safe and timely manner.

Experience gained with esophageal stents has revealed that major complications, most notably bleeding and perforation, are more likely to occur in patients who have undergone prior radiation therapy because of inherent tissue weakness and poor vascularity [31–33]. Experience suggests that the same increased potential for complications would be likely when stents are used in the colon. Care must be taken to inquire about a history of prior radiation therapy to the abdomen and/or pelvis (for prostate or testicular cancer in males, for gynecologic cancers in females) before the decision to place a colonic stent can be made. If the patient has had radiation therapy, this risk must be weighed in light of the possible benefits from stent placement.

Colonic stents may become impacted with stool. Stool impaction is typically seen when long stents are used, or if multiple devices are placed in a stent-within-stent fashion (Fig. 3) [25,30]. To avoid stool impaction, we recommended that patients should consume a low-residue diet and maintain indefinitely a regimen of a daily laxative or stool softener after the stent has been placed.

Other less common complications include postprocedure pain, bleeding, and tenesmus. This last problem is occasionally seen in patients with rectal lesions who require stent placement. Rarely, the device must be removed if tenesmus is intractable.

Multimodality therapy in the palliation of colon cancer

Given the different advantages afforded by both stents and lasers, it is not surprising that some investigators have combined these two treatment modalities. Tack et al [34] used nitinol SEMS in 10 patients with metastatic rectal or sigmoid adenocarcinomas presenting with left-sided obstruction. In 6 of these 10 patients, Nd:YAG laser therapy was used prior to stent placement to debulk the tumors and allow passage of the colonoscope and guidewire. Four of 6 patients had undergone earlier laser therapy as a palliative measure.

Among the patients who underwent dual therapy, an average of 2 ± 0.4 sessions of laser therapy were required before SEMS placement was undertaken. Overall, stent placement was successful in 9 of 10 patients. The only technical failure occurred in a patient in the dual-therapy group. This patient had undergone laser therapy on three prior occasions and experienced a large bowel perforation during stent deployment that required surgical intervention. Mean

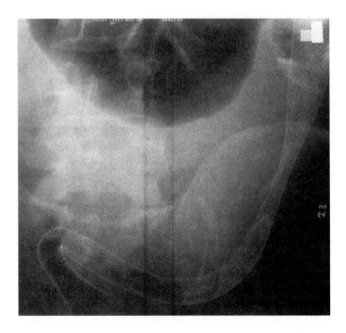

Fig. 3. Demonstration of multiple overlapping stent-within-stent in a patient with an extrinsically compressing pelvic malignancy.

survival for all 10 patients was 204 ± 43 days. Five patients died with patent stents a mean of 180 ± 38 days after placement, and the other 5 patients had either experienced stent migration or had their stents removed at the time of surgical resection.

The advent of dedicated colonic stents that are deployed over hydrophilic biliary guidewires and through-the-scope delivery systems obviates the need to debulk the tumor prior to attempted stent deployment. Indeed, passage of a guidewire across the strictured lumen is often all that is needed to allow proper stent placement and deployment. Still, the study by Tack et al highlights the combined use of lasers and stents. Lasers can be used to ablate tumor tissue that threatens to cause tumor obstruction by ingrowth or overgrowth. Lasers can also be used to coagulate bleeding sites on tumors that have been previously treated with SEMS.

Placement of a colonic SEMS in patients with advanced disease does not preclude the subsequent use of more traditional therapies such as radiation, chemotherapy, or both. Although experience is limited in this realm, the experience of the authors would seem to indicate that patients with colonic SEMS tolerate subsequent radiation and chemotherapy without an increased incidence of complications [35].

Summary

Multiple endoscopic options exist for physicians seeking to provide palliative therapy for patients with colorectal cancer. Endoscopic decompression tubes can allow urgent stabilization for patients with malignant obstruction requiring some form of surgical palliation. Patients who are not candidates for palliative surgery can experience good symptomatic relief from malignant large bowel obstruction via laser therapy or placement of a colonic stent. Laser therapy can be used in conjunction with SEMS to recanalize and decompress large bowel in certain situations. The use of colonic stents is rapidly becoming more commonplace as acceptance of the technique becomes more widespread. Patients with unresectable disease may be able to avoid surgery altogether and achieve successful and lasting palliation of large bowel obstruction. Overall, they provide effective and durable palliation in patients with malignant obstruction, have an excellent risk/ benefit profile, and are within the technical means of both gastroenterologists and interventional radiologists.

References

[1] Dean GT, Krukowski ZH, Irwin ST. Malignant obstruction of the left colon. Br J Surg 1994; 81:1270–6.
[2] Baron TH, Dean PA, Yates III MR, et al. Expandable metal stents for the treatment of colonic obstruction: techniques and outcomes. Gastrointest Endosc 1998;47:277–86.
[3] Valerio D, Jones PF. Immediate resection in the treatment of large bowel emergencies. Br J Surg 1978;65(10):712–6.

[4] Arnell T, Stamos MJ, Takahasi P, et al. Colonic stents in colorectal obstruction. Am Surg 1998; 64:986–8.

[5] Gandrup P, Lund L, Balslev I. Surgical treatment of acute malignant large bowel obstruction. Eur J Surg 1992;158:427–30.

[6] Lelcuk S, Merhav A, Klausner JM, et al. Rectoscopic decompression of acute rectosigmoid obstruction. Endoscopy 1987;19:209–10.

[7] Lelcuk S, Ratan J, Klausner JM, et al. Endoscopic decompression of acute colonic obstruction. Avoid staged surgery. Ann Surg 1986;203:292–4.

[8] Rattan J, Klausner JM, Rozen P, et al. Acute left colonic obstruction: a new nonsurgical treatment. J Clin Gastroenterol 1989;11:331–4.

[9] Horiuchi A, Maeyama H, Ochi Y, et al. Usefulness of dennis colorectal tube in endoscopic decompression of acute, malignant colonic obstruction. Gastrointest Endosc 2001;54:229–32.

[10] Cello JP, Gerstenberger PD, Wright T, et al. Endoscopic neodynium-YAD laser palliation of nonresectable esophageal malignancy. Ann Intern Med 1985;102:610–2.

[11] Fleischer D, Kessler F. Endoscopic ND:YAG laser therapy for carcinoma of the esophagus: a new form of palliative treatment. Gastroenterology 1983;85:600–6.

[12] Lightdale C, Zimbalist E, Winawer S. Outpatient managmnet of esophageal cancer with endoscopic Nd:YAG laser. Am J Gastroenterol 1987;82:46–50.

[13] Naveau S, Poynard T, Chaput J. Endoscopic Nd:YAG laser therapy as palliative treatment for esophageal and cardial cancers: parameters affecting long-term outcome. Dig Dis Sci 1990; 35:294–301.

[14] Liozou LA, Grigg D, Boulos PB, et al. Endoscopic Nd:YAG laser treatment of rectosigmoid cancer. Gut 1990;31:812–6.

[15] Daneker GWJ, Carlson GW, Hohn DC, et al. Endoscopic laser recanalization is effective for prevention and treatment of obstruction in sigmoid and rectal cancer. Arch Surg 1991;126: 1348–52.

[16] Mandava N, Petrelli N, Herrera L, et al. Laser palliation for colorectal carcinoma. Am J Surg 1991;162:212–4.

[17] Tan CC, Iftikhar SY, Allan A, et al. Local effects of colorectal cancer are well palliated by endoscopic laser therapy. Eur J Surg Oncol 1995;21:648–52.

[18] Brunetaud JM, Maunoury V, Cochelard D. Lasers in rectosigmoid tumors. Semin Surg Oncol 1995;11:319–27.

[19] De Gregorio MA, Mainar A, Tejero E. Acute colorectal obstruction: stent placement for palliative treatment: results of a multicenter study. Radiology 1998;209:117–20.

[20] Akle CA. Endoprostheses for colonic strictures. Br J Surg 1998;85:310–4.

[21] Camunez F, Echenagusia A, Simo G, et al. Malignant colorectal obstruction treated by means of self-expanding metallic stents: effectiveness before surgery and in palliation. Radiology 2000; 216(2):492–7.

[22] Mainar A, Ariza M, Tejero E, et al. Acute colorectal obstruction: treatment with self-expanding metallic stents before scheduled surgery: results of a multicenter study. Radiology 1999;210: 65–9.

[23] Law WL, Chu KW, Ho JW, et al. Self expanding metal stent in the treatment of colonic obstruction caused by advanced malignancies. Dis Colon Rectum 2000;43:1522–7.

[24] Mauro M, Koehler RE, Baron TH. Advances in gastrointestinal intervention: the treatment of gastroduodenal and colorectal obstruction with metallic stents. Radiology 2000;215:659–69.

[25] Binkert CA, Ledermann HP, Jost R, et al. Metallic stenting of gastroduodenal and colonic stenoses. Abdom Imaging 1998;23:580–6.

[26] Wholey MH, Levine EA, Ferral H, et al. Initial clinical experience with colonic stent placement. Am J Gastroenterol 1998;175:194–7.

[27] Soonwalla Z, Thakur K, Boorman P, et al. Self-expanding metallic stents in the management of obstruction of the sigmoid colon. Am J Gastroenterol 1998;171:633–6.

[28] Lamah M, Mathur P, McKeown B, et al. The use of rectosigmoid stents in the management of acute large bowel obstruction. J R Coll Surg Edinb 1998;43:318–21.

[29] Turegano-Fuentes F, Echenagusia-belda A, Simo-Muerza G, et al. Transanal self-expanding metal stents as an alternative to palliative colostomy in selected patients with malignant obstruction of the left colon. Br J Surg 1998;85:232–5.

[30] Binkert CA, Ledermann H, Jost R, et al. Acute colonic obstruction: clinical aspects and cost-effectiveness of preoperative and palliative treatment with self-expanding metallic stents— a preliminary report. Radiology 1998;206:199–204.

[31] Kinsman KJ, DeGregorio BT, Katon RM, et al. Prior radiation and chemotherapy increase the risk of life-threatening complications after insertion of metallic stents for esophagogastric malignancy. Gastrointest Endosc 1996;43:196–203.

[32] Siersema PD, Hop WC, Dees J, et al. Coated self-expanding metal stents versus latex prostheses for esophagogastric cancer with special reference to prior radiation and chemotherapy: a controlled, prospective study. Gastrointest Endosc 1998;47:113–20.

[33] Wengrower D, Fiorini A, Valero J, et al. EsophaCoil: long-term results in 81 patients. Gastrointest Endosc 1998;48:376–82.

[34] Tack J, Gevers A, Rutgeerts P. Self-expandable metallic stents in the palliation of rectosigmoid carcinoma: a follow-up study. Gastrointest Endosc 1998;48:267–71.

[35] Adler DG, Baron TH. Preoperative chemoradiation therapy following placement of a self-expanding metal stent in a patient with an obstructing rectal cancer: clinical and pathologic findings. Gastrointest Endosc 2002;55:435–7.

Hematol Oncol Clin N Am
16 (2002) 1031–1040

HEMATOLOGY/
ONCOLOGY
CLINICS OF
NORTH AMERICA

Index

0889-8588/02/$ – see front matter © 2002, Elsevier Science (USA). All rights reserved.
PII: S 0 8 8 9 - 8 5 8 8 (0 2) 0 0 0 7 2 - 2

Changing Your Address?

Make sure your subscription changes too! When you notify us of your new address, you can help make our job easier by including an exact copy of your Clinics label number with your old address (see illustration below.) This number identifies you to our computer system and will speed the processing of your address change. Please be sure this label number accompanies your old address and your corrected address—you can send an old Clinics label with your number on it or just copy it exactly and send it to the address listed below.

We appreciate your help in our attempt to give you continuous coverage. Thank you.

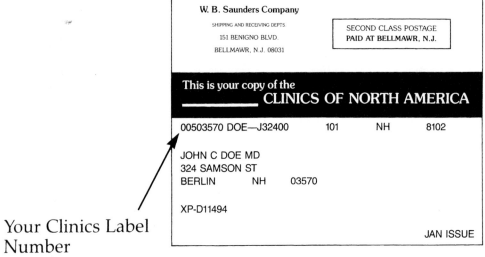

W. B. Saunders Company

SHIPPING AND RECEIVING DEPTS.
151 BENIGNO BLVD.
BELLMAWR, N.J. 08031

SECOND CLASS POSTAGE
PAID AT BELLMAWR, N.J.

This is your copy of the
_____ CLINICS OF NORTH AMERICA

00503570 DOE—J32400   101   NH   8102

JOHN C DOE MD
324 SAMSON ST
BERLIN   NH   03570

XP-D11494

JAN ISSUE

Your Clinics Label Number

Copy it exactly or send your label along with your address to:
W.B. Saunders Company, Customer Service
Orlando, FL 32887-4800
Call Toll Free 1-800-654-2452

Please allow four to six weeks for delivery of new subscriptions and for processing address changes.